# IN DEFENSE OF THE CONCEPT

One of the most controversial contemporary debates on the concept of health is the clash between the views of naturalists and normativists. Naturalists argue that, although health can be valued or disvalued, the concept of health is itself objective and value-free. In contrast, normativists argue that health is a contextual and value-laden concept, and that there is no possibility of a value-free understanding of health. This debate has fueled many of the, often very acrimonious, disputations arising from the claims of health, disease and disability activists and charities and the public policy responses to them.

In responding to this debate, Ananth both surveys the existing literature, with special focus on the work of Christopher Boorse, and argues that a naturalistic concept of health, drawing on evolutionary considerations associated with biological function, homeostasis, and species-design, is defensible without jettisoning norms in their entirety.

# Ashgate Studies in Applied Ethics

Scandals in medical research and practice; physicians unsure how to manage new powers to postpone death and reshape life; business people operating in a world with few borders; damage to the environment; concern with animal welfare – all have prompted an international demand for ethical standards which go beyond matters of personal taste and opinion.

The *Ashgate Studies in Applied Ethics* series presents leading international research on the most topical areas of applied and professional ethics. Focusing on professional, business, environmental, medical and bio-ethics, the series draws from many diverse interdisciplinary perspectives including: philosophical, historical, legal, medical, environmental and sociological. Exploring the intersection of theory and practice, books in this series will prove of particular value to researchers, students, and practitioners worldwide.

*Series Editors:*

Ruth Chadwick, Cardiff Law School, Cardiff University, UK
Dr David Lamb, Honorary Reader in Bioethics, University of Birmingham, UK
Professor Michael Davis, Illinois Institute of Technology, USA

*Other titles in the series include:*

Edited by Nikolaus Knoepffler, Dagmar Schipanski and Stefan Lorenz Sorgner
*Humanbiotechnology as Social Challenge*
*An Interdisciplinary Introduction to Bioethics*

Michael W. Austin
*Conceptions of Parenthood*
*Ethics and The Family*

Michael Hauskeller
*Biotechnology and the Integrity of Life*
*Taking Public Fears Seriously*

Sandra L. Borden
*Journalism as Practice*
*MacIntyre, Virtue Ethics and the Press*

# In Defense of an Evolutionary Concept of Health
Nature, Norms, and Human Biology

MAHESH ANANTH
*Indiana University-South Bend, USA*

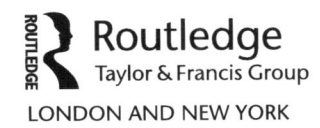

Routledge
Taylor & Francis Group
LONDON AND NEW YORK

First published 2008 by Ashgate Publishing

Reissued 2018 by Routledge
2 Park Square, Milton Park, Abingdon, Oxon OX14 4RN
605 Third Avenue, New York, NY 10017

First issued in paperback 2021

*Routledge is an imprint of the Taylor & Francis Group, an informa business*

© Mahesh Ananth 2008

Mahesh Ananth has asserted his moral right under the Copyright, Designs and Patents Act, 1988, to be identified as the author of this work.

All rights reserved. No part of this book may be reprinted or reproduced or utilised in any form or by any electronic, mechanical, or other means, now known or hereafter invented, including photocopying and recording, or in any information storage or retrieval system, without permission in writing from the publishers.

A Library of Congress record exists under LC control number: 2007005498

Notice:
Product or corporate names may be trademarks or registered trademarks, and are used only for identification and explanation without intent to infringe.

Publisher's Note
The publisher has gone to great lengths to ensure the quality of this reprint but points out that some imperfections in the original copies may be apparent.

Disclaimer
The publisher has made every effort to trace copyright holders and welcomes correspondence from those they have been unable to contact.

ISBN 13: 978-0-815-38967-5 (hbk)
ISBN 13: 978-1-351-15584-7 (ebk)
ISBN 13: 978-1-138-35608-5 (pbk)

DOI: 10.4324/9781351155847

*For Rekha, Kathan, and Rohan*

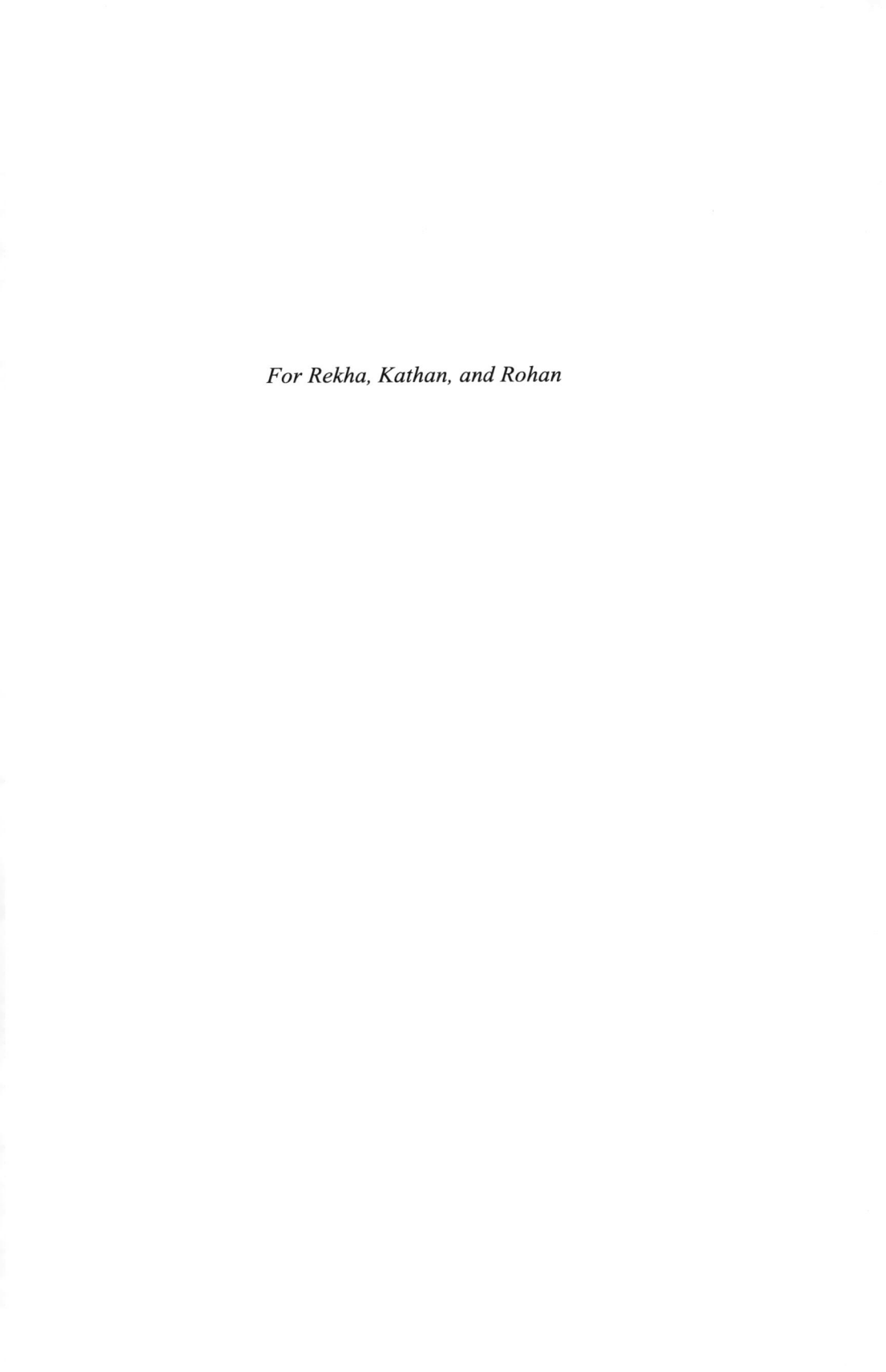

# Contents

| | | |
|---|---|---|
| *List of Figures* | | *ix* |
| *Foreword* | | *xi* |
| *Preface* | | *xiii* |
| *Acknowledgements* | | *xv* |
| 1 | Introduction to the Concept of Health: Topic of Study: The Importance and Priority of a Concept of Health | 1 |
| 2 | Boorse's Critique of Naturalist Concepts of Health | 13 |
| 3 | Boorse's Critique of Normative Concepts of Health | 39 |
| 4 | The Function Debate and the Emergence of Boorse's Concept of Function | 57 |
| 5 | Boorse's Concept of Health | 95 |
| 6 | Boorse and His Critics | 125 |
| 7 | An Evolutionary Concept of Health | 173 |
| *Conclusion* | | *217* |
| *Bibliography* | | *219* |
| *Index* | | *231* |

# List of Figures

| | | |
|---|---|---|
| 2.1 | Divisions of the Normal Distribution of Serum Albumin | 17 |
| 5.1 | Efficiency of the Functioning of the Thyroid | 117 |
| 7.1 | Standard Homeostatic System | 190 |

# Foreword

H. Tristram Engelhardt, Jr.

Health and disease are concepts upon which much in our culture turns. How we think of health and disease lies at the very core of medical practice, reflections on bioethics, and the formation of health care policy. How one understands these concepts bears on how one understands justice in health care and the proper allocation of medical resources. These concepts are cardinal for the philosophy of medicine as a whole and for bioethics in particular. In this very important book, Mahesh Ananth has brought together an ingeniously critical re-appraisal of debates bearing on concepts of health and disease through developing an evolutionary-homeostatic account of physical health. He focuses his energies on the controversies separating what have come to be termed naturalist versus normativist accounts of disease. For the purpose of this volume, (1) naturalists are those who argue that concepts of health, and for that matter of disease, are not socially constructed but objective and value-free, even though one may value or disvalue in different ways being healthy or being diseased, and (2) normativists are those who argue that concepts of health, and for that matter of disease, are socially constructed and in themselves value-laden, even though one may value or disvalue being healthy or being diseased. Other debates in the philosophy of medicine loom in the background. Aristotelians are naturalists, but not neutralists, in recognizing intrinsic values in health. There is also in the background the clash between nominalists and realists, who dispute as to whether the border identified between health and disease is an independent fact of the matter, or represents primarily a useful line to draw, but not one anchored in the way things are. This clash was reflected in the history of medicine in disputes about the nature of disease entities and was expressed in the early nineteenth century in the disagreements between ontologist (i.e., realist) and physiologist (i.e., nominalist) theories of disease.

The central figure in the book's analysis is Christopher Boorse, whose work has served as one pole in the debates between naturalists and normativists, and who is the most prominent defender of the naturalist position. My work in this area has been in dialectical interchange with Christopher Boorse for nearly a third of a century. Much of the debate has taken shape around various responses to Christopher Boorse's arguments, and this book is no exception.

Ananth's work draws extensively and fruitfully on the last half-century's complex literature regarding concepts of health and disease. The reader finds in this book a balanced exploration of this battleground of philosophical argument. Both sides in the debate will appreciate the care with which Ananth has developed his analyses and arguments, even though he comes down clearly on one side by defending a naturalistic concept of disease, although still taking norms seriously and recognizing the context-dependent (that is, environment-dependent) character of the concept of health. He advances his account by developing a forward-looking version of evolutionary functional naturalism that identifies functions in terms of their conferring an enhancing propensity on creatures that possess them, so that this propensity contributes to an increased individual survival or reproductive success. In this way, he seeks to free himself in part from etiological accounts that are backward-looking through being tied to evolutionary causal history.

In all of this, a key question remains for future debate and reflection, namely, whether there are quite different clusters of concepts of health and disease nested within different kinds of practices, in particular, the practices of the unapplied versus the applied sciences. One must wonder whether one cluster of understandings may be embedded in a biological-scientific context that presupposes the defining importance of individual survival and reproductive success, and the other embedded in the clinical practice of medicine with foci of concern beyond mere survival and reproductive success. Did Boorse attempt to reconstruct accurately the concepts of health and disease as these function in the unapplied science of human biology, while failing to attend to the value-laden character of these concepts within the applied context of clinical medicine? The need remains to explore these issues carefully in the light of a philosophical history of medicine that can aim us better to gauge how concepts of health and disease have actually done their work in clinical medicine over time.

Wherever one stands in these debates now and in the future, one will find in Ananth's work a well-developed fabric of arguments that must be taken seriously by all subsequent literature in the field. Although this is Ananth's first major work, it is an opus magnum; it is a work of serious depth and substance. It has significant implications for core debates in the fields of the philosophy of medicine, philosophy of biology, and for that matter in bioethics.

Rice University/Baylor College of Medicine<br>
Houston, Texas

# Preface

When I was searching for a dissertation topic in graduate school, the concept of health was suggested to me by my soon-to-be dissertation advisor, Fred D. Miller, Jr. I decided to review some of the literature on the debate and quickly became engrossed with the topic. I soon discovered that my interests in Philosophy of Science (especially Philosophy of Biology), Bioethics, and Ancient Greek Philosophy could all be satisfied by this one topic. Although much of the Ancient Greek philosophical debates about the nature of health are not included in this book, I was deeply inspired by those debates. Broadly speaking, moreover, many of the contemporary debates on the concept of health are (in part) a repeat performance of the philosophical toil of Ancient Greek thinkers like Empedocles, Plato, Aristotle, Hippocrates, Galen, and others.

The philosophy of health belongs to a genre that intersects philosophy of science (specifically philosophy of biology), philosophy of medicine, sociology, history, value theory, metaphysics, bioethics, and philosophy of psychology. Given the range of disciplines that intersects the health literature, philosophers of health would not only have philosophers as their target audience, but also those in the fields of biology, medicine, history (of science and medicine), psychology, and many other specialties within the field of health care. No doubt, it would be a near-impossible task to be able to speak persuasively and intelligibly to all of these audiences in a single book and I do not attempt to do so here. The focus of this book is the contemporary philosophical battle between "naturalists" and "normativists." Even so, there is an enormous literature on this circumscribed region of the philosophy of health. For example, both physical health and mental health are discussed within this particular debate.

After struggling to locate my "domain of discourse," I had a wonderful exchange with Michael Bradie, my Philosophy of Science/Biology mentor and dissertation committee member, who suggested focusing on the work of Christopher Boorse—a leading contemporary proponent of a naturalistic concept of health. Upon examining Boorse's works, which spans over twenty years, I was able to locate a project that not only satisfied my interests, but was both manageable and could still engage the debate between the "naturalists" and the "normativists." Moreover, David Copp, a member of my dissertation committee, offered much guidance on the normativity dimension of the debate and L. Fleming Fallon, Jr. (M.D.), the external reviewer of my dissertation, was kind enough to suggest many of disease topics that make up the final chapter of this work.

In summary, through a critical examination of the work of Christopher Boorse, this book (which is a modified version of my dissertation) attempts both to adjudicate the debate between the naturalists and the normativists regarding the concept of health and to defend an evolutionary concept of health, which draws on concepts of biological function, species, and homeostasis. Although, at the end of the day, there may be objections to my defense, I submit that the evolutionary-homeostatic concept of health developed within these pages is a reasonable account of the concept of physical health.

# Acknowledgments

I am grateful to Fred D. Miller, Jr., Michael Bradie, David Copp, and L. Fleming Fallon, Jr. Their assistance, guidance, and encouragement on the dissertation version of this project continue to be inspiring. Indeed, Fred Miller, the chair of my dissertation committee, was unwavering in his support and his copious feedback—a mile was never taken because an inch was never given! Michael Bradie was always available to debate my arguments with lively exchange. David Copp's critical feedback always reminded me of what it means to do philosophy. And L. Fleming Fallon's medical training was a source of much insight.

Of course, I acknowledge my family. First my parents, Santha and P.V. Ananthakrishnan, whose love and support were always unwavering and still palpable. Some debts can never be repaid fully. Moreover, I thank my sisters, Jayanthi and Vasanthi, for keeping an eye on me through the many tough times.

Notably, I appreciate the late night discussions of this project with Ben Dixon, Radha Murthy and Uma Ayer (M.D.) who pushed me to clarify and rethink a number of my arguments. Their patience and thoughtful criticisms were both helpful and motivating.

I am also appreciative of the many years of professional assistance and convivial relief from the Social Philosophy and Policy Center.

Finally, I would like to thank my wife, Rekha, for her love and support. Her willingness to follow me around from New York to Ohio and to Chicago speaks for itself. She and our sons, Kathan and Rohan, have been the source of much strength. I dedicate this book to them.

# Chapter 1
# Introduction to the Concept of Health

**Topic of Study: The Importance and Priority of a Concept of Health**

This work is a contribution to the extensive philosophical literature on the concept of health. Given that a concept of health is indispensable to (1) the practices of medicine,[1] (2) the many debates surrounding public policy issues,[2] and (3) the ethical concerns that loom over the decisions made by medical practitioners,[3] it might be presumed that much progress has been made with regard to the concept of health. In fact, there is still a notable lack of consensus concerning the concept of health among scholars and healthcare professionals. Lennart Nordenfelt offers the following summation of this problem:

> The entire medical enterprise—theoretical and clinical research as well as medical practice—has human health as its ultimate end. Health, as well as disease and illness, must be in the focus of medical attention ... In spite of their central place, however, and in spite of numerous efforts directed to the clarification of the concepts of health and disease, there is far from universal agreement about their nature. In fact, the controversies are quite profound ... [O]ne encounters anthropological, sociological, psychological, and

---

[1] Robert Mordacci emphasizes just this point when he claims that "the very end of medicine depends in great part on our understanding of the nature of health and illness both as objects of medical intervention and as experiences of the person." Robert Mordacci, "Health as an Analogical Concept," *The Journal of Medicine and Philosophy*, 20/5 (1995): 477. See also Leon R. Kass, "Regarding the End of Medicine and the Pursuit of Health," *Public Interest*, 40/1 (1975): 11–42, and Arthur Caplan, "Does the Philosophy of Medicine Exist?" *Theoretical Medicine*, 13/1 (1992): 67–77.

[2] See *The Price of Health*, eds George J. Agich and Charles E. Begley (Dordrecht, 1986), Norman Daniels, *Just Health Care* (Cambridge, 1985), Victor R. Fuchs, "Concepts of Health—An Economist's Perspective," *The Journal of Medicine and Philosophy*, 1/3 (1976): 229–37, Susan Giaimo, *Markets and Medicine: The Politics of Healthcare Reform in Britain, Germany, and the United States* (Ann Arbor, 2002), Jeffrey D. Milyo and Jennifer M. Mellor, "Is Inequality Bad for Our Health?" *Critical Review*, 13/3–4 (2000): 359–72, and David T. Ozar, "What Should Count as Basic Health Care?" *Theoretical Medicine*, 4/2 (1983): 129–41.

[3] For some of these moral problems, see *Contemporary Issues in Bioethics*, 5th edn, eds Tom L. Beauchamp and LeRoy Walters (Belmont, 1999), Thomas M. Garrett, Harold W. Baillie, and Rosellen M. Garrett, *Health Care Ethics: Principles and Problems*, 3rd edn (Upper Saddle River, 1998), and *Intervention and Reflection: Basic Issues in Medical Ethics*, 5th edn, ed. Ronald Munson (Belmont, 1996).

biological theories, as well as combinations of these. The contents of the various theories are quite different and often quite difficult to compare.[4]

Despite the pressing need for a cogent concept of health across disciplines, no single account has been agreed upon to address adequately the many practical and theoretical difficulties associated with (1)–(3) above. The problem, thinks Nordenfelt, is that the assumptions and agendas of different disciplines come into conflict, rendering "consilience" near impossible.[5]

Therefore, the goal of this project is to provide a *naturalistic* concept of health that is able to parry some of the difficulties encountered by previously proposed concepts. Before turning to a sketch of this naturalistic approach, the general problem under consideration in this project needs to be made clear.

*The Concept of Health Debate: Naturalists Versus Normativists*

The problem with offering a definitive account of health is apparent in the World Health Organization's (WHO) definition. In 1947, the WHO offered the following statement about health: "Health is a state of complete physical, mental, and social well-being, and not merely the absence of disease and infirmity."[6] There is a great deal that must be unpacked in this rather broad definition of health. What does the WHO mean by "complete"? Moreover, what does it mean by the use of "physical," 'mental,' and the supposed distinction between these two terms? Further, what does the WHO have in mind when it employs "social" and "well-being" to define "health?" Finally, what is the meaning of "disease" and "infirmity" in the WHO's definition of health? These terms need to be explained carefully so that a detailed account of health can be made manifest.

Indeed, many contemporary scholars, who have offered their own theories of health, have, in effect, refined, supplemented, and, in some cases, abandoned or accepted entirely the WHO's definition of health. Specifically, in the last few decades, philosophers, sociologists, psychologists, and scientists (chemists, biologists, ecologists, neuroscientists, etc.) have provided accounts of health that pick out one or more of the above terms as definitive constituents of a concept of health. As a result of this scholarship, the following two schools of thought with respect to the concept of health have emerged:

1. Health as a Natural Concept
2. Health as a Normative Concept

---

[4] Lennart Nordenfelt, "Introduction," in Lennart Nordenfelt and B. Ingemar B. Lindahl (eds), *Health, Disease, and Causal Explanations in Medicine* (Dordrecht, 1984), p. xii.

[5] Edward O. Wilson defines "consilience" as "literally the 'jumping together' of knowledge by the linking of facts and fact-based theory across disciplines to create a common groundwork of explanation." See Edward O. Wilson, *Consilience: The Unity of Knowledge* (New York, 1998), p. 8.

[6] World Health Organization, "Constitution of the World Health Organization," *Chronicle of the World Health Organization*, 1/1–2 (1947): 3.

The contemporary debate on the concept of health is basically between *naturalists* and *normativists*. The fundamental issue concerns the role of values with respect to the scope of medicine.

On the one hand, although health may be valued or disvalued, naturalists argue, the concept of health is itself a value-free concept. For example, naturalists contend that whether a heart is healthy or diseased is an *objective* matter to be determined by relevant medical scientists. It is entirely a separate matter, they argue, whether or not such a condition is of value. Michael Ruse describes the naturalist perspective as follows:

> The naturalist approach...attempts initially to approach matters in a nonvalue-laden fashion. In particular, the notion of disease, the concept of disease, is defined without respect to the implications for the bearer—whether they be good or bad, happiness-generating or otherwise, or anything else of this emotive nature. Essentially, a healthy state is taken to be one of proper functioning, that is to say, proper functioning for the species *Home sapiens*. A diseased state is taken to be one that, in some sense, interferes with this proper functioning.[7]

Thus, naturalists deny that values are part of the concept of health, on the grounds that health essentially involves only the *functional* activities of organisms and their parts.

In contrast, normativists argue that the concept of health is value-laden. Their justification is two-fold. First, they claim that, since science itself is littered with values, medical scientists (e.g., pathologists or physiologists) cannot escape incorporating values into their concepts. For example, in response to those who think that concepts of health and disease can be understood from a value-neutral scientific perspective, George Agich offers the following reply:

> This approach is based on an unacceptably simplistic view of science as value-free. In these terms, medicine appears value-laden and is often criticized for that reason. Work in philosophy of medicine, however, has helped question this view and aided in the recognition that science, too, is a practice laden with particular value as well as conceptual commitments.[8]

Second, normativists claim that the scope of the concept of health is ultimately tethered to diagnosis *and* treatment of patients within a cultural/social context. Talcott Parsons defends this normativist position from a social context perspective as follows:

> Health may be defined as the state of optimum *capacity* of an individual for the effective performance of the roles and tasks for which he has been socialized. It is thus defined with reference to the individual's participation in the social system. It is also defined as

---

[7] Michael Ruse, "Defining Disease: The Question of Sexual Orientation," in James M. Humber and Robert F. Almeder (eds), *What is Disease?* (Totowa, 1997), p. 143.

[8] George J. Agich, "Disease and Value: A Rejection of the Value-Neutrality Thesis," *Theoretical Medicine*, 4/1 (1983): 36–7. Agich's argument will be discussed in detail in Chapter 6.

*relative* to his "status" in the society, i.e. to differentiated type of role and corresponding task structure, e.g., by sex or age, and by level of education which he has attained and the like.[9]

Similarly, H. Tristram Engelhardt offers the following assessment of the concept of disease within the context of diagnosis and treatment:

> Clinical medicine is not developed in order to catalogue diseases *sub specie aeternitatis*, but in order for physicians to be able to make more cost-effective decisions with respect to considerations of morbidity, financial issues, and mortality risks, so as to achieve various goals of physiologically and psychologically based well-being. Thus, clinical categories, which are characterized in terms of various warrants or indications for making diagnosis, are at once tied to the likely possibilities of useful treatments and severity of the conditions suspected.[10]

Given the above account, it is clear why Engelhardt thinks that "there will not be the possibility to elaborate either univocal or value-neutral, culture free concepts of disease…"[11] Thus, normativists, like Agich, Parsons, and Engelhardt, think that the idea of a value-free concept of health is fundamentally misguided because science is value-laden, or because the concept of health includes values associated with medical practice and the broader social environment in which people find themselves.[12]

A barrier to a generally accepted concept of health is this fundamental tension between normativists and naturalists. Normativists, who include societal concerns and goals within the scope of medicine, insist that norms are an ineliminable part of the concept of health. Naturalists, in contrast, restrict the scope of medicine to the somatic condition of the human body. In response to this controversy, this book will defend a modified naturalistic concept of health. It will argue that, although *epistemic norms* (e.g., predictive power, replicability, parsimony, etc.) are an integral part of a naturalistic account, *non-epistemic norms* (e.g., social, moral, desirability, etc.) are not.[13]

## Plan of Study: Method

There are several different ways of approaching the concept of health and identifying the problems it raises. Philosophers, from antiquity until the present age, have

---

[9] Talcott Parson, "Definitions of Health and Illness in the Light of American Values and Social Structure," in Arthur L. Caplan, H. Tristram Engelhardt, Jr., and James J. McCartney (eds), *Concepts of Health and Disease: Interdisciplinary Perspectives* (London, 1981), p. 69. [italics in original]. A variation on Parson's account is offered by Joseph Margolis, "The Concept of Disease," *The Journal of Medicine and Philosophy*, 1/3 (1976): 238–55.

[10] H. Tristram Engelhardt, Jr., "Clinical Problems and the Concept of Disease," in Lennart Nordefelt and B. Ingemar B. Lindahl (eds), *Health, Disease, and Causal Explanations in Medicine* (Dordrecht, 1984), p. 36.

[11] Ibid., p. 33.

[12] Also see H. Tristram Engelhardt, Jr., "Ideology and Etiology," *The Journal of Medicine and Philosophy*, 1/3 (1976): 256–68.

[13] It may seem that this discussion begs the question against "value naturalists" who claim that evaluative discourse is both normative and naturalistic. This is a legitimate concern and it will be discussed in Chapter 3 under the label of "weak normativism."

written at length about the concept of health.[14] One way, then, to understand the concept of health would be to start by following the course laid out by philosophers old and new. Alternatively, the concept of health could be approached through the writings of those practitioners of the special sciences and/or medical professionals. A list of definitions of health offered by those in each of these sub-disciplines could be compiled and seen as definitive within each domain of inquiry. Of course, a compatabilist approach, incorporating fruitful insights from both philosophers and scientists, could be a better approach to the concept of health. For surely the analytical skills of the philosopher would be of great assistance with respect to conceptual analysis. So, if it is the *concept* of health that is of interest, then philosophers could be of great service.

Yet, an argument could be advanced against the idea of looking to analytic philosophers for guidance. The main concern is expressed by Jay Rosenberg:

> While an analytic philosopher may in fact be an advocate of some grand world-conception, in his professional capacity, he is not so much concerned with articulating and defending any one such worldview as he is with articulating and defending criteria according to which the intelligibility, clarity, coherence, rationality, cogency, or plausibility of various theses and systems ought properly to be assessed. This aim puts his questions "at one remove from the facts." Rather than asking "Is this or that thesis true?" or "What evidence is there in favor of this or that belief?" an analytic philosopher of this persuasion will more likely pose such questions as "How are we to understand this thesis?" and "What is meant by it?" and "What sorts of grounds or reasons could there be for believing it?"[15]

If the above account is an accurate depiction of contemporary analytic philosophers, then it seems that their professional duty is to make sure that other disciplines (and their own) are using terms appropriately and advancing arguments that are governed by the rules of logic. No doubt, there are many scientists, bioethicists, and healthcare professionals who share Rosenberg's view of contemporary analytic philosophers and find it quite troubling.[16] They fear that analytic philosophers—whose concerns

---

[14] For this history, see Paul Carrick, *Medical Ethics in Antiquity* (Dordrecht, 1985) and *Western Medical Thought from Antiquity to the Middle Ages*, ed. Mirko D. Grmek (Cambridge, 1997). For contemporary discussions, see George Khushf, "Why Bioethics Needs the Philosophy of Medicine: Some Implications of Reflection on Concepts of Health and Disease," *Theoretical Medicine*, 18/1–2 (1997): 145–63, J.B. Scadding, "Health and Disease: What Can Medicine Do for Philosophy?," *Journal of Medical Ethics*, 14/3 (1988): 118–24, and David Seedhouse, "The Need for a Philosophy of Health," in David Lamb, Teifion Davies, and Marie Roberts (eds), *Explorations in Medicine Volume 1* (Aldershot, 1987), pp. 123–51.

[15] Jay F. Rosenberg, *Thinking Clearly About Death*, 2nd. edn (Indianapolis, 1998), p. 8.

[16] For example, Donald Light and Glenn McGee state the following: "Analytic philosophy, with its insistence on linguistic strictures and universal moral duties, tends to reduce the complexities of the clinic to the most benign details…As a result of their training, bioethicists are inclined to take an anecdotal approach to the basic 'principles' of bioethics. Or, even worse, analytic philosophers turned bioethicists will insert here and there, as suits their argument, a few facts or assertions about the real world. The full range of variables present in a clinical context will be ignored, as will the implications of these variables for defining the issues and finding solutions." See Donald W. Light and Glenn McGee, "On the Social

are "at one remove from the facts"—do not place enough emphasis on the details of the practice of science and medicine. Rather, they suspect that analytic philosophers favor technicalities regarding the use of language. This lack of concern by analytic philosophers for the details of how science works or how the doctor-patient relationship functions, argue their critics, vitiates their pronouncements on the concept of health. So, again, why should the insights of philosophers be entertained seriously within any discussion concerning the topic of health?

A reply to the above objection is that the topic of health is ideally suited for the conceptual analysis found in philosophy as a second-order discipline. For analytic philosophers are in the business of providing both analysis and synthesis concerning particular topics that may not have been recognized by those in a particular specialized discipline. In the words of Peter Caws: "Philosophy ... examines critically everything that may be offered as grounds for belief or action, including its own theories, with a view to the elimination of inconsistency and error."[17] For instance, the contribution made by those practitioners of the special sciences regarding the concept of health are of interest to philosophers because these accounts of health often include claims about (1) what we are as humans when we are thought to be healthy, (2) how we are able to come to be in a state of health, and (3) how we relate to the world when we are in a certain state of health. Claims that fall within the purview of (1)-(3) are just the kind of claims that are of great interest to philosophers. It is just this ability to pay attention to such claims and examine them that uniquely distinguishes philosophy as a second-order discipline from other first-order disciplines.[18] Indeed, in response to their critics, analytic philosophers can justifiably reply: why should only the ruminations of medical practitioners and the custodians of the special sciences be considered with respect to the concept of health?

The resolution as to which discipline, philosophy or the special sciences or both, has the authority to investigate the concept of health can be resolved in favor of the compatabilist approach in the following way. Although the first-order disciplines are indispensable, philosophy *qua* second-order discipline can provide a valuable service by clarifying the concepts employed by first-order disciplines. For example,

---

Embeddedness of Bioethics," in Raymond DeVries and Janardan Subedi (eds), *Bioethics and Society: Constructing the Ethical Enterprise* (Upper Saddle River, 1998), p. 1.

[17] Peter Caws, *The Philosophy of Science: A Systematic Account* (Princeton, 1965), p. 5. I am also quite sympathetic to Edmund Pellegrino's articulation of the role of philosophy in medicine. He says: "It is the critical, reflective, systematic study of concepts and presuppositions of the healing encounter between human persons as individuals or societies that is the domain of philosophy of medicine ..." See Edmund D. Pellegrino, "What the Philosophy *Of* Medicine Is," *Theoretical Medicine and Bioethics*, 19/4 (1998): 332. See also Khushf, "Why Bioethics Needs the Philosophy of Medicine: Some Implications of Reflection on Concepts of Health and Disease."

[18] In his lucid account of the role of analytic philosophers in the field of medicine, David Thomasma argues that it is precisely this sensitivity to concepts that reveals the benefit analytic philosophers can provide medical practitioners. See David C. Thomasma, "The Role of the Clinical Medical Ethicist: The Problem of Applied Ethics and Medicine," in Michael Bradie, Thomas W. Attig, and Nicholas Rescher (eds), *The Applied Turn in Contemporary Philosophy* (Bowling Green, 1983), vol. 5, pp. 136-57.

a physiologist might offer a list of properties that *uniquely* distinguishes a healthy organism from an unhealthy one with respect to the species to which it belongs. A philosopher of biology might ask the physiologist what he means by this: has he offered an essentialist account of what it means to be a healthy token of a type? The philosopher of biology is trying to impress upon the physiologist the question of whether he has taken a standard philosophical position about natural kinds. In this case, the philosopher of biology can explain to the physiologist that an essentialist account implies that tokens of a type have a unique immutable cluster of properties that are possessed by *all and only* those tokens of that type. The philosopher of biology may go on to inform the physiologist that viewing species as historical entities is another alternative that he may do well to entertain.[19] This alternative to the essentialist position suggests that two organisms belong to the same group as a result of their historical relationship to each other, not in virtue of an immutable set of physical properties shared by the group.

The above biology/philosophy example is offered not to resolve the debate about what a species is, but to make clear that philosophers can provide valuable insights and suggestions to those researchers in other areas of inquiry. Moreover, note that the concepts (e.g., species) evaluated by philosophers will have been formed to fit the phenomena (e.g., healthy humans or healthy mice) discovered by researchers. In the above example, if the field biologist were to offer additional empirical evidence to buttress his essentialist position, then it would be incumbent upon the philosopher of biology to assess whether this additional evidence helps resolve the problem under consideration. It may very well be the case that the new evidence reveals that the essentialist position is more plausible than the alternative historical position. Most importantly, it should be clear that there is a general "give-and-take" between philosophers and the researchers of specific disciplines. Conceptual analysis, then, is a sort of "two-way street" between philosophy and other primary disciplines; that is, both philosophers and other researchers of specific areas of inquiry engage in an exchange of information that is indispensable to the precision and clarity of their respective enterprises.

If the above account is correct, then neither the custodians of the special sciences nor the philosophers may monopolize an analysis of the concept of health. Rather, a joint effort between these researchers and scholars is necessary to provide a careful and insightful analysis of the concept of health. Thus, the compatabilist methodology is the most promising of the methodologies to address adequately the concept of health. This compatabilist methodology will be employed throughout the analysis of the concept of health that is to follow.

---

[19] As Kim Sterelny and Paul Griffiths explain: "Contemporary views on species are close to a consensus in thinking that species are identified by their histories. According to these views, Charles Darwin was a human being not by virtue of having the field marks—rationality and an odd distribution of body hair...but in view of his membership in a population with a specific evolutionary history." See Kim Sterelny and Paul E. Griffiths, *Sex and Death: An Introduction to Philosophy of Biology* (Chicago, 1999), p. 8. Also, for a critical reply to the "histories" approach to understanding the concept of a species, see Philip Kitcher, "Species," *Philosophy of Science*, 51/3 (1984): 308–33.

**Focus of Study: Narrowing the Topic**

A survey of a handful of introductory health texts reveals that (1) physical health, (2) mental health, (3) social health, (4) environmental health, (5) spiritual health, and (6) emotional health are some of the commonly discussed dimensions of health.[20] To the extent that there is a definitive concept of health, such a definition is thought by many to be circumscribed to each of the different specializations associated with (1)–(6). For example, there may be a definitive account of mental health within psychology or social health within sociology or environmental health within environmental science, but there is not thought to be an authoritative account of health that ranges over all these different dimensions of health.

The focus of this project is on the naturalistic concept of *physical* health that ranges over humans and non-human animals. It is possible that the arguments advanced in this analysis may be of assistance in making sense of the other dimensions of health noted above. However, this possible connection between the concept of physical health and the other dimensions of health will not be broached in this project except with respect to normativism. Thus, for the sake of this discussion, the concept of health refers to the concept of physical health, unless stated otherwise.

The claim that the focus of this project is the naturalistic concept of health is still rather vague. To try to explore the contemporary debate between the normativists and the naturalists through a catalogue of the various concepts of health offered by specific theorists would still be too ambitious and massive a task. So, as a way of navigating through this debate between the normativists and the naturalists, the primary focus of this project is on the widely discussed naturalistic concept of health offered by a particular philosopher, namely Christopher Boorse.

Boorse is one of the most ardent and discerning defenders of a value-free naturalistic concept of health, which places an emphasis on the concept of function. His account provides an excellent entry point into the debate between the normativists and the naturalists. In fact, many of the contemporary normativists and naturalists have developed their own concepts of health after launching an assault on Boorse's "radical" account. In the spirit of this approach, the details of Boorse's concept of health and the reply of his critics will be the major focus of this work.[21] This analysis will argue that, although Boorse can defend his account against most of the criticisms

---

[20] Willard Dalrymple, *Foundations of Health* (Boston, 1959); William Fassbender, *You and Your Health*, 3rd edn (New York, 1984); Jerrod S. Greenberg and George B. Dintiman, *Exploring Health: Expanding the Boundaries of Wellness* (Englewood Cliffs, 1992); Wayne A. Payne and Dale B. Hahn, *Understanding Your Health*, 3rd edn (St. Louis, 1992). If one were to think that the dimensions of health include a sort of progression from physical health to mental health to spiritual health (and everything in between), then an exemplar is Deepak Chopra, *Creating Health: Beyond Prevention, Toward Perfection* (Boston, 1987).

[21] Boorse's concept of health will be drawn from the following material he has published over the years: "On the Distinction Between Disease and Illness," *Philosophy and Public Affairs*, 5/1 (1975): 49–68; "What a Theory of Mental Health Should Be," *Journal of the Theory of Social Behavior*, 6/1 (1976): 61–84; "Health as a Theoretical Concept," *Philosophy of Science*, 44/4 (1977): 542–73; "Concepts of Health," in Donald Van DeVeer and Tom Regan (eds), *Health Care Ethics: An Introduction* (Philadelphia, 1987), pp. 359–93; "A Rebuttal on

from the normativists, he is unable to deflect particular criticisms concerning his handling of biological and environmental factors. Nonetheless, after resolving these difficulties with Boorse's concept of health, this work will argue positively that a modified version of his account is defensible. Thus, the goal of this work is to show that a naturalistic concept of health, which makes room for epistemic norms, is worthy of pursuit despite the concerns of many of its critics.

*A Brief Guide to the Rest of This Work*

Boorse devotes a great deal of effort to evaluating various concepts of health and function before offering his own naturalistic concept of health. So, this work begins by providing the context of Boorse's own concept of health. Chapters 2–4 discuss and evaluate Boorse's critical analysis of various naturalistic and normative concepts of health and the emergence of his own concept of function through his careful discussion of the function debate. With this preliminary background in place, Chapter 5 provides the details of Boorse's concept of health. Then, Chapter 6 discusses the critical replies to Boorse's concept of health, his rejoinder to them, and the extent to which he is successful in his rejoinder. Finally, in an attempt to overcome some of the difficulties with Boorse's account, Chapter 7 offers a modified version of Boorse's concept of health.

The contents of this work have been organized so as to begin, in Chapter 2, with Boorse's understanding of some of the influential naturalistic concepts of health and his reasons for rejecting them. Specifically, Boorse focuses on the following three naturalistic concepts of health: (1) the *statistical*, (2) the *adaptation*, and (3) the *homeostatic*. This chapter reveals that Boorse is successful in his rejection of (1), partially successful against (2), and actually endorses a version of (3).

Chapter 3 examines Boorse's various arguments against the thesis that the concept of health is normative. Boorse's strategy is to reject two general versions of normativism—*strong normativism* and *weak normativism*—that he thinks handle most normative accounts. Moreover, Boorse charitably discusses two additional normative concepts of health—*moral normativism and functional normativism*—that he thinks pose specific challenges that require special attention. This chapter makes clear that, although Boorse is (for the most part) persuasive in his rejection of *strong normativism, weak normativism,* and *moral normativism,* additional support is required to show that he is justified in rejecting *functional normativism*.

In Chapter 4, the central element of Boorse's naturalistic concept of health— namely his concept of function—is discussed. Since the details of Boorse's own concept of function emerge as a response to Larry Wright's account,[22] a detailed description of Wright's concept of function and Boorse's reasons for rejecting it

---

Health," in James M. Humber and Robert F. Almeder (eds), *What is Disease?* (Totowa, 1997), pp. 3–134.
  [22] Larry Wright, "Functions," in Elliott Sober (ed.), *Conceptual Issues in Evolutionary Biology* (Cambridge, 1994), pp. 27–47. This article was published originally in *Philosophical Review*, 82/1 (1973): 139–68; Christopher Boorse, "Wright on Functions," *The Philosophical Review*, 85/1 (1976): 70–86.

are explained. What emerges out of this discussion is Boorse's *part-functional contextualist* concept of function. The critical assessment of Boorse's analysis concludes that it is able to overcome some of the difficulties with Wright's account, but still faces some difficulties of its own.

Chapter 5 offers the fine points of Boorse's concept of health. First, upon providing two separate argument reconstructions of Boorse's concept of health, the details of the numerous technical terms in those arguments are explained. The initial set of technical terms includes "mechanism," "part-functionalism," and "organic functional holism." After explaining these terms, it will be argued that Boorse is best understood as a *part-functionalist*. Second, Boorse claims to be offering an *objective* concept of health. To make sense of this term, different senses of "objectivism" are distinguished. This section argues that Boorse should be understood as both a *metaphysical objectivist* and a *disciplinary objectivist*. Finally, the other technical terms that make up the core of Boorse's concept of health are explicated. These terms are "reference class," "normal function," and "disease." The conclusion is that, after explaining these various technical terms, it is reasonable to understand Boorse to be offering a *non-normative ideal part-functional/contextualist* concept of health.

In Chapter 6, the focus shifts from Boorse's concept of health to the reply of his critics. Broadly, the four major types of objections to Boorse's concept of health are as follows: (1) the charge of circularity, (2) the charge of covert normativism, (3) the charge of bad biology, and (4) the charge of bad medicine. The critical assessment of Boorse's rejoinder to his critics concludes that he is successful in his reply to (1), mostly successful in his reply to (2), partly unsuccessful in his reply to (3), and successful in his reply to (4). The general conclusion this chapter draws is that Boorse's reply to his critics is, for the most part, a success, but that there are a few glaring difficulties with his concept of health related to evolutionary biology and environmental factors.

In an attempt to address the difficulties with Boorse's account, Chapter 7 develops a modified version of his naturalistic concept of health. First, drawing on the concept of function in the philosophy of biology literature, an evolutionary propensity concept of function is defended. The reason for drawing on evolutionary considerations is that Boorse has a problem in justifying the claim that health and disease are to be understood in terms of *objective* functions. So, as a way of justifying the goal-directed nature of biological functions, this section argues that both the goals of biological systems and the means that bring about these goals are the product of natural selection.[23] Second, following Boorse's lead, the next section offers a detailed account of homeostasis, which includes both an *internal* sense and an *organism* sense. Third, the evolutionary concept of function and the concept of homeostasis are brought together to argue that health is best understood

---

[23] This is not to suggest that all of nature is replete with goal-directed activities. Rather, the claim is that biological systems (as opposed to rocks) reveal a complex hierarchical structure of interdependence that requires an explanation. This section argues that evolution by natural selection is the appropriate framework from which to make sense of this complex organization.

as an evolved homeostatic propensity of both the parts of organisms and organisms as a whole to ensure survival and reproductive success. This concept of health is further qualified with respect to species, gender, and age groups. Fourth, as a way of revealing the fruitfulness of this modified account and handling possible objections to it, the following cases of "diseases" are discussed: (1) tuberculosis, (2) allergies, (3) Down's syndrome, (4) sickle cell anemia, and (5) osteoporosis. This section argues that the concept of health defended in this chapter helps to make sense of these cases. Finally, in order to handle one lingering objection, the last section briefly argues that it is possible to defend the claim that the individual organism is the unit of selection. The conclusion of this study is that, after making necessary modifications to Boorse's account, the naturalistic concept of health defended in this chapter is a reasonable account of physical health.

Chapter 2
# Boorse's Critique of Naturalist Concepts of Health

**Introduction: The Many Faces of Naturalism**

Christopher Boorse argues that the concept of health is best understood from a *naturalistic* perspective.[1] Although Boorse does not offer a sustained analysis of "naturalism," he suggests that "naturalism" with respect to the concept of health should refer to the concepts of *body design* and *function* discussed by contemporary biologists. Boorse recommends just this account of naturalism in the following account of what it means for an organism to be healthy:

> The state of an organism is theoretically healthy, i.e., free of disease, insofar as its mode of functioning conforms to the natural design of that kind of organism … Contemporary biology employs a version of the idea of natural design that seems ideal for the analysis of health … The crucial element in the idea of a biological design is the notion of a natural function … The health of an organism consists in the performance by each part of its natural function.[2]

The details of Boorse's own naturalistic/functional concept of health will be discussed in Chapter 5. For now, it is enough to know that Boorse claims that the concepts of health and disease are *value-free* scientific concepts in the sense that "the classification of human states as healthy or diseased is an objective matter, to

---

[1] I will not attempt an analysis of the concept of naturalism. "Naturalism" is a very complicated term that is used in many different ways by different disciplines. For example, a naturalistic approach in the field of physics is frequently contrasted with a naturalistic approach in biology or the social sciences. The reason that "naturalism" is understood differently in different fields is that it masks different assumptions and concerns of distinct disciplines. For instances, "naturalism" can refer to (1) concerns about the limits of human knowledge in different subject matters, (2) the appropriateness of certain methods of inquiry, or (3) the extent to which there are essential similarities or differences of the subject matters of distinct disciplines. Since Boorse does not provide a systematic account of how he understands naturalism, it would be an arduous task (and one that would move the discussion considerably away from the concept of health debate) to determine how he understands this term. For a concise account of some of the senses of naturalism, see David Copp, "Why Naturalism?" *Ethical Theory and Moral Practice*, 6/2 (2003): 179–200.

[2] Christopher Boorse, "On the Distinction Between Disease and Illness," *Philosophy and Public Affairs*, 5/1 (1975): 57–8.

be read off the biological facts of nature without need of value judgments."[3] Boorse recognizes that he has two preliminary tasks that he must complete in order to give credence to his value-free naturalistic concept of health. First, he acknowledges that there are other competing naturalistic concepts of health that he must consider. Second, he sets out to argue against those who claim that the concept of health is a value-laden or a *normative* concept.

Chapter 2 will focus on the first task, namely, Boorse's explanation and rejection of three *naturalistic* concepts of health: the *statistical*, the *adaptation*, and the *homeostatic*. (Chapter 3 will examine Boorse's second task of rejecting the idea that the concept of health is value-laden.) There are two distinct versions of the adaptation concept of health: (1) *evolutionary-adaptation* and (2) *acclimation-adaptation*. The acclimation-adaptation concept of health includes (i) a positive and (ii) a negative version. This second chapter will argue that Boorse is successful in his critiques of the statistical concept of health, to some degree of the homeostatic concept of health, and of the positive version of the acclimation-adaptation concept of health. Moreover, this chapter will reveal that, although there may be some difficulties with the evolutionary-adaptation concept of health and the negative version of the acclimation-adaptation concept of health, Boorse is not very successful in his reply to them.

## Naturalism and the Concept of Health

*The Statistical Concept of Health*

An explanation is thought to be naturalistic in one sense if it abides by some (if not all) of the methodology employed by contemporary scientists. Specifically, one of the central requirements of a scientific explanation is that it must render phenomena under investigation mathematically analyzable. Within the concept of health literature, this demand of *scientific naturalism* is met by the statistical concept of health. Boorse begins his discussion by noting the following:

> It is safe to begin any discussion of health by saying that health is normality, since the terms are interchangeable in clinical contexts. But this remark provides no analysis of health until one specifies the norms involved. The most obvious proposal, that they are pure statistical norms, is widely recognized to be erroneous.[4]

Although Boorse does not target a specific author's statistical concept of health, it is still possible to provide a general description of what he has in mind. Basically, a statistic is a numerical quantity that characterizes some specific aspect of a subgroup

---

[3] Christopher Boorse, "A Rebuttal on Health," in James M. Humber and Robert F. Almeder (eds), *What is Disease?* (Totowa, 1997), p. 4. The other works of Boorse that will be discussed in this chapter include: "What a Theory of Mental Health Should Be," *Journal of the Theory of Social Behavior*, 6/1 (1976): 61–84; "Wright on Functions," *The Philosophical Review*, 85/1 (1976): 70–86; and "Health as a Theoretical Concept," *Philosophy of Science*, 44/4 (1977): 542–73.

[4] Boorse, "On the Distinction Between Disease and Illness," 50.

drawn from a specified sample.[5] Statistical analysis aims to summarize and describe the characteristics of a large set of data. For example, imagine an allergist who has given 1000 allergy tests ranging over 49 distinct allergens and has computed the total score of each patient's test. In order to assess and interpret this information, the allergist needs a way of organizing this large quantity of data. Employing techniques such as (1) frequency distributions and graphs, (2) measures of central tendency, (3) measures of variability, and (4) transformed scores, the allergist is able both to summarize and to describe large quantities of data.[6]

Boorse describes the statistical concept of health as follows:

> In clinical language, diseases or pathological conditions are also called abnormal, and healthy conditions normal. An obvious idea that fits some features of medicine well is to interpret this normality statistically. Textbook normals for clinical variables like height, weight, pulse and respiration, blood pressure, vital capacity, basal metabolism, sedimentation rate, and so on are... statistical means surrounded by some range of normal variation ... [T]here is a persistent intuition that the average person—or at least the average heart, lung, kidney, thyroid, etc.—must be normal, or we would have no way of telling what the normal person or organ should be like.[7]

Three points are relevant to a statistical concept of health as described by Boorse. First, clinicians label disease states as "abnormal" and healthy conditions as "normal." Second, clinicians justify their use of such terms (e.g., "normal" and "abnormal") on the basis of information provided through statistical analysis. Third, clinicians understand "statistical" to mean "a range of normal variation." Specifically, "statistical normality" refers to the mean (average value) of a distribution. These three points imply that clinicians understand the concept of health to be closely connected to the concept of normal distribution or average value. Thus, according to Boorse's account, it is not uncommon for clinicians to think that a person (or parts of a person) is healthy to the extent that the person (or the parts of a person) falls within a certain range of normal limits or common variation/distribution.

---

[5] Joan Welcowitz, Robert B. Ewen, and Jacob Cohen, *Introductory Statistics for the Behavioral Sciences*, 4th edn (San Diego, 1991), p. 6.

[6] These elementary technical aspects of descriptive statistics can be found in Jan W. Kuzma, *Basic Statistics for the Health Sciences*, 2nd edn (Mountain View, 1992).

[7] Boorse, "Health as a Theoretical Concept," 546. A very similar description of statistical normality is discussed in C. Daly King, "The Meaning of Normal," *Yale Journal of Biology and Medicine*, 17 (1945): 494 and Lila R. Elveback *et al.*, "Health, Normality, and the Ghost of Gauss," *Journal of the American Medical Association*, 211/1 (1970): 69–75. Indeed, Lila Elveback *et al.*, offer the following assessment that is in line with Boorse's description of the statistical concept: "Even today, regrettably, many medical students graduate from their medical schools firmly convinced that if a sample is large enough, the distribution will be 'normal,' regardless of the measurement under study, and that 95% of the measurements will be included in $x \pm 2\sigma$." See Elveback *et al.*, "Health, Normality, and the Ghost of Gauss," 69.

Still, there is a legitimate concern as to why the idea of normal variation should be relevant to the concept of health. Jan Kuzma's account of the usefulness of the normal distribution provides a possible answer:

> There are a legion of reasons why the normal distribution plays such a key role in statistics. For one thing, countless phenomena follow (or closely approximate) the normal distribution. Just a few of them are height, serum cholesterol, life span of light bulbs, body temperature of healthy persons, size of oranges, brightness of galaxies...Another reason for the normal distribution's popularity is that it possesses certain mathematical properties that make it attractive and easy to manipulate. Still another reason is that much statistical theory and methodology was developed around the assumption that certain data are distributed approximately normally.[8]

First note that "normal distribution" refers to a distribution of values of a particular characteristic (e.g., height, weight, length, etc.) in the form of a bell-shaped graph (see figure 2.1 on p. 17). Most of the values of such a distribution fall between the two extreme "tails" of the bell-shaped curve. Those values that fall between the two extremes are considered normal. Kuzma observes that a normal distribution is employed to make sense of particular phenomena because, in general, (1) so many phenomena follow the normal distribution pattern, (2) the mathematical distribution is easy to manipulate, and (3) there is a long-standing assumption in the history of statistics that certain kinds of data follow a normal distribution pattern.

Yet, a clear account of the details of "a range of normal variation" is crucial to understanding the statistical concept of health. The following example will be of assistance in understanding the concept of normal variation/distribution. Consider the protein serum albumin (also called albumin). It has been established that serum albumin is chiefly responsible for the maintenance of blood pH. Albumin, which is synthesized in the liver, is also the most abundant protein in the circulatory system and is crucial to the maintenance of blood pressure.[9] For any sample population, the concentrations of serum albumin tend to follow a *normal distribution*; that is there is a middle range of concentration levels of serum albumin that is thought to be normal (approximately 95% of the sample population fall into this range of a normal distribution). Moreover, a normal distribution also has two distinct ranges that are thought to be abnormal (approximately 5%—2.5% above the middle range and 2.5% below the middle range—of the sample population fall outside of the range of a normal distribution). This middle range, in a normal distribution, captures the normal limits for albumin. This middle range is calculated by adding and subtracting two *standard deviations*[10] from the *mean*[11] of a large set of observations obtained from a sample

---

[8] Kuzma, *Basic Statistics for the Health Sciences*, 81.
[9] Georges-Louis Friedli, *Interaction of Deamidated Soluble Wheat Protein (SWP) with Other Food Proteins and Metals*, http://www.friedli.com/research/PhD/PhD.html#contents?
[10] A *standard deviation* is a statistic that reveals the distance a particular datum is from *the mean* of a set of data.
[11] The *mean* is the average of a set of N numbers. If all possible observations of the data are included, then the mean refers to the *population mean*. If, however, a proportion of observations is taken from the whole, then the mean refers to the sample mean.

population. A given concentration level of serum albumin is considered normal as long as it falls within two standard deviations of the mean. Hence, according to Boorse's explanation of a statistical concept of health, a clinician would consider concentration levels of serum albumin that fall within two standard deviations of the mean to be normal and therefore healthy concentration levels. If, however, a given concentration level is either greater or less than two standard deviations from the mean, then such a concentration level will be considered abnormal and not healthy. Thus, within any standard distribution, approximately 95% of a population will be considered normal and healthy, but approximately 5% will be considered abnormal and not healthy.

The following numerical example should help to illustrate normal variation. For the sake of simplicity, assume that the serum albumin level of a given population is normally distributed in the following way:

Mean ($\mu$) = 100g
Standard Deviation ($\sigma$) = 15g

The normal distribution curve for serum albumin is as follows (Figure 2.1):

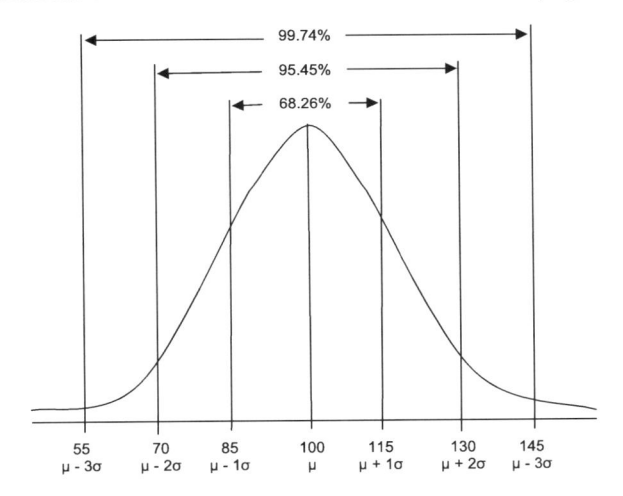

Figure 2.1 Divisions of the Normal Distribution of Serum Albumin[12]

Three points can be gleaned from the above graph. First, the normal distribution/ variation has the appearance of a symmetrical bell-shaped curve extending infinitely in both directions. Second, the normal distribution is a theoretical distribution defined by two parameters: the mean $\mu$ and the standard deviation $\sigma$. Third, all normal distributions have a particular internal distribution for the area under the curve. Regardless of whether the standard deviation and the mean are large or small, the relative area between any two designated points is always the same. For example, the 68.26% of the area are contained within +/- 1$\sigma$, 95.45% within +/-2$\sigma$, and 99.74% within +/− 3$\sigma$. As it happens to be the case, approximately 95% of

---

[12] This graph is from Kuzma, *Basic Statistics for the Health Sciences*, 82.

the serum albumin levels fall between 70g and 130g. Finally, close to 2.5% of the population is above 130g and 2.5% is below 70g.[13]

*Boorse's critical reply to the statistical concept of health*   Boorse offers the following criticism of the statistical concept of health:

> [S]tatistical normality fails as a necessary or sufficient condition of health. It cannot be necessary because unusual conditions, e.g., type *O* blood or red hair, may be perfectly healthy. It cannot be sufficient because unhealthy conditions may be typical. No doubt the average person or organ is healthy in a practical sense of displaying no indications for treatment, but that is not the same as complete freedom from disease. Some of what medical texts consider disease processes are at work in virtually everyone below the level of clinical detection. There are also particular diseases—atherosclerosis, minor lung inflammation, perhaps tooth decay—that are nearly universal. *In spite of these difficulties we will give statistical normality an important role in our view, which shows that necessary and sufficient conditions are not the only possible components of an analysis.*[14]

Boorse does not think that the statistical concept of health provides either a necessary condition or sufficient condition for health. First, he denies that it provides a necessary condition, because it is possible for some people to have a certain physiological or phenotypic feature that is quite outside of the mean, although they are entirely healthy. For example, it is possible for there to be a person who has exceptional functioning kidneys or excellent eyesight (two standard deviations from the mean) beyond that which is present in the average person. According to Boorse's explication of the statistical concept of health, such a person with exceptional kidneys or excellent eyesight would not be considered healthy. Thus, he concludes that deviating considerably from the mean with respect to a certain condition is not a necessary condition for health.

Furthermore, Boorse argues that the statistical concept of health also does not provide a sufficient condition for health, because there are many physiological states

---

[13] Note that to determine how many standard deviations away from the mean a particular observation is or what proportion of people fall within a certain range (e.g., 100–130), a *Z score* would be required. A Z score is a standardized unit that gives the relative position of any observation in the distribution. For example, the proportion of people who have serum albumin levels greater than 130 could be determined using a Z score analysis.

[14] Boorse, "Health as a Theoretical Concept," 546–7 [my italics]. As will be made clear in the next chapter, Boorse will argue that providing both necessary and sufficient conditions for a complete concept of health will not be possible because of the vexing problems associated with the concept of function. This rejection of a necessary-and-sufficient-conditions analysis of health may reflect a lack of charity on Boorse's part. For he wishes to show the inadequacies of other theories based on the inability of these theories to render a concept of health that meets both necessary and sufficient conditions. Yet, he is unwilling to offer such an account himself. I think there is something to this concern. Boorse may very well be unfair to the theories that he is criticizing, since he is not willing to allow his own concept of health to be scrutinized by the same critical standards that he requires of other theories. Still, the reasons for Boorse's rejection of a necessary-and-sufficient-conditions analysis of the concept of health will be made clear in the next chapter.

which are within two standard deviations from the mean, that are typical but not healthy. According to Boorse, those who employ the statistical approach, however, would have to claim that all states at or near the mean are healthy states. For example, tooth decay is a common condition for most all people in the world. Tooth decay is also thought to be a degenerative disease state by most doctors.[15] Assuming that tooth decay is a condition that is not healthy, then it would be a mistake to use statistical normal limits to claim that tooth decay is a healthy state. Thus, Boorse concludes that being near the mean with respect to a certain condition is not sufficient to be deemed healthy.[16]

This section has shown that, although the statistical concept of health involves a kind of naturalistic explanation of health, Boorse rejects it. Specifically, he persuasively argues that statistical normality provides neither a necessary condition nor a sufficient condition for health. Thus, he reasonably concludes that the statistical concept of health offers little in terms of a defensible naturalistic concept of health.

**Adaptation and the Concept of Health**

The term "naturalism" can also refer to the accounts of biological systems offered by biologists, psychologists, chemists, physiologists, or anthropologists. With reference to these accounts, healthy organisms are understood as those that are well *adapted* to their environments. The adaptation concept of health takes two main forms: (1) evolutionary-adaptation and (2) acclimation-adaptation. The acclimation-adaptation concept of health also has both a positive and a negative version. In what follows, a brief explanation of each concept will be given, along with Boorse's reasons for rejecting each one. Immediately following each of Boorse's replies, an assessment will be offered. This section will argue that, although Boorse is mostly successful in his reply to (2), his critique of (1) is unpersuasive.

*Evolutionary-Adaptation Concept of Health*

Although it may be true that all biological properties are physical properties, many scholars insist that biological organisms have a hierarchical complexity that requires a distinct sort of explanatory foundation.[17] This foundation, they argue, can be found in evolution theory. Specifically, evolutionary theory acknowledges the fact that biological entities are complex hierarchically organized entities designed to solve problems posed by the environment, problems of internal integration, and

---

[15] See S.R. Prabhu, D.F. Wilson, D.K. Daftary, and N.W. Johnson, *Oral Diseases in the Tropics* (New York, 1992).

[16] A variation on these criticisms to statistical normality can be found in Jerome C. Wakefield, "The Concept of Mental Disorder: On the Boundary Between Biological Facts and Social Values," *American Psychologist*, 47/3 (1992): 377–8.

[17] For example, see William C. Wimsatt, "The Ontology of Complex Systems: Levels of Organization, Perspectives, and Causal Thickets," in M. Mathen and R. X. Ware (eds), *Biology and Society: Reflections on Methodology* (Calgary, 1994), pp. 207–74.

the problems associated with reproduction.[18] Notably, biological evolution explains the presence of many of the traits organisms possess in terms of survival and reproductive success; that is, an organism is considered *fit* to the extent that it is able to survive and reproduce through the use of its many evolved physical traits. A striking example of such adaptive traits is the echolocation system of bats. This system enables certain species of bats to produce high-energy, high frequency sound waves. Also, echolocating bats have mechanisms that protect their ears when they produce such powerful sounds and both facial and neural structures that assist in detecting return echoes. These structures are evolved adaptations for flight guidance, pursuit of prey, and avoidance of predators. All in all, these different interacting features represent a fairly efficient evolved adaptive system that is crucial to survival and reproductive success.[19]

William Bechtel offers the following account of the health status of complex biological systems from an evolutionary perspective:

> Darwinian natural selection ... is uniquely capable of revealing the importance of organized systems, for it shows that such systems have been selected because of their ability to meet environmental demands ... [Such evolved systems] are those that can survive and replicate in the face of fluctuations in their environments. A healthy state of the system is one in which it makes best use of its physiological endowments in responding to selection pressures.[20]

Two points can be gleaned from Bechtel's account. First, an organism is fit and therefore in a healthy state to the extent that its physical traits operate the way they have evolved to operate within certain environmental parameters. Second, meeting environmental demands is typically understood in terms of survival and reproduction. Thus, from the evolutionary-adaptation perspective, an organism is in a state of health to the extent that its evolved traits assist in keeping the organism alive and helping it to reproduce.

*Boorse's reply to the evolutionary-adaptation concept of health*   Boorse responds to the evolution-adaptation concept of health by noting that many writers in diverse fields have "identified health with a biological notion of fitness and reproduction."[21]

---

[18] For a more detailed analysis of the concept of adaptation, see Richard M. Burian, "Adaptation: Historical Perspectives," in Evelyn Fox Keller and Elisabeth A Lloyd (eds), *Keywords in Evolutionary Biology* (Cambridge, 1992), pp. 7–12.

[19] The adaptation of bat echolocation systems is briefly discussed in Kim Sterelny and Paul E. Griffiths, *Sex and Death: An Introduction to the Philosophy of Biology* (Chicago, 1999), pp. 29–30.

[20] William Bechtel, "A Naturalistic Concept of Health," in James M. Humber and Robert F. Almeder (eds), *Biomedical Ethics Reviews 1985* (Clifton, 1985), p. 149 and p. 154 [bracketed addition mine]. Note that the positive account in Chapter 7 will include some of Bechtel's analysis.

[21] Boorse, "Health as a Theoretical Concept," 548. Boorse is referring to the following writers: J.A. Ryle, René Dubos, and Heinz Hartmann. Bechtel's evolutionary account is basically a variation on these accounts.

From this claim, Boorse then goes on to point out that if "being healthy" refers solely to the biological notion of genetic fitness, then it is misguided, because

> [p]arents hardly become healthier with each successive child, nor would anyone maintain that the healthiest traits are the ones that promote large families. Fitness or adaptation here must be a relation between organism and environment *only indirectly* related to bearing progeny.[22]

There are two parts to Boorse's criticism. First, he notes that an evolutionary version of adaptation that focuses only on genetic fitness is misguided, because it is possible for parents to be genetically fit by producing many children, but unhealthy in terms of caring for many children. Second, given this difficulty with the evolution-adaptation concept of health, Boorse claims that the genetic aspect of the evolutionary account should be marginalized in favor of how well organisms interact with their specific environments. Boorse's point is that reproductive success cannot be either a necessary or a sufficient condition for health, because producing more children can reduce the health of parents from (presumably) both the additional energy expended to care for each additional child and the "wear and tear" of childbearing on mothers. Rather, as Boorse notes in the last sentence of the above passage, "adaptation" or "fitness" must refer primarily to how well organisms interact with their environments, and secondarily to reproduction. This means, for Boorse, that the evolutionary aspect of "adaptation" or "fitness" is not of primary concern when determining the health status of an organism.

Boorse's reply to the evolutionary-adaptation concept of health is reasonable to a degree. Some scholars paint a picture of evolution that obscures the organism-environment relationship in favor of focusing exclusively on genes. For example, József Kovács remarks:

> Biologically, the "purpose" of our organs is not our survival, but the survival of our genes and our organs help our survival only in so far, as this contributes to the survival of our genes. Thus, the purpose of adaptation is the spread of our genes.[23]

Kovács's account of adaptation is partially correct, but it ignores or discounts nongenetic factors (e.g., the environment) that are crucial to genetic retention and transmission. It is important to note that natural selection is generally understood as an interaction between (1) phenotypic variation, (2) differential fitness, and (3) heritability. To focus on only one of these aspects of evolution is to obscure the fact that features of organisms are the product of both genetic and nongenetic factors related, in part, to phenotypes interacting with the environment. As Kim Sterelny and Paul Griffiths note,

> All traits have both genetic and nongenetic causes. The development of any trait can be blocked by some genetic modification. Equally, barring mutation-induced disaster, nongenetic modifications can stop any trait from developing. Social deprivation of young

---

[22] Ibid. [my italics].
[23] József Kovács, "The Concept of Health and Disease," *Medicine, Health Care and Philosophy*, 1/1 (1998): 33.

rhesus monkeys will prevent them from displaying their "innate" sexual behaviors as adults ... So it is universally accepted that all biological traits develop as a result of the interaction of genetic and nongenetic factors.[24]

Thus, Boorse is quite correct in pressing those "gene-centered scholars," who think of evolution only in terms of genetic reproduction, to take the organism-environment relationship seriously.

Nonetheless, Boorse's reply to the evolution-adaptation concept of health fails to take reproduction/genetic fitness seriously enough. As Boorse states in the first blocked quotation above, "Fitness or adaptation here must be a relation between organism and environment *only indirectly* related to bearing progeny." Yet this is not an accurate account of biological evolution. For evolutionary theory must not only take seriously the fact that non-genetic factors contribute to the success of an organism in interacting with its environment, but it must also emphasize the genetic or reproductive success (either directly or indirectly) of the individual organism. In this context, "reproductive success" refers to the extent to which an organism is able to survive and reproduce through the use of its many evolved physical traits; that is, the ability of an individual organism to produce a certain number of offspring under normal environmental conditions. On this view of biological evolution, it is not appropriate to emphasize the organism-environment relationship over reproductive success or vice versa. Boorse has done the former. Thus, Boorse has underemphasized the role of reproduction in his attempt to block the overemphasis of genetic fitness by some scholars.

Admittedly, there is much attention given to genes because of their information-carrying capacity. Once all the "genes-eye view" rhetoric is cast aside, however, it is clear that most reasonable evolutionary theorists assume that the organism-environment relationship is an integral part of genetic fitness.[25] Drawing on Boorse's own example, reproductive success and child rearing in many species are closely connected. For example, if the average number of offspring for a particular type of organism is two, then it is usually the case that there is selection pressure in favor of a certain amount of energy expenditure to raise two children to a certain level of maturity. Parents will be considered healthy to the extent that they are not only able to produce two children, but also rear two children. Of course, if there is selection pressure in favor of expending a certain amount of energy to care for two children, then the expenditure of additional energy on a third child (or more) could prove deleterious to the parents and the family as a whole.[26] Thus, an evolutionary

---

[24] Sterelny and Griffiths, *Sex and Death*, p. 98.

[25] See Kenneth J. Halama and David N. Reznick, "Adaptation, Optimality, and the Meaning of Phenotypic Variation in Natural Populations," in Steven Hecht Orzack and Elliott Sober (eds), *Adaptationism and Optimality* (Cambridge, 2001), pp. 242–72.

[26] Producing fewer young and giving each a high level of investment is known as *K selection* (as opposed to the strategy of producing many children with little rearing, which is known as *r selection*). Usually, *K selection* occurs in predictable and competitive environments, while *r selection* usually occurs in rapidly fluctuating environments. For further details about these different sorts of mating and rearing strategies, see Chapter 5 of Alison Jolly, *Lucy's Legacy: Sex and Intelligence in Human Evolution* (Cambridge, 1999).

perspective with respect to reproduction and child rearing does take seriously the idea that the organism-environment interaction is crucial to the concept of health. The further upshot is that there is no need to insist, as Boorse does, that an evolutionary sense of "adaptation" with respect to the concept of health must treat reproduction as a subordinate element to the organism-environment relationship.

In fact, it is clear that Boorse does endorse the close connection between reproductive success and the organism-environment relationship as part of his account of species design. Consider the following passage:

> It would be a mistake to think that this notion of a species design is inconsistent with evolutionary biology, which emphasizes constant variation. The typical result of evolution is precisely a trait's becoming established in a species, only rarely showing major variations *under individual inheritance and environment* … biological designs have a massive constancy vigorously maintained by normalizing selection.[27]

Putting to one side Boorse's account of species design (see Chapters 4 and 5 for this discussion), it is clear from the above passage that Boorse takes seriously evolution, specifically a particular version of natural selection. As he notes, natural selection has helped to maintain various traits in species. Since Boorse thinks that (for the most part) bodily activities "are contributions to individual survival and reproduction,"[28] it is unnecessary for him to minimize the role of reproductive success in his reply to the evolution-adaptation concept of health. First, Boorse accepts the view that a trait is healthy if it is able to achieve its goal. Moreover, given Boorse's acceptance of natural selection as the "fixer" of traits and body design, it follows that he accepts that the goals of traits and bodies are also fixed by natural selection. Thus, rather than minimizing genetic fitness as part of the evolution-adaptation concept of health, Boorse's account of traits and body design suggests he endorses it as an integral part of the concept of health. Thus, Boorse's criticism of the evolutionary-adaptation concept of health is successful only in response to those who maintain a "genes eye" view of evolution.[29]

This section argues that in his attempt to give prominence to the environment-organism relationship, Boorse has somewhat obscured the evolution-adaptation concept of health. Although Boorse is correct to note the importance of the environment-organism relationship with respect to the evolution-adaptation concept of health, he is mistaken to give it explanatory prominence over reproductive success. In fact, his own account of species design gives equal weight to environmental and genetic factors.

---

[27] Ibid., p. 557 [my italics].
[28] Ibid., p. 556.
[29] This point about evolution will be explored in greater detail in Chapters 5 and 6, where it will be argued that the role of evolution in Boorse's concept of health is unclear. Also, in these chapters and Chapter 7, further criticisms of the evolutionary concept of health will be considered.

## Acclimation-Adaptation Concept of Health

An alternative approach to evolutionary-adaptation is the view that an organism is healthy to the extent that it is well acclimated to its current environment irrespective of any Darwinian considerations. On this account, an organism can be healthy in one environment to which it is well acclimated, but be unhealthy in another environment to which it is not well acclimated. Thus, an organism is healthy or unhealthy to the extent that is it either successful or unsuccessful in coping with and adjusting to its present environment. Boorse summarizes two variations of the acclimation-adaptation concept of health as follows:

> Adaptation may be made a positive ideal of maximum enhancement of the abilities useful in each person's unique circumstances. Or one may develop the negative theme that conditions which would be intolerable in one person's situation may be tolerable or beneficial in another's.[30]

Boorse notes that there are two versions of the acclimation-adaptation account—a positive and a negative version. The positive version of the acclimation-adaptation concept of health is the idea that people are considered healthy if they are able to develop skills at a very high level to the point where such skills assist them in living well in their local environments. A close advocate of this view is Talcott Parsons, who claims that health is "the state of optimum capacity of an individual for the effective role and tasks for which he has been socialized."[31] If it is accepted that "acclimated" and "socialized" are related terms, then Parsons's account is very similar to the one offered by Boorse.

For example, imagine that Mary is a physically gifted (that is, she is tall, quick, strong, and has tremendous jumping ability) athlete. As a result of her socialization, she is of the view that being a good basketball player is crucial to her success. Thus, she accepts that she needs to use her physical skills and become an excellent basketball player. Given that Mary plays basketball in an environment that has many excellent basketball players, she devotes most of her energy to perfecting the various skills required to excel in this environment of fierce basketball competition. As a result of her relentless pursuit of being the best basketball player in her county, Mary receives many awards and much praise by her peers. Mary, on this account, is healthy as a result of her near "maximum enhancement" of her abilities in her current environment.

The negative version of the acclimation-adaptation account stresses the idea that being able to tolerate certain environmental conditions better than others distinguishes healthy from unhealthy individuals. J.A. Ryle, to whom Boorse is responding, describes the negative view by way of the following example:

---

[30] Boorse, "Health as a Theoretical Concept," 548.
[31] Talcott Parsons, "Definitions of Health and Illness in the Light of American Values and Social Structure," in Arthur L. Caplan, H. Tristram Engelhardt, Jr., and James J. McCartney (eds), *Concepts of Health and Disease: Interdisciplinary Perspectives* (London, 1981), p. 69.

The small stocky Durham miner—poor though his general physique may appear to be from the combined effects of heredity, malnutrition in childhood, and occupational stress in adolescence—is probably better adapted to underground work and life than would be the more favored and robust candidate from the Metropolitan police force.[32]

Ryle is claiming that people **X** with all sorts of physical, genetic, and occupational difficulties can be healthy to the extent that they are able to tolerate the demands of their environment **E** better than people **Y** (who do not have poor physical, genetic, and occupational influences and are from a different environment) could tolerate **E**. It is this comparative approach between people from different environments that distinguishes the negative version of the acclimation-adaptation concept of health from the positive version.

*Boorse's reply to the acclimation-adaptation concept of health*   Boorse rejects both versions of the acclimation-adaptation concept of health. With respect to the positive version, he argues as follows:

> All sorts of abilities—violin playing, tightrope walking, impersonating a President—may enhance people's ability to live well in their particular environments. But that does not mean that the lack of these abilities would be pathological for them or anyone else.[33]

Boorse's reply above is quite reasonable. Imagine that Mary's friends are the products of the same socialization as she is, but they are not very good at basketball. Assume further that they are not able to excel in any activity—they are simply mediocre at all that they do. It seems very odd to call these people unhealthy because they do not excel at a certain range of skills that are advantageous in their social environment(s). The point is that excelling at a skill in one's environment is not a necessary condition for health.

In fact, one could excel at a particular skill in one's environment and be quite unhealthy. For example, a world champion chess player, who has lung cancer, is unhealthy despite his remarkable chess-playing skills. Thus, being highly proficient at a particular activity in a particular environment is not sufficient for being healthy. Boorse's point is that the positive sense of acclimation-adaptation notion of health is neither necessary nor sufficient condition for health.

In reply to the negative version defended by Ryle, Boorse argues as follows:

> The thesis that a condition is not a disease if it helps you on the job would hardly make a good principle of labor law. On the contrary, it is a medical truism that symptoms of disease, e.g. inflammation, may be adaptive responses to environmental insult. As we saw, on the usual view of disease it is quite possible for diseases like cowpox or myopia to be advantageous in special environments. They do not thereby cease to be diseases, for

---

[32] J.A. Ryle, "The Meaning of Normal," *The Lancet*, 249/6436 (1947): 3. [Note that all variables to follow in this manuscript are emboldened to distinguish them from the rest of the text. In some cases, the font of quoted text has been altered for the sake of consistency.]

[33] Boorse, "Health as a Theoretical Concept," 549.

the judgment that they are is a judgment about the types of condition and mentions no particular environment.[34]

Boorse's rejoinder to the negative version is somewhat on the mark, but requires further explanation to make sense of how it is reasonable. The initial problem is that the negative acclimation-adaptation account is not so much, as Boorse suggests, about whether a particular not-so-debilitating-disease is successful in a particular environment at blocking some other debilitating disease in the same environment. Rather, the negative account assumes that there are two people (e.g., **A** and **B**) from two distinct environments (**E1** and **E2**) doing two distinct types of jobs (**J1** and **J2**). That is, **A** does **J1** in **E1** and **B** does **J2** in **E2**. Although it might appear that **B** is healthier than **A**, it turns out that this is not the case because **B** cannot do **J1** in **E1** as well as **A**. For Boorse's criticism to have greater force than it does he must show that this cross-environment comparison method of understanding health is misguided. As it is articulated, his cowpox example does not specifically tell against the negative account, because cowpox is present in a smallpox victim *in the same environment*.[35]

Still, there is little doubt that this negative account is misguided. The fact that a particular set of features allows people to excel in their environments relative to those in other environments is not sufficient for that feature to be healthy. The problem is with the comparison itself. There is no basis for comparison between a physically fit accountant from New York and a mineworker with deteriorating lungs from North Carolina. Indeed, the comparison could have just as well been made with the use of a newborn baby. That is, a miner from North Carolina with lung deterioration is better at mining than a newborn baby from New York. Anyone, who employs this cross-environment method, could argue that the miner is healthier than the baby.

Notice, however, that nothing about the activities of the baby or the New York accountant has any bearing on the miner's ability to mine. The point is that an implication of the negative account is that it is possible for a person **A** with many physically debilitating diseases to be considered healthy so long as a person **B** from a different environment cannot do what **A** can do in his environment. Thus, in principle, the only way a person could be unhealthy on the negative account is if a person is incapable of doing or greatly limited in doing those activities he is acclimated and trained to do. For as long as **A** can do **J1** in **E1**, it is possible to find some **B** who cannot do **J1** in **E1** like **A** can. The point is that the negative account is misguided because it compares "apples with oranges."

The appropriate comparison would be between the miner with lung deterioration and a similar miner, who does not have any substantial lung deterioration, is in the same environment, is around the same age, and is in possession of similar work-related experiences. Then, a comparison of their abilities as miners can be made. The point is that, even if one granted the claim that job efficiency or success is

---

[34] Ibid.

[35] The point is not that the cowpox-smallpox victim is healthy. On the contrary, the cowpox-smallpox victim is still unhealthy, but not as unhealthy as he might have been if the cowpox was not present. Rather, the point is that the negative account emphasizes different environments, not different diseases interacting at the same time in the same environment.

the criterion for health, drawing comparisons between the activities of individuals in distinct environments provides little or no basis from which to make health judgments. Thus, the negative version of the acclimation-adaptation concept of health is not very plausible.

Imagine, however, that the miner with the deteriorating lungs turns out to be more productive in the mines than the miner without the deteriorating lungs. Also, assume that it is determined that deteriorating lungs are better suited to handle the levels and mixture of oxygen at certain depths within the mine. Would not the miner with deteriorating lungs be deemed healthier than his fellow worker? The answer would be "no." The reason for this answer is that people's health cannot be determined by how well they perform their professional tasks in a given environment, because people are able to perform all sorts of professional activities while in a poor state of health (recall the champion chess player example). Even if arthritic fingers are conducive to good guitar playing, it does not follow that arthritic fingers are healthy fingers. Thus, the ability to perform well those activities to which one is acclimated is neither a necessary nor a sufficient condition for health.

It is at this point that Boorse's criticism is warranted. That is, Boorse's cowpox example shows that, even if a particular condition **X** helps alleviate or eliminate the presence of another condition **Y**, it does not follow that **X** is no longer the condition that it was. For example, if a bank robber prevents a murderer from killing a person, it does not follow that the bank robber is any less of a thief. Similarly, a deteriorating lung may assist a miner in being able to perform certain tasks, but it dos not follow that the lung is not deteriorating. Likewise, having cowpox can greatly reduce the deleterious effects caused by smallpox, but cowpox is still a disease that renders a person unhealthy.[36]

In summary, this section explained the different senses of the adaptation concept of health, Boorse's reply to each sense, and a rejoinder to each of Boorse's replies. Moreover, this section made clear that Boorse is not entirely successful against the evolution-adaptation concept of health. Furthermore, although Boorse's reply to the positive sense of acclimation-adaptation concept of health is persuasive, his rejoinder to the negative acclimation-adaptation concept of health is reasonable only in the light of where it is located in the broader discussion.

---

[36] Still, one might ask why is it the case that a condition is not able to change based on how it affects other conditions. The obvious answer is that it is an empirical question with respect to the disease under scrutiny. As Boorse hints above, poorly functioning states do not change in terms of their functional ability by virtue of their influence on other states. The exception, of course, is if the influence of poorly functioning states on other states actually modifies the poorly functioning states to function well. If this occurs, then the state that was once a disease will no longer be considered a disease. Thus, even if poorly functioning lungs are useful in mines, the lungs are still dysfunctional *qua* unhealthy, unless the mining environment actually improves the functioning of the lungs. Thus, whether or not a state can change from a state of disease to a healthy state will be an empirical matter.

## The Homeostatic Concept of Health

"Naturalism" also refers to those explanations that exclude mention of occult entities and speaks instead in the language of physical processes. These processes are ascertained through various observational means of trained scientists. Within this framework, organisms can be viewed as healthy to the extent that they are able to maintain a kind of balance between their *internal environment* (i.e., internal physiological processes) and the *external environment* (i.e., processes outside the organism's body) of which they are a part. *Homeostasis* is the term frequently used to describe this balance between the internal environment and the external environment. It is George Engel's specific version of the homeostatic concept of health (with which Boorse takes issue) that will be the focus of this section. The conclusion to be drawn from this analysis is that Boorse has not offered a very cogent reply to Engel's account, even though Engel's homeostatic concept of health is less than persuasive.

The idea of *homeostasis* is the linchpin in the concept of health for the physiologists Claude Bernard[37] and Walter B. Cannon.[38] As Boorse notes, "Bernard looked at physiological processes as serving to maintain equilibrium in the *milieu intérieur*, while disease processes were disruptions of the equilibrium, or homeostatic failures."[39] It is the work of Bernard and Cannon that influenced Engel to defend a homeostatic concept of health.[40] In order to understand Engel's homeostatic concept of health, a brief explanation of Bernard's and Cannon's ideas about homeostasis will be useful.[41]

Bernard made a distinction between an organism's "internal environment" and its "external environment." Cells and organs live within an organism in what he called its "internal environment," while the "external environment" is the outside world of which the organism is a part. In his study of the internal environment of organisms, Bernard observed that the chemical composition and physical properties of blood and other body fluids were generally constant. Although Bernard acknowledged that there is a close relationship between the internal environment and the external environment,[42] his research focused on how the constancy of body fluids maintains

---

[37] Claude Bernard, *Introduction to the Study of Experimental Medicine*, trans. H.C. Green (New York, 1957). Note that this was originally published in 1865.
[38] Walter B. Cannon, *The Wisdom of the Body* (New York, 1939).
[39] Boorse, "Health as a Theoretical Concept," 549.
[40] George L. Engel, "Homeostasis, Behavioral Adjustment and the Concept of Health and Disease," in Roy R. Grinker (ed.), *Mid-Century Psychiatry* (Springfield, 1953), pp. 33–59.
[41] A more detailed account of homeostasis will be provided in the positive account developed in Chapter 7.
[42] Although Bernard took the environment seriously, he downplayed its importance to some extent. He says: "A living body, especially in the higher animals, never falls into chemico-physical indifference to the outer environment; it has ceaseless motion, an organic evolution apparently spontaneous and constant; and though this evolution requires outer circumstances for its manifestation, it is nevertheless independent in its advance and modality." This passage is taken from Engel, "Homeostasis, Behavioral Adjustment and the Concept of Health and Disease," p. 36. Engel is clearly emphasizing the internal-external environment relationship

the internal environment. As a result of his research efforts, Bernard offered the following conclusion: "It is the fixity of the '*milieu interieur*' which is the condition of free and independent life," and that "all the vital mechanisms, however varied they may be, have only one object, that of preserving constant the conditions of life in the internal environment."[43]

Years later, as a result of his study of hormones, Cannon offered the following summary judgment:

> The coordinated physiological processes which maintain most of the steady states in the organism are so complex and so peculiar to living beings—involving, as they may, the brain and nerves, the heart, lungs, kidneys and spleen, all working cooperatively—that I have suggested a special designation for these states, *homeostasis*. The word does not imply something set and immobile, a stagnation. It means a condition—a condition which may vary, but which is relatively constant.[44]

Drawing on the insights of Bernard (and indirectly Cannon), Engel remarked that "Bernard pointed out that the conditions necessary to life are found neither in the organism nor in the outer environment, but in both at once."[45] In the spirit of Bernard's account, Engel offered his own rendition of the homeostatic concept of health:

> [H]ealth and disease are relative concepts, so that at times no clear distinction between the two is possible. This formulation takes into account the processes existing between and within the total organism and the total environment. The needs of the organism have a biologically determined source in instinctual energy, but satisfaction of the needs is achieved through biological, psychological, and social devices. *The aim is to maintain a condition of stable dynamic equilibrium between the internal and external environments...* If the capacity of the organism to deal with the stimulus is adequate, no disruption or equilibrium occurs and a state of health persists. If the stimulus cannot be dealt with, we recognize it as a stress which now upsets the previous homeostatic balance and disease is the consequence.[46]

Engel's homeostatic concept of health can be summarized in three steps.[47] First, Engel argues that health involves an organism's ability to maintain a balance

---

much more than Bernard. Nonetheless, he does draw this insight from Bernard as he moves to his own positive account of homeostasis.

[43] Claude Bernard quoted in Cannon, *The Wisdom of the Body*, p. 38.

[44] Cannon, *Wisdom of the Body*, p. 24.

[45] Engel, "Homeostasis, Behavioral Adjustment and the Concept of Health and Disease", p. 36.

[46] Ibid., p. 50 and p. 54 [my italics]. Note that Engel does explicitly mention the work of Cannon in ibid., p. 38. A similar version of homeostasis can be found in René Dubos, *Mirage of Health* (New York, 1979), pp. 110–28.

[47] It should be noted that this overall summary does not provide all of the details of Engel's account of homeostasis. The purpose of this summary is to provide the framework of Engel's account so that it is clear what version of homeostasis Boorse is rejecting. In what is to follow, it will be clear why certain elements of Engel's account cannot be explained in detail. Primarily, the role of *psychology* and the *social environment* are the two parts of his version

between the various biological and psychological processes *within* its body and to maintain a balance between biological and psychological processes and the external forces *outside* of the body. According to Engel, an organism is in a state of health (i.e., is able to satisfy *instinctual biological and psychological needs*) if and only if it is able to maintain a balance between both internal and external environmental stress. In contrast, the failure of an organism to respond to both internal and external stress (i.e., not be able to satisfy *instinctual needs*) will result in being "thrust" out of homeostasis and into a state of disease.

Second, it is the satisfaction of *instinctual needs*—physical, psychological, and social—that reveals a state of health for Engel. As he notes,

> The various adaptive devices, old and new, chemical, physiological, psychological and social which come into play to cope with stresses ... [contribute] to restore equilibrium and to assure satisfaction of instinctual needs. These may best be illustrated by an example, such as the invasion of a man by virulent bacteria. Here we see the specific and non-specific biologic responses to the bacteria, in the immuno-chemical reaction, the local inflammatory response, and the general change in bodily economy in the service of defense against the parasite. But we also see psychologic defenses, illustrated by such phenomena as regression, increased dependence, withdrawal of interest in the outer world, etc., as well as defences against these, such as denial of illness, which may be required to deal with old dangers revived by the regression itself or by the fact of being sick or by the particular psychological meaning of the disease itself. And finally social means may be utilized in the struggle, such as recourse to available medical resources, hospital care, social agencies, etc. ... The largest part of the disease picture is contributed to by this complex interaction of the adaptive devices in the service of homeostasis.[48]

Engel is arguing that physical, psychological, and social responses are necessary and sufficient to maintain homeostasis and satisfy instinctual needs. It is reasonable to infer from Engel's physical-psychological-social homeostatic concept of health that satisfying instinctual needs is both necessary and sufficient for health. Since being in homeostasis "assures" the satisfaction of instinctual needs, homeostasis (as understood by Engel) is a necessary and sufficient condition for being in a state of health.

Third, for Engel, a state of health will be relative to the social and physical environment in which the organism finds itself. For example, it may be healthy for an individual, who lives in a war-torn country, to maintain a defensive physical posture, a psychology of anxiety, and useful social alliances throughout much of every day. Such an overall defensive strategy would probably be crucial for survival. Alternatively, it may be quite unhealthy for a person living in an extremely safe surrounding to maintain a high-level defensive strategy. Thus, according to Engel, an organism is in a state of health if and only if it is able to assure the satisfaction of instinctual needs through a physical-psychological-social balance or equilibrium with respect to its internal and external environments.

---

of homeostasis that will be sketched here, because Engel himself concedes that only a broad sketch is possible.

[48] Ibid., p. 55 [bracketed addition mine].

Thus far, Engel's homeostatic concept of health has been discussed in general terms. It is important, however, to provide some details related to his account in order to understand it properly. To this end, the following three questions need to be answered:

1. To what specifically do "internal environment" and "external environment" refer?
2. What is required for the condition of homeostasis to be met with respect to the internal and external environments?
3. How does homeostasis work? That is, how is homeostasis maintained?

The answer to the first question is that "internal environment" refers to the surrounding area of the cells and organs and the individual organism's psychology.[49] *Intercellular fluid* is the term used to describe this area of cells and organs. This fluid provides the medium in which cells are able to live, reproduce, and engage in all sorts of activities necessary for life. For example, through this medium, "respiratory gases diffuse…, cells extract all their metabolites, and…[cells] shed unwanted substances."[50] Part of the answer to the first question, then, is that "internal environment" refers to the intercellular fluid in which parts of organisms (e.g., cells and organs) find themselves.

Engel thinks that the internal environment also includes both conscious and unconscious psychological processes. Drawing on the work of Sigmund Freud, Engel claims that the full development of the internal environment must include psychological forces. As Engel puts it, "Among higher organisms and man the development of the psychic apparatus allows for a psychological elaboration of the same [physical] process."[51] For example, with respect to unsatisfied needs, Engel offers the following assessment of the possible psychology of anger:

> [T]here may be any type of psychological representation of the affect, from conscious angry thoughts or phantasies, to all kinds of psychological processes which delay execution of the act or keep the affect or its object from consciousness, such as displacement, reaction formation, projection, turning against the self, etc.[52]

"External environment" refers to those elements external to the organism's body that can interfere with the basic needs or damage organs or parts of the body. Engel notes that these elements might include "such things as inadequate food, water, oxygen, as well as inadequate love, disruption of an interpersonal relation, or the restrictions of a society; it might include physical trauma, parasites, poisons, etc."[53] For Engel, the external environment not only includes the external physical

---

[49] Ibid., pp. 40–41. Of course, Engel is aware that not all species have psychological processes as part of their internal environment.
[50] M.B.V. Roberts, *Biology: A Functional Approach*, 4th edn (Surrey, 1986), p. 201.
[51] Engel, "Homeostasis, Behavioral Adjustment and the Concept of Health and Disease," p. 48 [bracketed addition mine].
[52] Ibid., p. 48.
[53] Ibid., p. 53.

environment, but also the social environment and its influences on individual psychology.

Second, what is required for the condition of homeostasis to be realized? The answer to this question is rather complicated and can only be broadly sketched. The general idea is that an individual organism's internal environment is in homeostasis if it responds appropriately to various stimuli from the external environment. Specifically, on the physiological level, the following physical states must be kept stable for the intercellular fluid to be in homeostasis:

(i) the chemical composition of the intercellular fluid (e.g., constant level of glucose in the bloodstream)
(ii) the osmotic pressure of the intercellular fluid (determined by the relative amounts of water and solutes)
(iii) the level of carbon dioxide in the intercellular fluid
(iv) the temperature of the intercellular fluid
(v) the elimination of waste from the intercellular fluid [54]

If the above five states of the intercellular fluid are held constant, then the internal environment is considered to be in homeostasis. As the biologist M.B.V. Roberts makes the point about these processes, "It is impossible to exaggerate their importance. Without them life would be impossible."[55] If any one of the five processes is not at its normal level or degree, then (depending upon the degree to which any one of the processes is above or below its normal level or degree) the body is unhealthy *qua* in a state of disease.[56]

The psychological aspect of the internal environment is much more difficult to explain. The problem is that there is no detailed account offered by Engel of what it means for the mind to be in homeostasis with respect to the external environment other than the brief homage he pays to Freud.[57] Part of the general answer, however, is that a certain balance between psychological needs is crucial to homeostasis. Engel notes the following with respect to anxiety: "The various systems of internal perception, unconscious and conscious, from chemoreceptors to the ego itself, are involved. If it achieves conscious representation, it may appear as feelings of anxiety, guilt, shame, remorse, as well as the more general feelings of malaise, weakness, fatigue, etc." Thus, a reasonable inference is that Engel's account of the psychological part of homeostasis is the achievement of a sort of equilibrium amongst a host of feeling states with respect to both the internal physiological environment and the various kinds of stress of the external physical and social environments.

---

[54] These five elements of intercellular fluid are taken from Roberts, *Biology: A Functional Approach*, p. 201.

[55] Ibid., p. 202.

[56] Engel categorizes these internal physical properties as "enzymatic constitution" and "physico-chemical composition." See Engel, "Homeostasis, Behavioral Adjustment and the Concept of Health and Disease," p. 41.

[57] Note that Engel lists nine concepts of how Freud's work has contributed to the concept of disease. These concepts range over both physical diseases and mental diseases. See ibid., pp. 38–40.

The third question, "How does homeostasis work?" can be answered in terms of physiological and psychological responses to bodily changes. When a change occurs in the body, there are two general ways that the body reacts to maintain both its intercellular fluid and its psychology. The first way is known as *negative feedback*—the body responds in such a way as to reverse the direction of change. For example, an important sugar the body uses for energy is glucose. The normal value of glucose in the bloodstream is approximately 90 mg/dL. The key to this constant amount of glucose in the bloodstream is the hormone insulin. When the bloodstream has too little glucose (a simple sugar the body uses as energy), the pancreas secretes less insulin than it normally does so that the liver converts glycogen and fat into glucose. Conversely, when the bloodstream has too much glucose, the pancreas secretes more insulin than it normally does. This increase in insulin production causes the liver to convert glucose into glycogen and fat in order to prevent gluconeogenesis (the wasting away of the tissues, which occurs in extreme starvation). The result is that glucose levels rise or fall back to the normal range. This example illustrates that fact that when certain chemicals in the body decrease or increase, there are a series of processes that are set in motion to return the chemicals to their normal levels. This reaction of reversing a change back to its normal levels, known as negative feedback, is part of the process of homeostasis that explains how homeostasis works.

The second way the body reacts to change is known as *positive feedback*—the body responds in such a way as to aid the direction of change. For example, pepsinogen is a protein-digesting enzyme that works in the stomach. When one pepsinogen molecule is activated, it triggers the activation of many such molecules nearby, which in turn activates other pepsinogen molecules. In this way, the number of active pepsin molecules increases rapidly, by using positive feedback.[58] The pepsinogen-pepsin system is thought to be one of the ways that the stomach avoids digesting itself. Pepsin is a powerful enzyme for breaking down proteins, and could damage the very cells that produce it. By secreting the inactive form (pepsinogen), the cells in the stomach's lining "play it safe" until it is necessary to bring about the active form. The point is that it is possible to have a positive feedback reaction that is beneficial to the body.[59]

Again, with respect to psychological homeostasis, it is difficult to determine what exactly constitutes positive and negative feedback. In his account of the various

---

[58] In a long footnote, Engel mentions (through the work of the biologist H.S. Jennings) both positive and negative ways that physiological processes maintain homeostasis. These terms are very close to the meaning of positive and negative feedback discussed here. See ibid., pp. 41–2.

[59] Of course, both negative and positive feedback processes are able to maintain homeostasis up to a certain point. For example, a fever is an example of positive feedback that can help maintain homeostasis by destroying bacteria. Beyond a certain temperature, however, high fever can cause permanent brain damage and even death. Also, an organism may attempt to satisfy reproduction or to care for its young in ways that go beyond satisfying instinctual needs (of course, this assessment is species specific). For example, an organism may engage in excessive life-threatening combat with others to secure a mate or to defend its children. Such reactions may very well compromise homeostasis. The point is that both positive and negative feedback have their limits.

defense mechanisms designed to maintain internal homeostasis, Engel includes both psychological and social factors. He includes such phenomena as:

> regression, increased dependence, withdrawal of interest in the outer world, etc., as well as defenses against these, such as denial of illness, which may be required to deal with old dangers revived by the regression itself or by the fact of being sick or by the particular psychological meaning of the disease itself. And finally social means may be utilized in the struggle, such as recourse to available medical resources, hospital care, social agencies, etc.[60]

For example, imagine a professional athlete who has a career ending injury (e.g., torn Achilles tendon). Getting medical treatment to care for both the physical injury and the psychological injury would require both a surgeon and a sports psychologist. Both forms of (social) therapy can be viewed as a sort of negative feedback (i.e., reversing the direction of both physical and psychological injury) in an attempt to achieve both physical and psychological homeostasis. Also, in the short term, increasing the amount of denial on the part of the athlete could be viewed as advantageous in terms of reducing psychological stress. Such an increase of denial in the short run could be considered analogous to positive feedback (i.e., aiding the direction of change). Admittedly, these psycho-social aspects of homeostasis are difficult to articulate clearly and in detail, because of how difficult it is to understand psychological phenomena in relation to social contexts. Engel himself concedes, "It is manifestly impossible in this paper to do more than present a broad conceptual scheme. We have neither the time nor the knowledge to elaborate all...the possibilities of contradiction between biological, psychological, and social adjustments. Much remains obscure and controversial and many chapters have yet to be written."[61]

In summary, Engel's homeostatic concept of health is the idea that crucial physiological, psychological, and social processes must be kept in an equilibrium or "steady state" in order that basic physiological and psychological needs can be met. This equilibrium is maintained through the processes of either (or both) positive or negative feedback.

*Boorse's reply to the homeostatic concept of health*   Although Boorse is well aware that many processes in the body are correctly explained by homeostasis, he rejects homeostasis as a sufficient account of health. He offers the following reply to Engel's homeostatic concept of health:

> Certainly many aspects of normal and abnormal physiology fit this model. Countless biological variables like blood temperature, acidity, speed of flow, and composition with respect to innumerable substances and organisms must be kept within narrow limits in a state of health...Homeostasis cannot, however, profitably be viewed as a general model of biological function. Many life functions are not homeostatic unless one stretches the concept to cover every goal-directed process. Perception, locomotion, growth, and reproduction upset equilibrium rather than maintain one. To say that their ultimate aim

---

[60] Engel, "Homeostasis, Behavioral Adjustment and the Concept of Health and Disease," p. 55.

[61] Ibid., p. 57.

## Boorse's Critique of Naturalist Concepts of Health　　　35

is internal equilibrium is unfounded; it is equally true, or truer, that the ultimate aim of internal equilibrium is perception, locomotion, growth and reproduction. Thus, there is no point in trying to view corresponding diseases such as deafness, limb paralysis, dwarfism, or sterility as homeostatic failures. One can see why various equilibria are crucial to life without confusing homeostasis with the broader idea of normal function.[62]

Boorse's criticism is that the concept of homeostasis is not the appropriate concept from which to understand physical health, because homeostasis is mistakenly thought of as a normal biological function. That is, if homeostasis is the normal biological function of the body, then it must be the case that *all* physiological processes aid to maintain homeostasis. Boorse replies that there are many physiological processes that disrupt equilibrium and that there are many disease states that are not connected to homeostasis. Thus, Boorse concludes that homeostasis is not the appropriate concept from which to explain health.

Given that Boorse is offering a reply to Engel's homeostatic concept of health, it is not very persuasive. Engel is clear that his concept of health is not limited to only physiological processes. Rather, he thinks that the correct sense of "homeostasis" includes not only physiological processes, but also psychological and social processes—that is, Engel thinks that the homeostatic concept of health should be understood in terms of the interaction between the internal and external environments. In order to offer a serious reply to Engel, Boorse must evaluate this tripartite (physical, psychological, and social) account.[63]

Also, even if Boorse's focus is on the physiological part of Engel's account, it is still not satisfactory, because Engel is clear that the physiological part of homeostasis is designed to secure instinctual needs. It is the maintenance of instinctual needs that reveals a state of physical health. The point is that Engel would agree with Boorse that the ultimate aim of internal physical homeostasis is the satisfaction of a host of other higher-end physical activities (e.g., reproduction, locomotion, growth, etc.). Thus, contrary to Boorse's reading, Engel thinks that physiological homeostasis is a necessary condition (not sufficient) for physical health *qua* the satisfaction of instinctual needs.[64]

Still, there are serious difficulties with Engel's homeostatic concept of health that Boorse should have noted. Two concerns will be mentioned here. First, as Engel himself concedes, a general theory of how to understand the mind and how it is in equilibrium is very complicated and speculative. The fact that Engel emphasizes a Freudian account would require much more justification than he has offered.

---

[62] Boorse, "Health as a Theoretical Concept," 549–50.

[63] It should be noted that Boorse is not replying to Bernard (or Cannon). For example, Bernard is clear that homeostasis is a means of maintaining life. That is, Bernard claims that the internal physical environment of the body is a goal-directed system that is distinguished by its tendency to sustain itself *by means of* homeostasis. To the point, Bernard would agree with Boorse that homeostasis of the intercellular fluid is a necessary condition for life, not that all life-sustaining activities are necessary conditions for homeostasis.

[64] No doubt, Engel would object to separating the physical dynamics from the psychological and social ones. Still, it is important to note that Engel is not making as strong a claim as Boorse suggests.

Restated, a behaviorist, reductionist, functionalist or emergentist account of the mind could also be defended within a homeostatic framework. Thus, even if Engel's tripartite account were to be taken seriously, it does not follow that his account of the psychological part must be accepted.[65]

Second, the social part of Engel's homeostatic concept of health implies a version of cultural relativism that must, at the very least, be critically defended. Imagine a society in which living a hedonistic lifestyle is praised (the city of Hedon). In order for people to be in homeostasis in Hedon, according to Engel's account, they would have to conform to the social norms of Hedon. If a citizen of Hedon does not embrace a hedonistic lifestyle, then he would be considered unhealthy, even if he did not have any physical disease. Yet, such a view leads to a type of cultural relativism that requires considerable justification. The point is that it may not be the case that all cultural norms are worthy of accepting. Indeed, it may very well be the case that a hedonistic lifestyle is quite deleterious to a person's overall psychology. At the very least, it is this sort of objection that Engel would have to entertain and overcome in order for the social part of his account to be considered an integral part of his homeostatic concept of health.

Where does this leave Engel's account? Since (by his own admission) both the psychological and social aspects of his analysis are rather speculative, it is only the physical part of his concept of health that stands up to scrutiny. If this is correct, then the concern is whether or not physical homeostasis is sufficient for health. It is at this point that Boorse's criticism has some force. Recall that Boorse is arguing that homeostasis is not a sufficient condition for physical health because there are cases in which diseases are present in conjunction with homeostasis. That is, a part of an organism can be diseased even if the intercellular fluid is in homeostasis. For example, it is possible for an eye to be diseased in conjunction with the intercellular fluid being in homeostasis. That is, intercellular homeostasis can be satisfied even with a diseased eye. Thus, Boorse is correct to reject the view that homeostasis is a sufficient condition for physical health.

Does Boorse, nonetheless, think that homeostasis is a necessary condition for health? After noting that he had not stressed homeostasis (which he calls "dynamic equilibrium") in his own naturalistic concept of health, he makes the following concession:

---

[65] There is a deeper metaphysical problem with Engel's account (and the mental health literature in general) in that he assumes *mental causation*. This is the idea that mental events and properties (e.g., someone desiring chocolate cake) participate in causal relations in bringing about actions. Yet, if mental properties are not neurophysiological properties, then it is not clear how they can be causally efficacious with respect to behavior. Of course, Engel could argue (as some have) that mental properties possess emergent causal powers of their own that explain behavior. Although such a suggestion still violates the so-called "causal completeness of physics," it is a possible strategy. The point is that any introduction of mental/psychological properties in an account of health must acknowledge and grapple with the problem of mental causation. Engel's account is wanting to the extent that he does not acknowledge the problem of mental causation with respect to his Freudian account of psychological forces.

Though I did not stress the dynamism [i.e., the process of homeostasis] of normal physiology in presenting [my naturalistic concept of health], I always assumed it ... Obviously, no fact is more pervasive than what is often called "dynamic equilibrium" of normal physiology: the normal functional variation within organisms acting and reacting to their environment. The normal level of almost all part-functions varies with what an organism is doing, what other part-functions are being performed, and the environment ... A common pattern is that environmental stress evokes short-term compensatory functions that maintain homeostasis up to a point, but beyond that point the coping mechanisms break down and a discontinuity, a discrete state of illness, results.[66]

It is clear from the above passage that Boorse does include homeostasis within his naturalistic functional concept of health. Setting to one side Boorse's concept of function, it is clear that homeostasis is an ineliminable part of his concept of health. To a certain degree, the body responds to all sorts of environmental stress. For example, when the temperature becomes too hot, the "coping mechanism" of sweating is activated to reduce overall body temperature. Beyond a certain temperature, however, the sweating mechanism is unable to maintain the body's regulated temperature level. In Boorse's own words, these coping mechanisms "are normal variation up to the point of breakdown; the homeostatic breakdown is pathological."[67] That is, Boorse's considered view is that homeostasis is a necessary condition for health, even though it is not a sufficient condition. Thus, homeostasis is a necessary element of Boorse's naturalistic concept of health.

**Conclusion**

En route to his naturalistic concept of health, Boorse took the task of evaluating and rejecting alternative naturalistic concepts of health. In terms of a final assessment, Boorse was successful in rejecting the statistical concept of health, but conceded that it was relevant to his naturalistic concept of health. With respect to the adaptation concept of health, this section revealed that Boorse was (for the most part) successful in his reply to the positive and negative versions of the acclimation-adaptation concepts of health, but was not very persuasive in his reply to the evolutionary-adaptation concept of health. In fact, this analysis revealed that he accepts an evolutionary sense of "adaptation" as part of his own naturalistic account of species design. Finally, in his reply to Engel's homeostatic concept of health, Boorse's critique is only partially successful. Although he is correct to reject homeostasis as a sufficient condition for physical health, he does, in the end, agree that homeostasis is a necessary part of his own naturalistic concept of health. Thus, although the statistical, adaptation, and homeostatic concepts of health are problematic when taken independently, Boorse concedes their importance to his naturalistic concept of health. How all of these elements fit into his own account will be the focus of Chapter 4. Forthwith, however, the next chapter will provide an assessment of Boorse's critique of the role of values with respect to the concept of health.

---

[66] Boorse, "A Rebuttal on Health," pp. 78–9 [bracketed additions mine].
[67] Ibid., p. 79.

Chapter 3

# Boorse's Critique of Normative Concepts of Health

**Introduction: Setting the Stage for Boorse's Critique**

The previous chapter included an explanation and critical assessment of Boorse's critique of specific naturalistic concepts of health. Recall that, as part of his attempt to defend his own naturalistic concept of health, Boorse also takes on the challenge of denying that the concept of health is *normative* or value-laden. This chapter will provide a critical analysis of Boorse's attempt to meet this challenge. Boorse begins his analysis by locating most normative accounts in either the *strong normativist* camp or the *weak normativist* camp. He also discusses two more specific normative theories of health, *moral normativism* and *functional normativism*, as a way of being charitable to specific accounts. This chapter will critically evaluate Boorse's arguments against these different normative accounts. This analysis will reveal that Boorse is successful in his reply to *strong normativism*, *weak normativism*, and *moral normativism*, but not entirely successful in his reply to *functional normativism*.

To start, Boorse asserts that his arguments against *normativism* "will apply to *all* versions indiscriminately."[1] Although Boorse does use "all" here, the domain of discourse must be made clear. There are many different kinds of normative or value-laden claims. As Boorse himself makes the point, "there are normative and nonnormative norms."[2] What he means is that "nonnormative norms" refers to values related to taking measurements. (Rather than using the peculiar phrase of "nonnormative norms," "metrical norms" will be used in its place.) For example, some scientists and philosophers of science speak of numerical symbols as having values in a quantitative or metrical sense.[3] Boorse is clear that such metrical norms,

---

[1] Christopher Boorse, "On the Distinction Between Disease and Illness," *Philosophy and Public Affairs*, 5/1 (1975): 51 [my italics]. It should be noted that Boorse's discussion of normativism covers many areas: (1) the relationship between the concept of illness and the concept of mental health, (2) the reason why the concept of illness (and not the concept of disease) has normative content, (3) the reason why mental health and physical health cannot be species of the same genus, and (4) the reason why the concept of physical health does not have normative content. This chapter focuses on (4), but will briefly make mention of (2).

[2] Ibid., p. 57.

[3] For example, Carl Hempel notes that: "Concepts such as length in centimeters, temporal duration in seconds, temperatures in degrees centigrade, etc., will be called *quantitative* or *metrical* concepts or, briefly, *quantities*: they attribute to each item in their domain of applicability a certain real number, the value of the quantity for that item. In addition to these so-called scalar quantities, whose values are single numbers, there exist

which are an integral part of the scientific enterprise, are not of *major* concern to him. Indeed, he begrudgingly concedes that "[i]f health and disease are only as value-laden as astrophysics and inorganic chemistry, I am content."[4] Thus, Boorse is not necessarily trying to offer a case against normativity in all of its guises.

The question, then, is with what sense(s) of "normativity" does Boorse take issue? He remarks:

> The orthodox view is that all judgments of health include value judgments as part of their meaning. To call a condition unhealthy is at least in part to condemn it; hence it is impossible to define health in nonevaluative terms. I shall refer to this orthodox view as *normativism*.[5]

Elaborating on the above account, Boorse continues:

> Normativism has many varieties, which are often not clearly distinguished from one another by the clinicians who espouse them ... It will ... be useful to make a minimal division of normativist positions into strong and weak. Strong normativism is the view that health judgments are pure evaluations without descriptive meaning; weak normativism allows such judgments a descriptive as well as a normative component.[6]

Thus, Boorse thinks that normativism can be divided into *strong normativism* and *weak normativism*. The former is the view that only value judgments (and not any descriptive element) are part of the concept of health. The latter is the view that the concept of health includes both descriptive and value-laden elements.

There is one concern that must be tackled immediately. As it was noted above, Boorse does think that there are metrical norms. These are quantitative norms. The concern is how do these sorts of norms fit within the weak versus strong distinction? The answer to this question is that metrical norms are part of the descriptive component in weak normativism, but are not at all a part of the value-laden component in strong normativism. So, weak normativism includes both metrical norms and other non-metrical value-laden elements, while strong normativism includes only non-metrical value-laden elements.

Since Boorse claims that he rejects both strong and weak normativism, does his own concept of health suggest an alternative to these two positions? The answer is yes. He thinks that there are judgments that admit of no values at all.[7] As Boorse

---

other metrical concepts, each of whose values is a set of several numbers; among these are vectors, such as velocity, acceleration, force, etc." Carl G. Hempel, "Fundamentals of Concept Formation in Empirical Science," 2/7, in Otto Neurath, Rudolf Carnap, and Charles Morris (eds), *International Encyclopedia of Unified Science: Foundations of the Unity of Science*, Volumes I–II (Chicago, 1952), p. 55.

[4] Christopher Boorse, "A Rebuttal on Health," in James M. Humber and Robert F. Almeder (eds), *What is Disease?* (Totowa, 1997), p. 56. Note that the debate as to whether or not scientific concepts are value-laden will be addressed in Chapter 6.

[5] Boorse, "On the Distinction Between Disease and Illness," p. 50.

[6] Ibid., p. 51.

[7] Of course, as it was mentioned, Boorse is willing to concede that if it can be shown that scientific concepts are value-laden (he is skeptical about this), then his scientific concept

clearly notes, "the medical conception of health as absence of disease is a value-free theoretical notion."[8] What he means by this claim is that there are health judgments that include only metrical norms (e.g., statistical values). These health judgments are those made by the scientist; that is, he thinks that scientific judgments include only metrical norms. This alternative to weak and strong normativism can be called *descriptive normativism*. This is the view that the concept of health includes only metrical norms. The three positions are as follows:

1. **Strong Normativism**→ The concept of health includes only non-metrical norms (i.e., desirability).
2. **Weak Normativism**→ The concept of health includes both metrical norms (e.g., statistical values) and non-metrical norms (i.e., desirability).
3. **Descriptive Normativism**→ The concept of health includes only metrical norms (e.g., statistical values).[9]

Again, this chapter will focus on 1 and 2 above. Whether or not scientific judgments have norms beyond the metrical norms of descriptive normativism will be explained and critically evaluated in Chapter 6, where Boorse's reply to his critics will be discussed.

*Strong Normativism*

An example will help to clarify Boorse's distinction between weak and strong normativism. People with allergies are hypersensitive to certain foreign substances called allergens. The immune system is compromised as a result of these allergens, which can take the form of dust, cat hairs, plant pollen, certain foods, the saliva or venom from insect bites or stings, etc. Upon exposure to certain allergens, some people display allergic reactions such as watery and swollen eyes, breathing difficulties, sneezing attacks, itchy throats, skin irritation, etc. Primarily, an allergic reaction results from the production by the immune system (mast cells located in the skin, intestines, and upper respiratory tract) of chemicals known as histamines (among others). These histamines constrict smooth muscle that results in the disruption of circulatory activity.[10]

Assume for the moment that people who have severe allergy attacks for an extended period of time are thought to be unhealthy. According to Boorse, the strong

---

of health will be just as value-laden. This issue of whether or not scientific concepts are value-laden will be examined in Chapter 6.

[8] Christopher Boorse, "Health as a Theoretical Concept," *Philosophy of Science*, 44/4 (1977): 542.

[9] Whether or not descriptive normativism should even be considered a version of normativism is debatable. It is included here, because it is part of the way Boorse attempts to handle the normativism debate within the concept of health literature. Still, descriptive accounts may be covertly value-laden. This concern will be addressed in Chapter 6.

[10] For more details on allergies and the immune system, see Arthur M. Silverstein, *A History of Immunology* (San Diego, 1989) and *Fundamental Immunology*, 4th edn, ed. William E. Paul (Philadelphia, 1999).

normativist would claim that severe allergic reactions are "unhealthy" only because they are not desirable. As Boorse claims, "The common feature of healthy conditions may, for example, be held to be either their desirability for the individual or their desirability for society."[11] He continues on to say, "Strong Normativism will be the view that health judgments are pure evaluations without descriptive meaning…"[12] As Boorse notes, these "pure evaluations" can come from an individual with a certain "healthy" or "unhealthy" condition or from society. Indeed, given this range, it is reasonable that the pure evaluations can come from family members and close friends of a person with an "unhealthy" or "healthy" condition or doctors. Boorse does not seem to be so concerned about who is making the evaluation. Thus, strong normativism (according to Boorse) is the view that a physical condition can be "unhealthy" or "healthy" entirely from the "pure evaluation" of a patient or a third party.

Boorse captures strong normativism by way of Judith Marmor's claims about homosexuality. Basically, Marmor is critical of those psychiatrists who insist that homosexuals are "deeply disturbed individuals." Marmor says: "…to call homosexuality the result of disturbed sexual development really *says nothing other than you disapprove* of the outcome of that development."[13] Marmor points out that it is *only* the value that one places on a certain stage and variation of ontogenetic development that captures one's use of "disturbed sexual development."[14] If "disapproval" and "not desirable" are thought of as synonymous, then Marmor can be understood as a strong normativist.

*Boorse's reply to strong normativism*   In response to Marmor's remarks, Boorse offers the following critical reply:

> Marmor is claiming that to call a condition unhealthy is only to *express disapproval* of it. In other words—to collapse a few ethical distinctions—for a condition to be unhealthy it is necessary and sufficient that it be *bad*. Now at least half of this view, the sufficiency claim, is demonstrably false of physiological medicine. It is undesirable to be moderately ugly or, for that matter, to lack the manual dexterity of Liszt, but neither of these conditions is a disease. In fact there are undesirable conditions regularly corrected by physicians

---

[11] Boorse, "On The Distinction Between Disease and Illness," p. 51.

[12] Ibid.

[13] Judith Marmor, "Homosexuality and Cultural Value Systems," *American Journal of Psychiatry*, 130/11 (1973), p. 1208; quoted from Boorse, "On the Distinction Between Disease and Illness," p. 51 [my italics].

[14] This version of strong normativism is somewhat echoed in Mark Twain's comments on tobacco. He says, "As concern tobacco, there are many superstitions. And the chiefest is this—that there is a *standard* governing the matter, whereas there is nothing of a kind. Each man's own preference *is the only* standard for him, the only one which he can accept, the only one which can command him. A congress of all the tobacco-lovers in the world could not elect a standard which would be binding upon you or me, or would even much influence us." See Mark Twain, "Concerning Tobacco," in Stuart Miller (ed.), *Essays and Sketches of Mark Twain* (New York, 1995), pp. 151–3 [my italics]. Although Twain uses "preference" instead of "value," he still implies a version of strong normativism that is rather similar to Marmor's version.

which are not diseases: Jewish nose, sagging breasts, adolescent fertility, and unwanted pregnancies are only a few examples. Thus, strong normativism is an erroneous account of health judgments ...[15]

In his reply to Marmor, Boorse argues that it is not the case that a particular physical feature of a person is unhealthy because a person judges that he does not desire the feature. For example, given that a person dislikes the appearance of muscles, it does not mean that my muscles are diseases *qua* unhealthy in any way. Extrapolating from Boorse's example above, the muscle example reveals that the sufficiency condition cannot be met.[16] The result of this criticism, thinks Boorse, is that strong normativism with respect to the concept of physical health is an untenable position.

The only difficulty with Boorse's reply to strong normativism is his choice of Marmor as its proponent. Marmor's comments about homosexuality are hardly substantive enough to determine her considered view on the top of normativity. For instance, what justification would a strong normativist give for thinking that the concept of health does not have descriptive meaning? Marmor offers no answer to this question in her brief comments about homosexuality. In order to evaluate strong normativism properly a richer argument wound need to be offered. For example, Peter Sedgwick offers the following justification for why "illness" and "disease" refer only to human interests:

> There are no illnesses or diseases in nature ... The fracture of a septuagenarian's femur has, within the world of nature, no more significance than the snapping of an autumn leaf from its twig; and the invasion of a human organism by cholera-germs carries with it no more the stamp of "illness" than does the souring of milk by other forms of bacteria...[17]

Sedgwick goes on to conclude that what counts as illnesses and diseases is only the result of people's "own anthropocentric self-interest."[18]

Sedgwick is arguing that there is no state of *illness* or *disease* in the natural world, because the natural world is simply a series of processes and activities of organisms. An HIV-filled body or bacteria-filled eye is, on Sedgwick's account, nothing more than physical processes of the natural world like planets moving around the sun. It can be inferred that Sedgwick is drawing a fundamental distinction between how things are (facts) and how one desires for them to be (values). Thus, according to Sedgwick, a body or the part of a body is healthy if and only if it is valued (i.e., there is an interest/desire in maintaining a certain physical state of the body) and

---

[15] Boorse, "On the Distinction Between Disease and Illness," p. 52 [my italics].

[16] Boorse offers a similar analysis in his "Health as a Theoretical Concept," pp. 545–6. He says that "[i]t is undesirable to be mildly below average in any valuable physical quality, e.g. height, strength, endurance, coordination, reflex speed, beauty, etc. It is undesirable to have such universal human weaknesses as a need for sleep and regular access to food and water. These conditions are not diseases. Yet one could never distinguish them from diseases on grounds of disvalue alone...It cannot be undesirability alone that makes a physical condition a disease."

[17] Peter Sedgwick, *Psycho Politics* (New York, 1982), p. 30.

[18] Ibid.

a body or part of a body is diseased (or a person is ill) if and only if it is disvalued (i.e., there is a interest/desire in eliminating a certain physical state of the body). If this interpretation of Sedgwick is correct, then he can be described as a strong normativist.

It is this sort of justification offered by Sedgwick that Boorse should have considered in his critique of strong normativism. Sedgwick's insistence on the *fact-value distinction* in support of strong normativism provides the sort of justification with which Boorse could take issue philosophically.[19]

Nonetheless, Boorse does have the resources to contend with a Sedgwick-type account. He would agree with Sedgwick about the fact-value distinction. He would disagree, however, that a disease state is not a fact. Rather, Boorse argues that "disease" refers to the fact of the property of physiological dysfunction. Boorse makes this point as follows:

> [T]here is no doubt that biological theory is deeply committed to attributing functions to processes in plants and animals. And the single unifying property of all recognized diseases of plants and animals appears to be this: that they interfere with on or more functions typically performed with members of the species.[20]

Thus, by way of his discussion of function and disease, Boorse is able to deflect this part of Sedgwick's criticism.

How is Boorse able to handle the illness aspect of Sedgwick's account? The answer is that he would disagree with Sedgwick on this point as well. Specifically, Boorse thinks that the distinction between disease and illness makes room for talk of values in the case of the latter, but not the former. Boorse articulates the distinction between disease and illness as follows:

> It is disease, the theoretical concept, that applies indifferently to organisms of all species. That is because ... it is to be analyzed in biological rather than ethical terms. The point is that illnesses are merely a subclass of diseases, namely, those diseases that have certain normative features reflected in the institutions of medical practice. An illness must be, first, a reasonably serious disease with incapacitating effects that make it undesirable.[21]

Boorse goes on to conclude that a disease is an illness "only if it is incapacitating, and therefore is (i) undesirable to the bearer, (ii) a title to special treatment; and (iii) a valid excuse for normally criticizable behavior."[22] For example, if a person has severe allergies that make it impossible for him carry on with his daily activities, then this might be diagnosed as a reasonably serious disease. Moreover, if this same allergy-ridden person requires special allergy shots on a weekly basis (ii), displays violent and uncontrollable sneezing attacks that resulted in constant absences from

---

[19] The fact-value distinction is the commonly regarded philosophical distinction between true claims (i.e., facts) and evaluative or normative claims (i.e., values). This distinction is briefly discussed by Joseph P. DeMarco, *Moral Philosophy: A Contemporary Overview* (Boston and London, 1996), pp. 249–51.

[20] Boorse, "On The Distinction Between Illness and Disease," pp. 57–8.

[21] Ibid., p. 56.

[22] Ibid., p. 61.

work (iii), and genuinely dislikes the fact that he has this allergy condition (i), then such a person would be deemed ill according to Boorse. Thus, according to Boorse, every case of illness is a disease, but not every case of disease is an illness.

In contrast to the concept of illness, Boorse is insisting that "disease" is a value-free term in its theoretical sense. His justification is that it has the science of biology as its foundation. The idea here seems to be that disease is value-free on the basis that biology is value-free. Yet, Boorse is well aware that value judgments (moral and otherwise) permeate the field of medicine. His response is that those judgments within medical practice belong to the concept of illness.

Understood as a reply to a Sedgwickian-type objection,[23] Boorse could argue that the concept of illness reflects a mixed normativist account rather than a strong normativist account. That is, on Boorse's account, a person who is "ill" must be physically incapacitated, find the physical condition undesirable, and need special attention. This means that both a descriptive element and a normative element are ineliminable to the concept of illness, according to Boorse. The point is that Sedgwick's account suggests that he is a strong normativist about both the concepts of disease and illness. This part of the rejoinder to Sedgwick makes clear that the concept of illness is actually part of weak normativism. Thus, Boorse can show that Sedgwick is incorrect in his analysis of both disease and illness.

In summary, this section has revealed that Boorse offers a reasonable criticism of Marmor's version of strong normativism. This section also noted that Boorse should have picked a more philosophically oriented account than the one offered by Marmor. Then, it was suggested that Sedgwick's account (or one like it) would qualify. In any case, this analysis showed that Boorse does have the resources to reveal the inadequacy of such an account. In conclusion, Boorse has offered a reasonable reply to strong normativism.

*Weak Normativism*

It could be argued that even if desirability is not a sufficient condition for health, at the very least, it is a necessary condition along with other descriptive features for health. Boorse is aware of such a rejoinder and offers a reply to it by way of his critique of *weak normativism*. Weak normativism, in contrast to strong normativism, is the view that descriptive and value-laden elements are both conjointly necessary and sufficient for health. The reason is that the weak normativist claims that "the physical" and "the evaluative" are both ineliminable constituents of a concept of health. H. Tristram Engelhardt in the following quotation offers a version of weak normativism as it relates to the concepts of health and disease:

> Health and disease are both normative and descriptive ... [D]isease in itself is in the end the disease as it exists for us who both experience illness and explain it. Disease as an explanatory account is bound to the circumstances of that account ... Health, though,

---

[23] Note that Boorse's distinction between disease and illness is not a direct reply to either strong normativism or Sedgwick's account. It is being used to show that Boorse could argue against this sort of objection put forth by Sedgwick.

represents a direction common to all the continua from particular diseases to well being ... Health is a common way away from the many ways of disease.[24]

A return to the allergy example will illustrate the above passage. A weak normativist, like Engelhardt, would claim that the physiological aspects of an allergic reaction capture the descriptive component of the immune system. Still, the weak normativist would insist that the disvalue of having a prolonged and sever allergy attack must not be overlooked.[25] Indeed, a healthy immune system, according to the weak normativist, is one that does not mistakenly attack harmless entities in the body and does not produce the symptoms common to an allergic reaction. Moreover, the weak normativist thinks that labels such as "awful," "frustrating," "bad," "mishap," "innocuous," and "erroneous" are used by doctors or patients partly because of the disvalue of enduring a severe allergy attack. As Boorse remarks, "the weak normativist thesis [is] that healthy conditions are good conditions which satisfy some further descriptive property as well."[26] So, weak normativism is the view that the concept of health has both descriptive and evaluative content.

*Boorse's reply to weak normativism* Boorse offers the following reply to defenders of weak normativism:

> [E]ven weak normativism runs into counter examples within physiological medicine. It is obvious that a disease may be on balance desirable, as with the flat feet of a draftee or the mild infection produced by inoculation. It might be suggested in response that diseases must at any rate be *prima facie* undesirable. The trouble with this suggestion is that it is obscure. Consider the case of a disease that has infertility as its sole important effect. In what sense is infertility *prima facie* undesirable? Considered in abstraction from the actual effects of reproduction on human beings, it is hard to see how infertility is either desirable or undesirable. Possibly those who see it as *prima facie* undesirable assume that most people want to be able to have more children. But the corollary of this position will be that writers of medical texts must do an empirical survey of human preferences to be sure that a condition is a disease. No such considerations seem to enter into human physiological research, any more than they do in standard biological studies of diseases in plants and animals. Here indeed is another difficulty for any normativist, weak or strong. It seems clear that one may speak of diseases in plants and animals without judging the conditions in questions undesirable. Biologists who study the diseases of fruit flies or sharks need not assume that their health is a good thing for us. On the other hand, there is not much sense in talking about the best interests of, say, a begonia. So it seems that normativists must

---

[24] H. Tristram Engelhardt, Jr., "The Concepts of Health and Disease," in Engelhardt, H. T., Jr., and S. F. Spicker (eds), *Evaluation and Explanation in the Biomedical Sciences: Proceedings of the First Trans-Disciplinary Symposium on Philosophy and Medicine Held at Galveston* (Dordrecht, 1975), p. 125, p. 136, and pp. 138–9 [bracketed addition mine].

[25] Though maybe not entirely, negative or positive desire is part of what Engelhardt must mean by "experience illness."

[26] Boorse, "On the Distinction Between Disease and Illness," p. 52 [bracketed addition mine].

interpret health judgments about plants and lower animals as analogical, in the same way as would be statements about the courage or considerateness of wolves and rats.[27]

An example will help make sense of Boorse's criticism. The weak normativist might claim that poorly formed feet or a poorly functioning circulatory system are both unhealthy conditions, because they are both undesirable and there is an underlying biological explanation to buttress the reason for the physiological mishaps. Suppose, however, the following case: the nation is engaged in a controversial war and a draft (involuntary conscription) is imposed, but persons with poorly functioning circulatory systems or flat feet are exempt from military service. In such a case, having poorly shaped feet or a poorly functioning circulatory system may prove to be very desirable for those who do not wish to go to war or very undesirable for those who do wish to go to war. The implication of Boorse's criticism is that the weak normativist, who is thought to maintain that disease states are always undesirable, would have to accept that people with the same physiological conditions would be healthy or unhealthy, depending on whether they desired to go to war. The further upshot of Boorse's criticism is that the desirability criterion is not able to do the work the weak normativist would like it to do. Such examples like involuntary conscription would disqualify certain disease states as being unhealthy. Thus, thinks Boorse, weak normativism should be abandoned as a legitimate contender in the concept of physical health debate, because the desirability criterion is not a necessary condition for determining whether or not a person is physically healthy or unhealthy.[28]

This criticism by Boorse is plausible, but as he remarks, weak normativism may be interpreted in different ways, depending on whether health must be desirable all things considered or only *prima facie*. These possibilities will be discussed in turn. First, it seems rather implausible to think that health judgments about physical bodily conditions require knowledge about whether or not the condition is or is not desirable all things considered. For example, imagine that two people, Joe and Jane, suffer the same sort of chronic back pain as a result of being struck by lightning. Joe finds the new condition desirable because he is able to secure an indefinite paid leave of absence from his job. In contrast, Jane is a professional tennis player. She finds the chronic back pain undesirable because she is unable to play the sport she

---

[27] Ibid., p. 53 [my italics]. Note that Boorse does shift from human "desires" to human "preferences" in the above passage. For the sake of this discussion, it is reasonable to assume that Boorse is not using "preferences" or "desires" in any technical sense. For example, some scholars within both the areas of practical reasoning and rational choice argue that preferences include only cognitive states (e.g., beliefs), only conative states (e.g., desires), or some combination of cognitive and conative states; see David Schmidtz, *Rational Choice and Moral Agency* (New Jersey, 1995) and Elijah Millgram, *Practical Induction* (Cambridge, 1997). The technical nature of preferences and desires, however, is not an issue for Boorse.

[28] In his "Health as a Theoretical Concept," p. 545, Boorse makes a similar criticism against weak-normativism. He says that "[i]t is clear that diseases can be desirable under some circumstances. Cowpox could save a person's life in the midst of a smallpox epidemic; myopia would be advantageous if it meant avoiding the infantry. Sterility, in a world without contraception, might be a heavenly blessing to parents of large families." Again, Boorse's point is that something can be a disease and still be desirable.

loves and is no longer able to earn a living. On the one hand, in Joe's case, the weak normativist would be forced to claim that he (or his back) is healthy. On the other hand, in the case of Jane, the weak normativist would have to claim that she (or her back) is unhealthy. Given that both Joe and Jane are in the same physical condition with respect their backs, it is extremely implausible to think that the health judgment about their backs could differ so dramatically. Thus, Boorse is correct to reject the version of weak normativism, if it is understood to claim that a healthy condition is desirable all things considered.

However, Boorse charitably offers a way out for the weak normativist: disease states are, at the very least, *prima facie* undesirable. For example, the HIV virus may be assumed to be undesirable until additional evidence can be shown to the contrary. This charitable move, however, is not considered fully. For there seems to be two distinct senses of *prima facie*, and Boorse has addressed only one of the two senses. One (more popular) sense of *prima facie* is that **X** is or is not the case *at first glance* or *before close inspection*. According to this sense, the claim that people do not desire a disease that results in infertility is an initial hunch, intuition, or what would *appear* to be the case prior to any sort of careful inquiry. A second (more legal) sense of *prima facie* is that **X** is or is not the case *based on preliminary evidence* or "evidence that would, if uncontested, establish a fact or the presumption of a fact."[29] According to this second sense, a survey of a certain sub-population may reveal that most people in this sub-population do not desire a disease that has infertility as its only effect, but such evidence could prove inconclusive in the light of further evidence.

Boorse's criticism is directed against this second (legal) sense. That is, he thinks that, based on preliminary evidence, it is not clear whether or not people desire a disease that has infertility as its only effect. Even preliminary findings (by polling people for example), according to Boorse, would result in desires both for and against being fertile based on people's circumstances.

If this second sense of *prima facie* is accepted, then Boorse's reply is reasonable. Depending on the population polled, all sorts of answers about infertility are possible. Yet, if the first sense of *prima facie* is the relevant sense, then it does not seem at all odd to think that most people do not desire, *at first glance*, a disease that has infertility as its only effect. This suggests that it is possible to be a weak normativist and not think that polling people is the way to determine whether or not a particular physical condition is or is not *prima facie* desired. Rather, it seems plausible that, *at first glance*, most people desire to be fertile. Moreover, diseases are reasonably (with respect to the first sense) *prima facie* undesirable. Hence, Boorse should have also considered the first more popular sense of *prima facie* in his criticism against weak normativism.

If Boorse would have considered the popular sense of *prima facie*, then he could have conceded that it is possible to be a weak normativist in this sense. Yet, he could have gone on to note that the plausibility of the popular sense of *prima facie* does not disturb his overall critique of normativism. Since he is primarily concerned with

---

[29] William Morris, ed., *The American Heritage Dictionary of the American Language: New College Edition* (Boston, 1978), p. 1039.

the concept of health within the philosophy of health literature, Boorse could argue that the popular sense does not disturb the analysis (i.e., necessary and sufficient conditions) of health. Moreover, Boorse could argue that this popular sense of *prima facie* is similar to strong normativism. Since this sense is concerned with only the desires people have prior to careful consideration, Boorse could rely on his criticism that desirability (even in the popular *prima facie* sense) is neither necessary nor sufficient for health. For example, even if a condition such as hypercholesteremia (the presence of a high amount of cholesterol in the cells and plasma of the blood) is not undesirable *prima facie* (in the first sense), research in the medical literature could reveal that it is not a healthy condition. So, Boorse has the resources to contend with the popular sense of *prima facie*.

Bringing together his critique of the desirability criterion in both weak and strong normativism, Boorse has clearly shown that desirability is neither necessary nor sufficient for health.[30] It is worth noting that Boorse's point is related to science and values. He is evidently assuming that a self-correcting empirical methodology is built into the activities of medical science. He argues (in the above quotation) that if it is possible to provide medical judgments concerning non-human organisms, then it is possible to proffer the same kind of judgments with respect to the human animal. Boorse appears to imply that both the replicability of experiments and the assessment of how certain procedures and tests are performed help to ensure the plausibility of final judgments rendered by particular specialists—be they field biologists or doctors/medical researchers housed in hospitals. There is no need, for example, to go out and poll people as to what gets to be classified as a physical disease. Disease classification and determination, Boorse argues, is the business of the scientific community, not the community of public opinion. Boorse concludes that such judgments made by scientists and medical practitioners concerning physical health do not include values (except the metrical values of descriptive normativism), despite the claims made by normativists to the contrary. Chapter 6 will examine the extent to which Boorse is correct in this claim.

To recapitulate, this section explained weak-normativism and Boorse's critique of it. This analysis revealed that Boorse's reply to weak-normativism is persuasive. It also made clear that desirability is neither necessary nor sufficient for health. So, thus far, Boorse has successfully argued against both strong and weak normativism.

---

[30] Two points need to be noted here. First, with respect to Boorse's analysis, he appears to be concerned with the *thick/thin distinction* through his own weak/strong distinction. Thick concepts have both descriptive and normative content, while thin concepts have only normative content. So, the strong normative concept of health could be understood as a *thin concept*, while the weak normative concept of health could be understood as a *thick concept*. Second, it may also be the case that Boorse could be interpreted as suggesting that strong normativists are *non-cognitivists*, while weak-normativists are *cognitivists*. Non-cognitivism is the view that normative judgments do not make assertions or propositions, while cognitivism is the idea that normative language reports something to be the case (that normative propositions are either true or false). Since Boorse is clear that he wants to ignore some of these subtle meta-ethical distinctions, it is not certain where he stands on the cognitivism/non-cognitivism issue. For the sake of this discussion, then, Boorse will not be pressed on how he categorizes both strong and weak normativists in terms of the cognitivist/non-cognitivist distinction.

## Moral and Functional Normativism

Boorse is aware that the foregoing criticisms against strong and weak normativism may not tell against other versions of normativism. In order to provide a more comprehensive reply to normativism than he has up to this point in the discussion, Boorse discusses two more specific versions of normativism—moral normativism and functional normativism—that are commonly defended in the health literature, both of which he thinks fail.[31] Both of these versions of normativism will be explained in this section along with Boorse's reasons for rejecting each of them.

*Moral Normativism*

Moral normativism is the view that moral values play an ineliminable role in determining what it means to be a healthy human. Boorse's target of this version of normativism is Joseph Margolis.[32] Margolis claims that psychoanalysts have erroneously thought that their therapeutic practices and judgments "escape moral scrutiny."[33] Margolis sets up the problem as follows:

> On the one hand, we have a picture of a scientific, value-neutral enterprise, pursuing professionally formulated goals in terms of causal efficacy; on the other, we have a picture of technically qualified workers, who in offering professional advice, are promoting what they conceive to be the good life. One may suspect, as an independent observer, that, given the general nature of debates of this sort, there is a measure of justice on both sides.[34]

Margolis goes on to argue in defense of the morally value-laden aspect of the judgments made by the psychoanalyst as follows:

> [G]rant that a therapist prescribes a line of conduct for his patient solely in terms of its probable advantage in promoting healing—for instance, he advises a female client not to reveal her extramarital affairs to her husband, at least through the present interval of therapy ... one may disagree about whether a therapist actually does, or ought to, *prescribe* such conduct; one may also disagree about the division, between therapist and patient, of responsibility for truth-telling in a given interval of time...What we have to see, very simply is that a therapist's professional practice is, in principle, morally debatable.[35]

As Margolis suggests in the first passage, there is the belief among some psychoanalysts that their therapeutic activities and judgments are value-neutral. Margolis, siding with the moral-values interpretation of psychoanalysis, argues

---

[31] Actually, Boorse considers a third version of normativism (health as an "ideal") that is very similar to the adaptationist account discussed in Chapter 2. For this reason it will not be discussed in this chapter.
[32] Boorse, "On the Distinction Between Disease and Illness," p. 54.
[33] Margolis, *Psychotherapy and Morality*, p. 13.
[34] Ibid., p. 15.
[35] Ibid., p. 17. Margolis is referring to Heinz Hartmann. Margolis claims that Hartman argues that "Freud's own conception of psychoanalysis is a value-free, scientific endeavor." Ibid., p. 13. See also, Heinz Hartmann, *Psychoanalysis and Moral Values* (New York, 1960).

that the activities and judgments of psychoanalysts definitely are (and ought to be) under the moral microscope.[36] Margolis goes on to conclude, "if, as we have already argued, it is reasonable to view therapeutic values as forming part of a larger system of moral values, it is not likely that we shall be able to make out a strong logical contrast between judgments of the two sorts."[37]

Margolis's point is that, since the professional therapeutic values of psychoanalysts are part of the larger system of moral values, it is impossible to distinguish judgments stemming from either set of values. Margolis is assuming that moral values somehow influence therapeutic values (and possibly vice-versa). The result is that moral and therapeutic judgments are similar. Since judgments about the health of patients are one of the sorts of judgments that psychoanalysts make, it follows that such judgments will include moral values.

For example, psychoanalysts may endorse, as part of their goals of healing their patients, the policy of refraining from any sort of intimate relations with their patients. Embracing such a policy, according to Margolis, commits psychoanalysts not only to certain values, but also to the broader moral codes in which they find themselves.[38] It is these moral codes that Margolis thinks also influences the health judgments of psychoanalysts. Margolis's point is that if the judgments surrounding the practices of psychoanalysts include moral values, then the judgments surrounding the goals of such practices will also necessarily include moral values. So, if psychoanalysts think that their therapeutic practices produce a healthy patient, then the judgment that one of their patients is healthy includes moral values, because their therapeutic practices include moral values.

*Boorse's reply to moral normativism*  Boorse thinks that a devastating blow to moral normativism takes the following form:

> But this inference is a non sequitur. From *the fact* that the promotion of health is open to moral review, it in no way follows that health judgments are *value judgments*. Wealth and power are also "values" in the sense that people pursue them in a morally criticizable fashion; neither is a normative concept. The pursuit of any descriptively definable condition, if it has effects on persons, will be open to moral review.[39]

Boorse's point is that, even if health-promoting actions can be morally scrutinized, it does not follow that the corresponding health judgments themselves are morally value-laden. Thus, it does not follow that health judgments include moral norms.

This criticism by Boorse suggests that moral values are neither necessary nor sufficient for health. Moral values are not necessary for health, because people can be physically unhealthy even if their therapeutic treatment is of the highest moral standards. Moreover, moral values are not sufficient for health, because people can

---

[36]  Here, Margolis refers to the work of Philip Rieff. Margolis thinks that Rieff believed that Freud was "heavily committed to certain preferred moral doctrines." Ibid., p. 14. See also, Philip Rieff, *Freud: The Mind of the Moralist* (New York, 1959).
[37]  Margolis, *Psychotherapy and Morality*, p. 37.
[38]  Boorse, "On the Distinction Between Disease and Illness," p. 54.
[39]  Ibid., p. 54 [italics and bracketed addition mine].

receive therapeutic treatment that is morally praiseworthy and still be physically unhealthy.

It is clear from Boorse's reply that health judgments are distinct from therapeutic-action judgments. Although judgments about therapeutic action may be filled with all sorts of moral values, such values do not "filter" into the health judgments. This strict separation between health judgments and therapeutic judgments is crucial to Boorse's criticism, as he remarks:

> [O]ne should always remember that a dual commitment to theory and practice is one of the features that distinguish a clinical discipline. Unlike chemists or astronomers, physicians and psychotherapists are professionally engaged in practical judgments about how certain people ought to be treated. It would not be surprising if the terms in which such practical judgments are formulated have normative content. One might contend, for example, that calling a cancer "inoperative" involves the value judgment that the results of operating will be worse than leaving the disease alone. But behind this conceptual framework of medical practice stands an autonomous framework of medical theory, a body of doctrine that describes the functioning of a healthy body, classifies various deviations from such functioning as diseases, predicts their behavior under various forms of treatment, etc. This theoretical corpus looks in every way continuous with theory in biology and the other natural sciences, and I believe it to be value-free.[40]

Boorse holds that health is a state of the body that can be understood through the theories of a value-free science of biology. The theoretical judgments of biologists are conceptually distinct from the practical therapeutic judgments made by clinical practitioners. Thus, granting this distinction between theory and practice, it is easy to see why Boorse thinks that moral normativism does "next to nothing to rule out the alternative view that health is a descriptively definable property which is usually valuable."[41]

Boorse's criticism is quite reasonable. If one insists that theory and practice with respect to the concept of health can be separated (as Boorse does), then it is not at all clear that moral values associated with the practice of medicine are part of the concepts that form the theoretical framework of medicine. For example, it may be true that electric shock therapy is a morally reprehensible practice of securing a person's health. Yet, it does not necessarily follow that the concept of electric shock therapy and the concept of health include moral values associated with the practice of electric shock therapy. Indeed, as a result of electric shock therapy, a person could very well be returned to a state of health. Alternatively, the nefarious use of electric shock therapy may have no deleterious effects on a patient's health. The point is that what makes shock therapy morally reprehensible is distinct from its causal relation to health and disease. Thus, by distinguishing moral concerns from causation, Boorse's critique of Margolis's moral concept of health is persuasive.[42]

---

[40] Ibid., pp. 55–6.
[41] Ibid., p. 54.
[42] In Chapter 6, another variation of moral normativism in the form of a criticism against Boorse will be discussed.

In this section, the moral normative concept of health was made clear through the work of Margolis, who argues that the health judgments of psychoanalysts are normative, because their therapeutic practices are value-laden. Boorse objects that this conclusion does not follow, because the moral values associated with therapeutic-action judgments are not part of health judgments. The overall analysis revealed that moral normativism provides neither necessary nor sufficient conditions for health.[43]

*Functional Normativism*

Functional normativism is the view that function statements are value-laden. The idea here is that function statements presume certain objectively valuable goals that a system pursues. It is further assumes that the goals pursued by the system can be achieved at varying degrees of success or failure. It is the success or failure of the system and the end at which the system aims that capture the sense of value on this version of normativism. Since Boorse does not offer a particular author's version of functional normativism, an excellent version defended by James G. Lennox will stand as an exemplar of this camp.[44] Lennox explains functional normativism and its relationship to the concept of health as follows:

> [T]he continued existence of a living thing is dependent upon its continuous performance of a species-specific and determinable set of functions within a certain determinable range. Unlike other changes, such functions are distinguished by reference to their goals. But it is of the essence of life that these functions may or may not be successful in achieving their goals. The most fundamental value concepts are based on that simple fact: any living function may, judged by the standard of their agent's life as its goal, be a success or a

---

[43] It might be argued that Boorse has chosen a poor version of moral normativism. That is, he should have considered whether or not a patient's moral life is part of the concept of health. This is a reasonable concern, but notice that Boorse's critique of Margolis's version would work just as well against this kind of version of moral normativism. The reason is that the moral character or moral way of life of a person is neither necessary nor sufficient for health. One could be a morally upright person in action and thought, but suffer from lung cancer. This shows the moral status of a person is not a necessary condition for physical health. Moreover, a person could be a morally degenerate person and have no physical dysfunction. It would be very odd to consider such a person physically unhealthy. Thus, moral values are not sufficient for health. The point is that, although Boorse would have done well to include such a version of moral normativism, his critical reply to it would have been straightforward. A variation on this discussion about normativity with respect to theory and practice will be examined in Chapter 6.

[44] Boorse mentions that both Joseph Margolis and Ronald B. de Sousa defend a version of functional normativism (see Joseph Margolis, "Illness and Medical Values," *The Philosophy Forum*, 8 (1959): 55–76, Ronald B. de Sousa, "The Politics of Mental Illness," *Inquiry*, 15 (1972), pp. 187–201). Yet, he is very quick to dismiss this whole discussion in footnote fashion, and does not critically evaluate their accounts. Upon examining these authors' views, they are very much concerned with issues of mental health and functionalism. Since Boorse thinks that mental health is a concept that is rather problematic and should be treated separately from a natural *qua* physical concept of health, the naturalistic version offered by Lennox is quite appropriate here. See Boorse, "On the Distinction Between Disease and Illness," p. 58.

failure ... "Health" is, I am claiming, one of this class of value concepts. It refers to that state of affairs in which the biological activities of a specific kind of living thing are operating within the ranges which contribute to continued, uncompromised living ... The standard by which one judges the successful functioning of a biological system, then—the organism's life—is also the goal of that system. The concept of "health" identifies, as a value, the state in which all of an organism's goal-directed systems are contributing to this goal. Implicit in this judgment is the core idea that life is the standard of such value judgments, that by which every organic process is judged to be operating successfully or unsuccessfully.[45]

Lennox thinks that value is an ineliminable element of any descriptive account of biological functions, because the way that biological activities maintain life (or fail to do so) requires that life be understood as a fundamental value-laden benchmark. Restated, according to Lennox, the only way to determine the success or failure of a part of an organism (e.g., successful pumping of blood by the heart) is to understand the activities of the part in relationship to the life of an organism. It is in this sense that life is an objective value or standard for Lennox.

To illustrate further both the normative and functional elements of his concept of health, Lennox offers the following:

To claim that the immune system, say, is functioning successfully presupposes (a) that it is possible for it to function unsuccessfully and (b) that there is an objective way of differentiating success and failure. When an immunologist makes this judgment, I want to suggest, it is based on a particular standard of value—the life of the organism.[46]

For example, the goal of the immune system is to defend the body against foreign entities that may wreak havoc to the body. To the extent that the immune system is able to accomplish this goal, it is thought to be operating successfully—that is, it is functioning to assist the organism continue with its life or "uncompromised living." So, according to Lennox, the concept of health includes values that are relevant to the successful or unsuccessful pursuit (i.e., function) of maintaining life.

*Boorse's reply to functional normativism* Boorse's only direct reply to functional normativism is the following remark: "I think philosophers of science have made too much progress in giving biological function statements a descriptive analysis for this argument to be very convincing."[47] However, this reply will not do. Since Boorse is trying to be sensitive to the possibility of other normative accounts, he must offer a persuasive reply against those who claim that function statements are normative. Relying on the claims of philosophers of science, without offering their arguments (or one of his own), is an insufficient response.

Nonetheless, in this case, it seems that Boorse does have a reply available. The reply would be that it is not at all clear why the goal(s) of a system is an *objective value* of a system. Lennox is correct that successful functioning of a part of an

---

[45] James G. Lennox, "Health as an Objective Value," *Journal of Medicine and Philosophy*, 20/5 (1995): 502–3 and 507–8.
[46] Ibid., p. 507.
[47] Boorse, "On the Distinction Between Disease and Illness," p. 58, fn. 13.

organism is understood in terms of the goal(s) to which it contributes, but the goal, Boorse would claim, is a physical feature of the organism. From the fact that the goal of living is useful in terms of determining how successful or unsuccessful parts are at maintaining an organism's life, it does not follow that the goal of living is an objective value. For example, survival and reproduction are goals of most evolved biological systems. These goals are also the product of natural selection. If a function is understood as an evolved trait, then it exists to bring about its proximal goals and to ensure its distal goals of survival and reproduction. Now, if an evolved trait is not able to bring about both its proximal and distal goals, it is dysfunctional or unsuccessful. But both "dysfunctional" and "unsuccessful" are understood in terms of the proximal and distal goals of the organism. These goals are not values, but evolved physical features of organisms. It is not at all clear what role value plays in such an account.

The point is that Boorse could grant Lennox all of his account except the insertion of value into the analysis. Indeed, Boorse hints at such a response (in a different context) when he claims, "What goals a type of organism in fact pursues, and by what functions it pursues them, can be decided without considering the value of pursuing them. Consequently health in the theoretical sense is an equally value-free concept."[48] Seen as a possible reply to Lennox, Boorse is claiming that even if **Y** is the goal of **X**, it does not follow that **Y** has a value that needs to be understood in order to understand **X**.

Perhaps, Lennox might reply that goal(s) **Y** is an objective value to the extent that living is an objective feature of organisms that scientists are valuing when they engage in quantitative analysis. But Boorse would reply that life is then a value, only in the sense of a metrical value for the physiologist. For example, an immune system is functioning well to the extent that it ensures survival and reproductive success. Clearly, reproductive success can be analyzed quantitatively—the immune system is healthy to the extent that it contributes to an organism producing and rearing the relevant number of offspring for its species. In a similar way, survival is the continued existence of the individual organism. This has the metrical value of a single (or one) entity staying alive—that is, the immune system is healthy to the extent that it contributes to the survival of the individual organism of which it is a part. Thus, if Lennox means that life is an objective value in this quantitative sense, then Boorse would be happy to include Lennox in the descriptive normativism club. If, however, Lennox has some other sense of "value" in mind, then Boorse has the resources to reject it.

This section has explained the functional normative concept of health and Boorse's reason for rejecting it. Although Boorse's reply to this version of normativism was

---

[48] Ibid., p. 58 [my italics]. None of this is to deny that the goals of survival and reproductive success are useful to scientists in their attempts to determine precise measurements. To this extent, the goals of survival and reproduction do have instrumental value for physiologists. Yet, it does not follow that the usefulness of the goals of biological systems for physiologists is part of the concept of healthy or unhealthy functioning. Indeed, that the goals of organisms are useful to the organism itself does not confer value on understanding how parts bring about their respective goals.

rather perfunctory, this section went on to show that Boorse has the resources for a cogent reply to a Lennox-type version of functional normativism. The upshot is either that Lennox's account is a version of descriptive normativism and is not really in tension with Boorse's views or it is a normative account that Boorse is able to reject.

**Conclusion**

This chapter provided a glimpse into the discussion of Boorse's account of normativism with respect to the concept of health. Specifically, weak and strong normativism, moral normativism, and functional normativism were explained along with Boorse's arguments for rejecting them. This analysis revealed that he is successful in his reply to weak normativism, strong normativism, and moral normativism. Although his brief reply to functional normativism was unsatisfactory, the last section argued that he has sufficient resources to reject or accommodate this last version of normativism, depending upon how it is understood.

Up to this point in the overall discussion, Boorse's criticisms of both naturalistic concepts of health and normative concepts of health are in place. It is now necessary to turn to his concept of function in Chapter 4, since it is central to his concept of health.

Chapter 4

# The Function Debate and the Emergence of Boorse's Concept of Function

**The Importance of Function for Boorse's Concept of Health**

Boorse's criticisms of some of the influential naturalistic and normative concepts of health were discussed in the previous chapters. Despite his criticisms, he is sympathetic to certain elements present in some of these accounts. Notably, he finds that there is something salvageable in both statistical analysis and the concept of function. This chapter will focus on a part of the function debate and will culminate in Boorse's concept of function.

The importance of the concept of function for Boorse's concept of health is evident from the following passage:

> The health of an organism consists in the performance by each part of its natural function[1]...From our standpoint, then, health and disease belong to a family of typological and teleological notions which are usually associated with Aristotelian biology and viewed with suspicion. Often this suspicion is excessive. Informal thinking in the life sciences constantly uses typological and teleological ideas with profit, and much recent philosophical work has been done on concepts of function and goal-directedness in modern biology. This work suggests that aseptic substitutes can be found for ancient notions that continue to have a scientific use. I think one should see that the analysis below is essentially just such a substitute for the idea that diseases are conditions foreign to the nature of the species. Our version of the nature of the species will be a functional design[2] ... In my view the basic notion of a function is of a contribution to a goal. Organisms are goal-directed in a sense that ... they are disposed to adjust their behavior to environmental change in ways appropriate to a constant result, the goal. In fact, the structure of organisms shows a means-end hierarchy with goal-directedness at every level.[3]

It is evident from the above passage that Boorse has given special attention to the idea of function with respect to the concept of health. Indeed, he thinks it is possible to offer a concept of function in terms of goal-directedness that is defensible within the confines of contemporary biology. This fourth chapter will provide an

---

[1] Christopher Boorse, "On the Distinction Between Disease and Illness," *Philosophy and Public Affairs*, 5/1 (1975): 58.
[2] Christopher Boorse, "Health as a Theoretical Concept," *Philosophy of Science*, 44/4 (1977): 554–5. Boorse makes similar claims about the concept of function in his "A Rebuttal on Health," in James M. Humber and Robert F. Almeder (eds), *What is Disease?* (Totowa, 1997), pp. 7–12.
[3] Ibid., pp. 555–6.

account of Boorse's concept of function. How his concept of function fits within his concept of health will be discussed in the next chapter. For now, since the details of Boorse's own concept of function emerge as a response to Larry Wright's concept of function,[4] this chapter will provide a detailed account of Wright's concept of function, Boorse's reasons for rejecting it, and a rejoinder to Boorse's critique.[5] Finally, the chapter will discuss Boorse's own version of function and the extent to which it is a viable alternative to Wright's account. The general conclusions of this chapter are that Boorse is partly successful in his reply to Wright, but that his own concept of function is not as fruitful as he maintains.

**Wright's Analysis of Functional Explanations: the Three Adequacy Conditions**

In his attempt to offer a plausible account of a function, Wright acknowledges three adequacy conditions that are generally recognized by function theorists:

1. The distinction between *function* and *accident* should be maintained.
2. The distinction between *conscious function* (artifact function) and *natural function* (organism function) should be maintained.
3. A general concept of function must exclude any divine element.[6]

According to Wright's considered view, a persuasive concept of function must ignore the distinction in (2), maintain the distinction in (1), and accept (3). Importantly, Wright thinks that accepting (1) and (3), and ignoring (2) are the relevant adequacy conditions for a persuasive concept of function. A brief summary of each of these adequacy conditions will prove helpful as this analysis unfolds.

*1. Function versus Accident*

Within the function debate, there is a deep concern that it is difficult to distinguish a genuine function from a side effect or accident. This concern ranges over both artifacts and biological entities. For example, is the function of a traditional can opener to leave sharp edges around the lid that it opens or is its function to open a can? In this example, which is the function and which is the side effect? Carl Hempel illustrates the problem in connection with biological entities such as the heart.[7] Although the function of the heart is to circulate blood, the heart also makes

---

[4] Larry Wright, "Functions," in Elliott Sober (ed.), *Conceptual Issues in Evolutionary Biology* (Cambridge, 1994), pp. 27–47. This article was published originally in *Philosophical Review*, 82/1 (1973): 139–68.

[5] Christopher Boorse, "Wright on Functions," *Philosophical Review*, 85/1 (1976): 70–86.

[6] Wright, "Functions," pp. 28–30. Note that Wright also mentions that the distinction between *function* and *goal* should be maintained and that the distinction between *a function* and *the function* should be ignored. These two sets of distinctions, which are of general importance to the technical debates on function and teleology, will be ignored for the sake of this discussion.

[7] Carl Hempel, "The Logic of Functional Analysis," in Carl Hempel, *Aspects of Scientific Explanation* (New York, 1965), pp. 297–330.

thumping or beating sounds. Given that the heart regularly produces both of these effects, how is it to be determined which of these effects is a mere accidental effect and which is the *bona fide* function of the heart? Consider the allergy example. Imagine that every time there is a production of histamines by the mast cells there is also a corresponding inflammation of bodily tissue. Again, how is it to be adjudicated which—the production of histamines or the inflammation of tissue—is a mere accidental effect and which is a genuine function? These questions underscore the importance of offering a concept of function that allows for a way of distinguishing genuine functions from accidental or side effects.

*2. Conscious versus Natural Function*

Wright distinguishes between natural function and conscious function in the following manner:

> Natural functions are the common organismic ones such as the function of the heart... Consciously designed functions commonly (though not necessarily) involve artifacts, such as the telephone and the watch's sweep hand..."[8]

Wright observes that many scholars have denied that natural functions are at all possible:

> Several schools of thought, for different reasons, want to deny that there are natural functions, as opposed to conscious ones. Or, what comes to the same thing, they want to deny that natural functions are functions in anything like the same sense that conscious functions are. Some theologians want to say that the organs of organisms get their functions through God's conscious design, and hence these things have functions, but not natural functions *as opposed* to conscious ones. Some scientists, like B. F. Skinner, would deny that organs and organismic activity have functions because there is no conscious effort or design involved.[9]

The above passage makes clear that some theologians think that functions of organs and conscious functions of artifacts are the same to the extent that both owe their existence to a conscious designer—artifacts are designed by humans and organs by God.[10] Moreover, some scientists reject the idea that the functions of artifacts are anything like the functions of organs on the grounds that the former are the product of conscious design, but the latter are not.

---

[8] As Beth Preston makes the point, "It is commonplace among function theorists to assume that a viable function theory will be equally applicable to biological traits, artifacts, and anything else to which functions can be ascribed." See Beth Preston, "Why is a Wing Like a Spoon? A Pluralist Theory of Function," *The Journal of Philosophy*, 95/5 (1998): 215.

[9] Both passages can found in Wright, "Functions," p. 29.

[10] Although Wright does not offer an example, William Paley (an Anglican priest) could definitely stand as an exemplar. Paley thought that organisms are the epitome of functional organization as a result of the workmanship of a divine creator. See William Paley, *Natural Theology, or Evidences of the Existence and Attributes of the Deity Collected from the Appearances of Nature* (London, 1802).

However, since Wright holds that natural functions exist independently of any sort of divine agency, although they are similar to artifacts, he must offer a reply to both of these types of critics. He argues as follows:

> Now it seems to me that the notion of an organ's having a function–both in everyday conversation and in biology—has no strong theological commitment. Specifically, it seems to me consistent, appropriate, and even common for an atheist to say that the function of the kidney is elimination of metabolic wastes. Furthermore, it seems clear that conscious and natural functions are functions in the same sense, despite their obvious differences. Functional ascriptions of either sort have a profoundly similar ring. Compare "the function of that cover is to keep the distributor dry" with "the function of the epiglottis is to keep food out of the windpipe." It is even more difficult to detect a difference in what is being requested: "What is the function of the human windpipe?" versus "What is the function of a car's exhaust pipe?" Certainly no analysis should begin by supposing that the two sorts are wildly different, or that one is really legitimate…[11]

Wright argues that "conscious and natural functions are functions in the same sense, despite their obvious differences." Function statements take the form of "the function of **X** is to do **Z**" for both natural functions and conscious functions. Moreover, function statements answer the sort of "why questions" that are bound to emerge in the case of both natural functions and conscious functions. Thus, Wright also argues that it is possible to state "what it is to be a function—even in the conscious cases—that does not rely on an appeal to consciousness."[12] Thus, Wright does not think that maintaining a sharp distinction between natural functions and conscious functions is necessary for the concept of function.

*3. Functions and the Divine*

The final adequacy condition is fairly straightforward. As noted in in the above quotation, part of what it means to offer a naturalistic analysis is that it must exclude any hint of godlike influence. So, Wright also wishes to offer a naturalistic concept of function that leaves out divine intervention.[13]

The three adequacy conditions that Wright acknowledges have been explained. It is now possible to turn to Wright's concept of function and how he thinks he is able to satisfy these conditions.

**Wright's Etiological Concept of Function**

As part of his positive account, Wright notes that the underlying problem with the concepts of function that he rejects is that they all neglect to observe that "functional

---

[11] Wright, "Functions," pp. 29–30.
[12] Ibid., p. 30.
[13] Note that this adequacy condition allows for compatible theistic accounts. It only claims that theism is not required to explain function, and a naturalistic account should not include any theistic element. This point will be made again toward the end of the chapter.

ascriptions are–intrinsically, if you will—explanatory."[14] Wright thinks that function ascriptions are explanatory for two reasons. First, the "in order to" in function ascriptions has the same sense as the goal-directedness notion of "in order to" in teleological statements. Wright thinks that when it is said, "**X** does *in order to* **Z**," it is being explained *why* **X** does **Z**. For example, if it is said that the antelope leaps away from the lion in order to avoid being its next meal, an explanation of why it is the case that the antelope (**X**) is leaping is being offered—that is, leaping has the goal of predator avoidance (**Z**).

Second, the way people ordinarily ask about the functions of things suggests that they are looking for explanations. Basically, Wright believes that people's everyday thinking about functions is captured in their (reasonable) request to know why it is the case that **X** does **Z**. Wright explains as follows:

> "What is the function of the heart?" "Why do humans have a heart?" "Why does the heart beat?" All are answered by saying, "to pump blood," in the context we are considering. Questions of the second and third sort, being "Why?" questions, are undisguised requests for explanations ... These are rather ordinary ways of asking for a function. And if that is so, then it is ordinarily supposed that a function explains why each of these things is the case. The function of quills is why porcupines have them, and so forth.[15]

Having made clear that function statements are explanatory and assume an answer to specific why/what questions, Wright offers his concept of function in the following way:

The function of **X** is **Z** means

(a) **X** is there because it does **Z**.
(b) **Z** is a consequence (or result) of **X's** being there.[16]

(a) is Wright's etiological claim about the current presence of **X**. Wright is claiming that **X** has the form it currently has or exists as it currently exists because it does **Z**. (b) is Wright's "consequence-etiological" analysis. As Wright makes clear, "When we say that teleological etiologies are consequence-etiologies, we are saying that the consequences of goal-directed behavior are involved in its own etiology: such behavior occurs *because* it has certain consequences."[17] For example, the reason why mast cells (**X**), which are part of the body's immune system, are present throughout the body is *because* they produce chemicals (**Z**) (histamines) to help protect the body from foreign invaders. Moreover, the production of histamines is a consequence of the presence of mast cells.

---

[14] Ibid., p. 37. Wright is responding to Morton Beckner, *The Biological Way of Thought* (New York, 1959), Morton Beckner, "Function and Teleology," *Journal of the History of Biology*, 2/1 (1969): 151–64, and John Canfield, "Teleological Explanations in Biology," *British Journal for the Philosophy of Science*, 14/56 (1964): 285–95.

[15] Ibid., pp. 37–8.

[16] Ibid., p. 42. To avoid confusion, I have eliminated the "(2)" that Wright places in front of "(a)."

[17] Larry Wright, *Teleological Explanations: An Etiological Analysis of Goals and Functions* (Berkeley and Los Angeles, 1976), p. 56.

Importantly, Wright thinks that an appeal to consequences necessarily includes the view that there is something about consequence **Z** that is crucial to the existence of **X**. As Wright emphasizes, "When we explain the presence or existence of **X** by appeal to a consequence **Z**, the overriding consideration is that **Z** must be or create conditions conducive to the survival or maintenance of **X**."[18] For example, fever in a body is properly understood as a defense mechanism against infection (see Chapter 7 for discussion). This idea of fever as a defense mechanism further suggests that it promotes the maintenance and the survival of the organism itself. For a fever produces the consequence of "foreign invaders being eliminated or reduced" and the maintenance and survival of the organism. These consequences are the beneficial conditions that allow for the existence of fever. Thus, Wright would agree that a fever has a function because of the consequences that allow for its continued existence.

*Wright's Concept of Function and the Three Adequacy Conditions*

Wright is quite clear that his analysis is able to resolve the concern associated with genuine functions and mere accidents. Primarily, those things produced by **X** that are deemed mere accidents, thinks Wright, are those that do not assist in explaining how it is the case that **X** came to be. As Wright states, "It is merely accidental that the chlorophyll in plants freshens breath. But what it does for plants when the sun shines is no accident—that is why it is there."[19] Wright's point is that when two explanations are offered in support of being the function of **X**, the one that provides the most plausible etiological justification for the presence of **X** is the superior explanation. For example, imagine that a sheriff is able to defeat a gunslinger in a duel. As it turns out, a crucial part of his victory was that he was able to compromise the gunslinger's vision by reflecting the sun's light off his badge and into the gunslinger's eyes. Having momentarily "blinded" the gunslinger, the sheriff shoots him dead. In this example, would it be reasonable to claim that the function of the sheriff's badge is to distract gunslingers in duels? Wright would reply in the negative to this question, because such a suggestion does not provide a plausible explanation for the existence of the sheriff's badge. The function of the badge is designed to signify law enforcement agents. It is the historical success of this signification that explains the current retention of such an item. Thus, according to Wright, it is the most plausible causal history of **X** (from which the function of **X** is to be determined) that allows for being able to distinguish genuine functions from accidental effects.

Moreover, Wright thinks he has offered a concept of function that is able to range over both conscious functions (i.e., artifacts) and natural functions (e.g., organisms). So long as the idea of divine-conscious intervention is purged from the discussion, he thinks that his etiological theory of function can explain both artifacts and organisms. This conclusion, thinks Wright, is evident from the following examples:

---

[18] Wright, "Functions," p. 42. Wright's emphasis on natural selection as the appropriate sort of etiology will be discussed in more detail when the discussion turns to Boorse's critique. Specifically, it will be made clear that Wright actually qualifies his account to incorporate natural selection as part of his concept of function with respect to organisms.

[19] Ibid., p. 44.

Not only is chlorophyll in plants *because* it allows them to perform photosynthesis, photosynthesis is a *consequence* of the chlorophyll's being there. Not only is the valve-adjusting screw there *because* it allows the clearance to be easily adjusted, the possibility of easy adjustment is a *consequence* of the screw's being there.[20]

It can be inferred from Wright's use of the above examples that if the presence of **X** can be shown to bring about **Z**, and **Z** is a consequence of **X** *because* **Z** represents certain effects in favor of the continued existence of **X**, then **Z**—whether **Z** is a natural entity or an artifact—is a function. Thus, Wright thinks that a sharp distinction between conscious functions (artifacts) and natural functions (organisms) can be ignored.

Finally, since Wright is offering a naturalistic concept of function, he believes he has offered an account of function that is free of theological commitments. Wright defends his position as follows:

> [I]t is quite clearly a unifying analysis: the formula applies to natural and conscious functions indifferently. Both natural and conscious functions are functions by virtue of their being the reason the thing with the function "is there" ... When we explain the presence or existence of **X** by appeal to a consequence **Z**, the overriding consideration is that **Z** must be or create conditions conducive to the survival or maintenance of **X** ... This analysis begs no theological questions. The organs of organisms could logically possibly get their functions through God's conscious design; but we can also make perfectly good sense of their functions in the absence of divine intervention.[21]

Wright thinks that his analysis is able to ignore divine intervention because his emphasis on consequences allows for ignoring any divine element that may be present in both natural and conscious functions. Thus, although it is logically possible that God could have designed natural functions, Wright thinks his analysis is able to discount the issue.

In summary, Wright hopes to have offered a naturalistic concept of function that meets the following adequacy conditions:

1. Keeps distinct genuine functions from accidental effects
2. Ignores the sharp distinction between conscious functions and natural functions
3. Eliminates the need of any divine element

This section not only provided Wright's concept of function, but it also makes clear some of the adequacy conditions relevant to Wright's analysis. It is now possible to turn to Boorse's critique of Wright's account.

### Boorse's Reply to Wright's Concept of Function and a Rejoinder to Boorse

As part of his attempt to offer his own naturalistic concept of function, Boorse furnishes four criticisms of Wright's etiological concept of function. In this section,

---

[20] Ibid., p. 41.
[21] Ibid., pp. 43–4.

each of Boorse's criticisms will be explained and assessed in turn. This section will argue that Boorse's first objection is successful, his second objection is not successful, the first part of his third objection fails, while the second part of his third objection is partly successful, and his fourth objection is partly successful. The upshot of this section is that, although Boorse is not successful with respect to all of his objections, parts of his analysis reveal important weaknesses in Wright's analysis.

*Objection Number 1: The Criticism of Tautology*

First, Boorse argues that Wright's concept of function is very close to a *tautology*. That is, Wright's account of function lacks explanatory power because, in his attempt to use one term ("function") to explain another term ("effect"), it turns out that both terms have the same meaning.[22] If a term is being used to explain another term, but the terms are synonymous in meaning, then neither term can be used to explain the other term in any interesting sense. It this concern about the lack of explanatory power through the use of synonymous terms that sparks the following criticism by Boorse:

> Wright's rendering is much closer to a tautology than one expects from an apparently substantive remark. From a different angle, the difficulty is that "**X** is there because it has a certain function," has been made synonymous with "**X** is there because it has a certain effect." The result is peculiar if, as Wright insists, "function" and "effect" are not synonymous. On his account there is clear content in a specific statement like "The heart is there because it pumps blood" or "The stomach is there because it digests food." But there is almost no content in the generalization that the presence of an organic character may be explained by its function. For this generalization reduces to the statement that organic characters may be explained by things they do *by which they may be explained*. One could wish that explanatory force might be accorded function statements at a lower price.[23]

Boorse's criticism appears to be that when you extract the general formula of Wright's concept of function from particular examples, what you find is that "function" and "effect" are synonymous. Thus, according to Boorse, Wright would have to accept the implication that the presence of a thing with a function, which is not different from its effect(s), is being explained by its effect(s). That is, each term is being used to explain the other, but, since both terms have the same meaning, there is no genuine explanation.

*A rejoinder to Boorse's objection number 1* Upon close inspection, Boorse's criticism is on the mark, but Wright could reply as follows. The fact that a function is present because it produces certain effects, which aid in the maintenance of the function, in no way entails that the function and its corresponding effects are one and the same. The problem, Wright could claim, is that Boorse thinks that "**X** *has* a certain function" is synonymous with "**X** *has* a certain effect." But "has" is used

---

[22] Boorse, "Wright on Functions," p. 71.
[23] Ibid., p. 71 [my italics].

quite differently in these two statements. In the first, "has" refers to an activity that **X** can actualize. In the second, "has" refers to some phenomenon that **X** can bring to fruition, not something **X** actualizes. For example, the heart possesses the function of pumping blood, and it brings about the effects of oxygen distribution and life preservation. The heart does not, however, possess the feature of oxygen distribution or life preservation. Rather, through the actualization of pumping blood, it brings about such effects. The effects are what sustain the presence of the blood-pumping function. Once the different senses of "has" are clear, Boorse's insistence that "function" and "effect" are being used synonymously is incorrect. Thus, Wright could conclude that his claims about function are not tautological.

The above reply is plausible, but only reveals the problem with Wright's original formulation. By distinguishing the actualization of certain activities and the effects they have, Wright would be introducing an additional variable, call it **Y**, that refers to activities that are distinct from their effects. This variable is not present in his original formulation. It is this missing variable that could allow Boorse to insist that functions and effects are synonymous. Thus, it is reasonable to think that Boorse's criticism is on the mark. However, Wright should simply modify his account as follows:

The function of **X** is **Z** means

(a) **X** is there because it brings about **Z** by way of activity **Y**.

(b) **Z** is a consequence (or result) of **X**'s being there and actualizing activity **Y**.

This new formulation, which keeps activities distinct from their effects, can avoid Boorse's tautology criticism, but at the cost of abandoning Wright's original formulation.[24] Still, it should be made clear that Boorse's criticism is reasonable given Wright's original formulation.

*Objection Number 2: The Criticism of Equivocation*

Boorse's second objection is that Wright's general concept of etiology masks two distinct senses of "etiology"—one for organisms and one for artifacts.[25] Once these two senses of "etiology" are made transparent, Boorse thinks that Wright's attempt to provide an account of function that ranges over both artifacts and biological entities is doomed to failure. Boorse states his concern as follows:

> A second difficulty with Wright's analysis is that it is clearly incomplete as it stands. His formulation of the etiology clause—"**X** is there because it does **Z**"—is quite general, as is dictated by the aim of univocality between organisms and artifacts. The only restriction on the clause is that "because" is to be taken "in its ordinary ... causal-explanatory sense." Thus one would assume that regardless of whether organisms or artifacts are in question, any ordinary sort of etiological explanation of **X** by **X**'s effects will support a function statement. But this is not the case. The fact fails to emerge in Wright's discussion largely

---

[24] The problem of adding an additional variable to Wright's account is discussed by Lowell Nissen, *Teleological Language in the Life Sciences* (Lanham, 1997), p. 156.

[25] Boorse, "Wright on Functions," p. 72.

because all his organic examples involve one pattern of etiological explanation and all his mechanical examples another. When organisms are in question, all cases are of an evolutionary sort: the trait **X** arises in the first place by chance and then survives by virtue of doing **Z**. With artifacts, however, Wright considers only etiological explanations that appeal instead to the intentions of the designer. As soon as one examines cases where the pairings are reversed, it becomes clear that the restrictions to specific etiology patterns must be regarded as part of the analysis itself.[26]

With respect to organisms, Boorse claims that the causal story is an evolutionary one. As a result of random variation, a feature is accidentally present (among other features) and becomes a trait **X** by being selected because it does **Z**. Artifacts, on the other hand, have an etiology that originates in the intentions of a designer. As a result of the intentions of a designer, a feature **X** is selected (among other features) and designed to do **Z**. Boorse's main point of contention is that, once the evolutionary account is used to explain artifacts and the intentional designer account is used to explain organisms, it becomes clear that Wright equivocates on two distinct senses of "etiology." The further implication of this criticism is that Wright's concept of function cannot be generalized over both artifacts and organisms.

This "role reversal" criticism by Boorse can be understood through the following two examples. The first example makes clear the use of evolution to understand artifacts. Boorse provides the following scenario and the conclusion that should be gleaned from it:

> Suppose that a scientist builds a laser which is connected by a rubber hose to a source of gaseous chlorine. After turning on the machine he notices a break in the hose, but before he can correct it he inhales the escaping gas and falls unconscious. According to Wright's explicit proposal, one must say that the function of the break in the hose is to release the gas. The release of the gas is a result of the break in the hose; and the break is there—that is, as in natural selection, it continues to be there—because it releases gas. If it did not do so, the scientist would correct it. This and similar examples suggest that Wright will have to insist on the intention interpretation for artifacts.[27]

The second example offers an intentional/conscious purpose etiology interpretation of organismic traits. The example and the lesson to be learned from it are as follows:

> A man who is irritated with a barking dog kicks it, breaking one leg, with the intention of causing the animal pain. The dog's pain is the result of the fracture, and the fracture is there because its creator intends it to have that result. Yet I doubt whether Wright would wish to say that the function of the fracture is to cause the dog pain. So in parallel fashion one suspects that only the evolutionary interpretation of "**X** is there because it does **Z**" is supposed to be relevant to organisms.[28]

In the first example, Boorse argues that the natural selection interpretation of artifacts is implausible. Although the break in the hose appears to satisfy the conditions

---

[26] Ibid., p. 75.
[27] Ibid.
[28] Ibid.

of natural selection, no reasonable person would seriously entertain the possibility that the break in the hose was naturally selected because it allows for gas to escape from the hose. Boorse's "role reversal" argument could be understood as follows:

P1. Either the break in the hose should be explained through an intentional designer interpretation (i.e., conscious functions) of function or through an evolutionary understanding of function.
P2. If an evolutionary interpretation of function is appropriate for understanding the break in the hose, then it must be the case that the break in the hose satisfies the conditions of natural selection.
P3. If the break in the hose is to be considered a trait in a natural selection sense, then it must be a feature that is selected for because it has the function of releasing gas—a function which confers a fitness advantage, is present in a number of future generations, and it is stable in the population as a whole.
P4. The break in the hose is not a feature that is selected for because it confers a fitness advantage, is present in a number of future generations, and is stable in the population as a whole.
P5. It is not the case that the break in the hose is to be considered a trait in a natural selection sense.
P6. It follows that it is not the case that an evolutionary interpretation of function is appropriate for understanding the break in the hose.

*  *  *

Therefore, the break in the hose should be explained through an intentional designer interpretation of function.

With respect to the above argument reconstruction, it is important not to lose track of Boorse's general criticism. This general criticism is that Wright takes himself to be offering a single concept of function that ranges over both artifacts and organisms, but the counter examples suggest that he is unable to accomplish such a feat. Rather, argues Boorse, Wright is employing two senses of "etiology"—natural selection etiology and intentional designer etiology—that cannot always be substituted for one another. The broken hose example, argues Boorse, shows that a natural selection etiology is not appropriate. Thus, Wright must accept an intentional designer etiological account of function in this hose example.[29]

In the second example, Boorse offers a similar disjunction as P1 above, but the concern is now about organisms. This time Boorse substitutes the intentional designer explanation for the evolutionary explanation to reveal that only the latter makes sense. Basically, Boorse's dog example is designed to show that Wright must see the fracture as having the intentional designer sense of "function," because the presence of the fracture is the result of the painful effect intended by the man. Since Wright would not want to commit himself to the highly implausible view

---

[29] Note that Boorse is not arguing that the break in the hose does not have a function. This might seem like a reasonable criticism, but it is not the criticism that Boorse is making at this juncture of his analysis. Rather, he is simply trying to show that Wright equivocates on his use of "etiology," and that such an equivocation forces Wright into accepting a sense of "etiology" with which he would not be comfortable.

that the fracture has the function of causing the dog pain, Boorse concludes that Wright would have to accept that only an evolutionary interpretation of "etiology" is relevant to organisms.

In summary, the hose example is designed by Boorse to show that an intentional designer explanation—and not an evolutionary explanation—is appropriate. In the dog case, Boorse's point is that an evolutionary explanation—and not an intentional designer explanation—is appropriate. The general upshot of these two examples, thinks Boorse, is that Wright is not able to satisfy one of his own criteria—the idea that a part of a cogent concept account of function is one that ranges over both artifacts and organisms.

*A rejoinder to Boorse's objection number 2* The following rejoinder to Boorse includes both praise and criticism. Boorse's two examples against Wright's analysis are quite persuasive, if one insists that there is a clear difference between the intentional designer explanation and the evolutionary explanation. Assuming such a clear difference, Boorse's examples do reveal that Wright's analysis cannot range over both artifacts and biological entities. Boorse's strategy of substituting an evolutionary explanation for an intentional designer explanation in the case of an artifact and substituting an intentional designer explanation for an evolutionary explanation in the case of a biological entity makes the problem for Wright strikingly clear. That is, in the light of Wright's own analysis, Boorse has convincingly revealed that evolutionary explanations are appropriate only for biological entities, while intentional designer explanations are appropriate only for artifacts.[30]

With respect to this criticism, Boorse's reply to Wright is premature. Specifically, Boorse does not examine Wright's own claim that the intentional designer explanation is quite similar to the evolutionary explanation. Recall that it was noted above that Boorse's criticism of Wright is on the mark so long as one concedes that both sorts of explanation are not similar. Yet, depending upon how natural selection is to be understood, it may be possible for Wright to concede that he must accept an intentional designer interpretation of artifacts, but still insist that such an interpretation is similar to the natural selection interpretation. In fact, Wright makes just this move. He says:

> I can say that I selected something, **X**, even though I cannot give a reason for having chosen it: I am asked to select a ball from among those on the table in front of me. I choose the blue one and am asked why I did. I may say something like, "I don't know; it just struck me, I guess." Alternatively, I could without adding much give something which has the form of a reason: "Because it is blue. Yes, I'm sure it was the color." In both of these cases I want to refer to the selection as "mere discrimination" ... On the other hand, there are a number of contexts in which another, more elaborate reply is possible and natural. I could say something of the form, "I selected **X** because it does **Z**," where **Z** would be some possibility opened by, *some advantage* that would accrue from, or some other result of having (using, and so forth) **X**. "I chose American Airlines because its five-across seating allows me to stretch out." Or "They selected DuPont Nomex because of

---

[30] Of course, this assumes that theological explanations are excluded from the discussion.

the superior protection it affords in a fire." Let me refer to selection *by virtue of resultant advantage* of this sort as "consequence-selection." Plainly, it is this kind of selection, as opposed to mere discrimination, that lies behind conscious functions: the consequence *is* the function. Equally plainly, it is specifically this kind of selection of which natural selection represents an extension.[31]

Wright is arguing that natural selection functions and intentional (i.e., conscious) designer functions are similar because what counts as a function for both sorts of explanation is that functions are understood in terms of advantageous consequences. Wright would claim, in response to Boorse, that it is possible to substitute the evolutionary explanation for the intentional designer explanation (and vice versa) because both rely on the crucial idea that something has a function so long as its presence is due to its advantageous effects (i.e., consequences). If it could be shown that the hole of the hose has advantageous effects, which account for its presence, then a functional explanation of the hole is appropriate. Alternatively, if it could be shown that the dog's fracture has advantageous effects, which account for its presence, then a functional explanation is appropriate for it. It is reasonable to think that both of Boorse's examples fail because neither the presence of the hole in the hose nor the dog's fracture is present because of any advantageous consequences. Thus, Wright would likely reject both of Boorse's examples. Furthermore, Wright would likely conclude that, since both forms of functional explanations have consequence selection in common, he has offered an account of function that not only avoids any sort of equivocation, but also ranges over both artifacts and organisms.[32]

In order for Boorse's criticism to tell against Wright's concept of function, it must include an evaluation of whether or not Wright's belief that natural selection and conscious consequence-selection (i.e., intentional designer selection) are similar is justifiable. Since Boorse has offered no such criticism, his hose example against Wright is not persuasive.

Boorse's second example, the barking dog example, also fails to tell against Wright's account. Recall that Boorse thinks that the dog example requires Wright to accept a natural selection (i.e., evolutionary) interpretation of organic entities as opposed to an intentional designer interpretation.[33] However, as with the previous criticism, since Wright thinks that natural selection and intentional designer selection are similar, this example by Boorse is not effective. Thus, Boorse's criticism that Wright equivocates on his use of "etiology" is unsuccessful, if it is true that the two forms of function explanations are similar.[34]

---

[31] Wright, "Functions," p. 43 [my italics].

[32] It is this emphasis on consequences that makes clear why Wright thinks that the distinction between conscious functions and natural functions should not be viewed as completely distinct.

[33] In this discussion, I will be using "conscious function" and "intentional designer function" interchangeably. Both refer to the role that a "minded-entity" (divine or otherwise) plays in the creation of natural functions and artifact functions.

[34] It is also questionable whether or not natural selection and conscious selection are similar in the way that Wright suggests. This would require a rather complicated discussion in what is known as "meme theory," the idea that the selection of ideas is analogous to the

## Objection Number 3: The Criticism of Necessary and Sufficient Conditions—Part I

Boorse's third objection is that Wright's concept of function is neither necessary nor sufficient with respect to either artifacts or organisms. First, Boorse points out that Wright thinks that the intentions of a designer can explain the function of artifacts and their parts. Boorse objects that the intentions of a designer are not necessary because history is replete with cases in which designers did not know the function of a part of their inventions, but they knew that the part was important. Boorse argues that the role of yeast in alcoholic fermentation is a classic example. It was known that yeast was an important part of the production of alcohol, but it was not known that yeast is able to produce enzymes that are able to convert sugar into both carbon dioxide and alcohol. Thus, Boorse concludes that the intentions of the designer are not necessary for an artifact or its parts to have a function.[35]

*A rejoinder to Boorse's objection number 3—part I* In reply, it is quite surprising that Boorse uses an *organism* (i.e., yeast) to argue against how Wright's analysis is not able to account for the function of *artifacts* and their parts. Indeed, his objection fails because he does not provide an example that is a true artifact. Thus, it appears that the intentions of a designer are ineliminable for an artifact or its parts to have a function.

It might be thought that the above reply to Boorse is too fast—surely there must be some sort of artifact that can fit the general concern behind Boorse's yeast example. That is, Boorse is arguing that it is possible for an artifact or part of an artifact **X** to do **Z** and continue to exist as a result of doing **Z**, even if the designer did not know this is how it would work. For example, imagine that a catapult turned out to be more useful as a ladder to scale high walls than as a weapon of mass destruction. If the continued use (i.e., existence) of the catapult was used for scaling castle walls, then the function of the catapult would be, much like a ladder, to climb or descend vertically. Since it is likely that the creator of the catapult did not intend its function to be that of ascending and descending heights, this artifact example captures the point of Boorse's yeast example. Thus, one could conclude that, upon providing the correct artifact example, Boorse's criticism is vindicated.

The problem with such examples is that they violate Boorse's own restriction that the goal of the artifact cannot change. As Boorse states, "Many ancient mechanisms achieved their desired goals without being understood by the people who built them."[36] Boorse is trying to show that even if the desired goals of a mechanism are unchanged it is possible to show that artifacts can have functions "wholly unknown to their makers."[37] Boorse's own claims make it the case that examples like the catapult cannot be used because the desired goal of being a weapon of mass destruction has

---

selection of genes. Given the scope of this issue, it is not possible to explore it here. Still, Wright is treading on shaky ground to suggest that the advantageous consequences of natural selection are similar to the advantageous consequences of conscious selection. For a detailed discussion of this, see Susan Blackmore, *The Meme Machine* (Oxford, 1999).

[35] Boorse, "Wright on Functions," p. 73.
[36] Ibid.
[37] Ibid.

been changed to an instrument for scaling or descending from heights. Indeed, upon reflection, it is no trivial task to find an example in which a part of an artifact or an artifact as a whole has a function, but how the artifact or its part is able to do what it does is unknown to the designer of the artifact.

Of course, if Boorse is simply suggesting that there are many artifacts whose chemistry and physics were unknown to their designers (like the chemical activities of yeast), then prior to the revolution in atomic chemistry, no designers knew the make-up of their artifacts. The concern, however, is not about the chemical structure of an artifact or the physics of its movements, but about how it is the case that a part does what it does and whether **X's** existence is dependent upon such activity. It is vital to Boorse's criticism that he offers an appropriate example. His yeast example will not do. The tentative verdict is that finding an artifact or its part that has a function that is not understood by its designer is rather difficult. This is partly why Boorse had to turn to an organism, like yeast, to make his case. Thus, it can tentatively be claimed that Boorse's assertion that Wright's concept of function is not a necessary condition for artifacts is not compelling.

Boorse also thinks that Wright's concept of function is not sufficient to understand artifacts. Boorse's main concern here is that there are cases in which an artifact or its part(s) stops performing its function, but Wright's analysis does not allow for nonfunctional artifacts.[38] Boorse is clear on this point in the following passage:

> Consider first the position adopted by Wright that pure intentions can make **Z** the function of **X** independently of whether **Z** is actually produced. On this interpretation a part which once acquires a function can never lose it after the designer finishes his work.[39]

Wright uses a windshield washer example to make his point. He says, "In some contexts we will allow that **X** does **Z** even though event **Z** never occurs. For example, the button on the dashboard activates the windshield washer system (that is what it does, I can tell by the circuit diagram) even though it never has or it never will."[40] According to Wright, thinks Boorse, the windshield washer button still (and always will) functions as a windshield washer button because that is the function the designer intended it to have. The problem, according to Boorse, is that Wright's concept of function does not allow for the possibility of an artifact to become nonfunctional. Boorse concludes that such an implication of Wright's analysis appears extremely counterintuitive, suggesting that Wright has not provided a sufficient condition for understanding function as it relates to artifacts.

Moreover, Boorse reminds his audience that Wright thinks it is possible for a body part (e.g., the appendix) to lose its function. The concern is that Wright appears to endorse inconsistently the view that parts of organisms can become nonfunctional, but artifacts or their parts cannot. Given that Wright is hoping to offer an account of function that ranges over both organisms and artifacts equally, he seems (according to Boorse) to be caught in a contradiction. So, according to Boorse, Wright is either

---

[38] Boorse is referring to Wright, "Functions," p. 45.
[39] Boorse, "Wright on Functions," p. 74.
[40] Wright, "Functions," p. 39

caught in an inconsistency or he has not provided a sufficient condition for what a function is.

This criticism by Boorse is partly on the mark. That is, Boorse is correct to note that Wright is caught in an inconsistency with respect to artifacts. A brief expansion of Wright's analysis will reveal the presence of this inconsistency. At the very end of his discussion, Wright concedes that there can be cases in which **X** can lose or cease to have a function. By way of his safety driving regulations example, Wright explains his considered view as follows:

> [I]f the ineffective safety regulations were superceded by another set, and were merely left on the books through legislative sloth or expediency, we would no longer even say that had the ... *function* of making driving less dangerous. But, of course, that would no longer be the reason they were there. The explanation would then have to appeal to legislative sloth or expediency. This is usually done with verb tenses: that *was* its function, but it is not any longer; that was why it was there at one time, but is not why it is still there. A similar treatment can be given vestigial organs, such as the vermiform appendix in humans.[41]

It is clear from the above passage that Wright does allow both artifacts and organic entities to become nonfunctional. His justification is that if the function of **X** is understood in terms of **X** doing or bringing about **Z**, then if **X** ceases to do or bring about **Z**, then **X** no longer has a function.

The relevant criticism that Boorse has levied against Wright is that he is inconsistent in his treatment of whether or not artifacts can become nonfunctional. This is clear from the following two passages noted earlier:

**Passage 1**: The button on a dashboard activates the windshield washer system (that is what it does, I can tell by the circuit diagram) even though it never has and never will. An unused organic or organismic emergency reaction might have the same status.[42]

Then, Wright goes on to claim in his driving regulations example that artifacts and organic entities can lose their function. He concludes as follows:

---

[41] Ibid., p. 46. Note that both Boorse and Wright may be ignoring the idea that **X** can *cease* functioning without *losing* its function. For example, with respect to natural entities, it may be true that the appendix has ceased or stopped functioning, but it does not necessarily follow that it has lost its function. It may be the case that the appendix may still be able to function if the environmental conditions make it conducive to do so. Restated, the appendix may be naturally selected to perform its past function in future generations. The point is that the appendix may have the potential to function in a way it once actually did. In order for the appendix to lose its function, it might very well be the case that the appendix must no longer exist or must be irreparably damaged. The same point can be made for artifacts. For example, an air conditioner could be turned off and no longer used during the winter season. In this case, the air conditioner ceases to function, but it has not lost its function. When the summer season arrives, the air conditioner can regain its function by being turned on. No doubt, taking seriously the distinction between "cease function" and "lose function" is controversial. Much more would be needed to justify it. Nonetheless, it is a distinction that may be relevant to the debate on function.

[42] Ibid., p. 39.

**Passage 2**: This is usually done with verb tenses: that *was* its function, but it is not any longer; that was why it was there at one time, but is not why it is still there. A similar treatment can be given vestigial organs, such as the vermiform appendix in humans.[43]

In the first passage, Wright claims that it is not possible for an artifact to lose its function even if the relevant activity of the artifact is never actualized. His justification is that the intent of the designer (in this case made manifest through the circuit diagram) determines the function of an artifact. He goes on to claim, more cautiously, that certain organismic activities could be understood in the same way.

In the second passage, Wright is clear that artifacts and organic entities can lose their functional ability. Both the driving regulations example and the human appendix example make this point clear. The problem is that in the first passage Wright does not allow artifacts (and possibly organic entities) to lose their functions if the relevant activities of the artifacts are never actualized, but in the second passage he does allow both artifacts and organic entities to lose their functions if the relevant activities for both sorts of entities are never actualized. Yet, this qualification in the second passage is in tension with the first passage. Thus, Boorse's charge of inconsistency is warranted in the light of Wright's revealed analysis.[44]

*Objection Number 3: The Criticism of Necessary and Sufficient Conditions—Part II*

Now, Boorse is well aware that Wright could get out of the apparent difficulty noted above by insisting that parts of artifacts must actualize the functions they were intended to perform. The problem with this reply, thinks Boorse, is that it leaves open the possibility that a part of an artifact can have a function, but not contribute to a goal. The reason why this is supposed to be a problem for Wright is that in order for **X** to be a function, it must do or bring about **Z**. If **X** does perform some activity, but such an activity does not contribute to or bring about **Z**, then, according to Wright's account, **X** does not have a function. For example, the "Maytag" symbol on a washing machine has the function the manufacturer intends it to have—maybe a sign of quality. This sign of quality, however, in no way contributes to the function of the washing machine (cleaning of clothes) or any of its parts. According to Boorse, Wright would be forced to conclude that the Maytag sign is nonfunctional, even though it has an intended function. Thus, Boorse is arguing that Wright's account is not sufficient to handle artifacts even after his possible amendment.

Boorse's next concern is about a further qualification Wright makes to his concept of function. In order to understand Boorse's objection, this qualification that Wright makes to his concept of function must be made clear. Wright thinks that an adequate account of function for organisms must not only answer "How **X** does **Z**?" but it

---

[43] Ibid., p. 46.
[44] Many authors have echoed Boorse's concern that Wright contradicts himself in numerous places. In fact, as part of his analysis of Wright's concept of function, Peter McLaughlin offers the following prefatory warning: "Although he is quite consistent in his pursuit of the consequence etiology, the various statements made along the way are not all entirely consistent with each other, some aspects are quite vague, and many others are simply idiosyncratic." See Peter McLaughlin, *What Functions Explain* (Cambridge, 2001), p. 95.

must also address "Why is **X** there?" In order to address adequately this second question and distinguish genuine functions from mere effects, Wright argues that the proper etiological account must include the notion of natural selection. Wright explains as follows:

> [F]unctional ascription-explanations are in some sense etiological, concern the background of the phenomenon under investigation ... [F]unctional explanations, although plainly not causal in the usual, restricted sense, do concern how the thing with the function *got there*. Hence are etiological, which is to say "causal" in an extended sense.[45]

Moreover, since Wright wishes to offer an account of function that keeps accidental effects distinct from genuine functions, he makes the following claim:

> [A]ll of the accident counter examples can be avoided *if we include as part of the analysis* something about how **X** came to be there (where-ever): namely, that it is there because it does **Z**—with an etiological because.[46]

As Wright makes clear in the above passage, in order to offer an account that acknowledges genuine functions from mere accidental effects, how **X** came to be must be included in the concept of function. Now, in the case of biological entities, Wright first criticizes his own concept of function, and then he continues to offer a qualification to his "formula." His somewhat lengthy assessment is as follows:

> It is easy to show that this formula does not represent a sufficient condition for being a function, *which is to say there is something more to be said about precisely what it is to be a function*. The most easily generable set of cases to be excluded is of this kind: oxygen combines readily with hemoglobin, and that is the (etiological) reason it is found in human bloodstreams. But there is something colossally fatuous in maintaining that the function of that oxygen is to combine with hemoglobin, even though it is there because it does that. The function of oxygen in human bloodstreams is providing energy in oxidation reactions, not combining with hemoglobin. Combining with hemoglobin is only a means to that end. This is a useful example. It points to a contrast in the notion of "because" employed here which is easy to overlook and crucial to an elucidation of functions.[47]

As I pointed out above, if producing energy is the function of the oxygen, then oxygen must be there (in the blood) because it produces energy. But the "because" in, "It is there because it produces energy," is importantly different from the "because" in, "It is there because it combines with hemoglobin." They suggest different *sorts* of etiologies. If carbon monoxide (CO), which we know to combine readily with hemoglobin, were suddenly to become able to produce energy by appropriate (nonlethal) reactions in our cells and further, the atmosphere were suddenly to become filled with CO, we could properly say that the reason CO was in our bloodstreams was that it combines readily with hemoglobin. We could not properly say, however,

---

[45] Wright, "Functions," p. 38.
[46] Ibid. [my italics].
[47] Ibid., p. 40 [my italics].

that CO was there because it produces energy. And that is precisely what we could say about oxygen, on purely evolutionary-etiological grounds.[48]

All of this indicates that it is the nature of the etiology itself which determines the propriety of a functional explanation; there must be specifically functional etiologies. When we say that the function of **X** is **Z** (to do **Z**) we are saying that **X** is there because it does **Z**, but with a further qualification. We are explaining how **X** came to be there, but only certain kinds of explanations of how **X** came to be will do.[49]

The main point Wright makes in the above passage is that the relevant etiology for the phenomenon under investigation must be part of the concept of function for that type of phenomenon. It is only when the specific etiology is included as part of the concept of function is it possible not to run afoul of the accident/genuine function distinction. Specifically, in the case of organisms, the appropriate etiology must include natural selection—**X** is where it is because it was naturally selected to do or bring about **Z**. It is the inclusion of natural selection to his concept of function for organisms that satisfies Wright's attempt to answer the question of "Why does **X** exist?" So, in the light of the above qualification, Wright's concept of function has the following structure for organisms:

The function of **X** is **Z** means

(a) **X** is there because it does **Z**.
(b) **Z** is a consequence (or result) of **X's** being there.
(c) **X** exists and does **Z** because it was *naturally selected* to do **Z**.

It is this qualification in (c) by Wright that Boorse thinks is irrelevant to an adequate account of function. Boorse says:

> The modern theory of evolution is of recent vintage; talk of functions had been going on for a long time before it appeared. When Harvey, say, claimed that the function of the heart is to circulate the blood, he did not have natural selection in mind. Nor does this mean that pre-evolutionary physiologists must therefore have believed in a divine designer. The fact is that in talking of physiological functions, they did not mean to be making historical claims at all. They were simply describing the organization of a species as they found it … Suppose we discovered, for example, that at some point the lion species simply sprang into existence by an unparalleled saltation. One would not regard this discovery as invalidating all functional claims about lions; it would show that in at least one case an intricate functional organization was created by chance.[50]

There are two points that can be drawn from Boorse's claims in the above passage. First, according to Boorse, a complete account of function can be silent on the origin of a function. All that is required, as Boorse suggests in the above passage, is a description of what it is the mechanism does for the system of which it is a part. For instance, a functional explanation of mast cells need only include a description of *how* these cells produce histamines as part of the body's overall immune defense

---

[48] Ibid., pp. 40–41.
[49] Ibid., p. 41.
[50] Boorse, "Wright on Functions," p. 74.

system. Boorse is suggesting here that evolution *qua* natural selection is not a necessary condition for what a function is.

Second, Boorse notes that there is enough randomness in the events that take place in the natural world such that a new species (he uses the example of a new spontaneously generated species of lion) could spontaneously emerge (or it is logically possible it could emerge) in a way that does not cohere with any of the tenets of evolution. Given such a scenario, no person would want to claim, thinks Boorse, that the activities of a new species of lion are not worthy of being functions simply because they lack the appropriate natural selection etiology. Rather, Boorse thinks that a new spontaneously generated species of lion would have functioning parts that could be accurately described. Thus, because organisms or their parts can be described without concern for their origin, and since non-evolutionary generated species are possible (at least, logically possible), Boorse thinks that Wright's qualified theory of function does not provide a necessary condition for what an organic function is.

*A rejoinder to Boorse's objection number 3—part II*  Recall that Boorse's third objection comes in two parts. First, Boorse criticized Wright for allowing **X** to have a function even if **X** did not bring about **Z**. Since Wright is committed to the view that the function of **X** is determined in part by way of **X's** doing or bringing about **Z**, it seems that Boorse's criticism that Wright allows for **X** to have a function, even when **X** does not contribute to the bringing about of **Z**, is on the mark. The concern, however, is that the force of Boorse's criticism depends on what **Z** is. For example, if **Z** is "washed clothing," then the Maytag sign will be nonfunctional, because it does not contribute to the bringing about of washed clothing. If, however, **Z** is "marketing a quality product," then the Maytag sign does bring about **Z**. In his own hood ornament example, Boorse understands **Z** to be "transportation" as the goal of a car. Since the hood ornament does not contribute to this goal, Boorse claims that Wright would have to accept that it has no function.

Boorse, however, fails to recognize that something can have a different function than the **Z** that determines the function of the whole to which it belongs. The designer of a car may think that the goal of a car is transportation, but the marketer of the car may very well think that the goal is the selling of a classy or sexy automobile. Since the hood ornament, which signifies quality, luxury, or sex appeal, does contribute to the goal of selling certain automobiles, it does have a function. Thus, Boorse has not offered a conclusive reply to the idea that Wright's concept of function is not a sufficient condition for artifacts.

Also, Boorse could be assuming an incorrect goal of certain cars. For instance, the designer of the car could argue that the goal of his car is not only transportation, but also luxurious or stylish transportation. The presence of the hood ornament, the designer could argue, contributes significantly to such a goal. In fact, makers of exotic sports cars (e.g., a Ferrari) and high-end luxury sedans (e.g., Mercedes or BMW) consider their hood ornaments to be an integral part of the overall goal of these cars. Thus, Wright can answer Boorse's criticism.

Second, Boorse criticizes the evolutionary aspect of Wright's concept of function both on historical grounds and by way of constructing a possible world scenario.

With respect to the historical criticism, from the fact that physiologists prior to the Darwinian and genetic revolutions were able to provide a rigorous account of what a biological entity does, it does not follow that such an account is thorough in the light of new information. At the time of William Harvey's insightful research on the heart, an account of how **X** does **Y** may have exhausted the conceptual analysis with respect to function, if divine notions were thought to be inapplicable. Restated, if an answer to the question of "Why is **X** there?" always produced an account that included divine intervention, then naturalists, like Harvey, may have resisted answering such a question. Yet, in the wake of Darwinism and modern genetics, the question "Why is **X** there?" can be answered without any appeal to divine intervention. Rather, this question can be answered by appealing to genetic selective advantage—the reason why **X** is there is because **X**'s doing or bringing about **Z** procures a fitness (reproductive) advantage for **X**. For example, the reason that the kidneys exist is that the activity of purifying blood and the effect of blood purification help to secure a reproductive advantage to the species to which the kidney-bearing organism belongs.

In the light of evolution, the concept of function includes not only the descriptive claim (**X** does activity **Y** in order to bring about **Z**), but it also includes an account of why it is the case that **X** is present. Thus, Boorse's reliance on the fact that historical figures did not include an answer to the "Why is **X** there?" question in no way excuses post-Darwinian physiologists from ignoring this question. Indeed, Karen Neander defends the importance of this Darwinian perspective on functions. She makes her point in the following way:

> The notion of a "proper function" is the notion of what a part is supposed to do. This fact is crucial to one of the most important theoretical roles of the notion in biology, which is that most biological categories are only definable in functional terms ... It is the/a proper function of an item (**X**) of an organism (**O**) to do that which items of **X**'s type did to contribute to the inclusive fitness of **O**'s ancestors, and which caused the genotype, of which **X** is the phenotypic expression, to be selected by natural selection.[51]

Ignoring some of the technical jargon in the above passage, Neander is arguing that evolutionary considerations are crucial to distinguishing certain physiological features from other physiological features. Restated, descriptive accounts, which do not make mention of how a feature contributes to reproductive success, are not sufficient to determine whether or not an entity has a function. At the very least, current evolutionary biology allows the possibility that natural selection is a necessary condition for a cogent concept of function. The upshot is that, contrary to Boorse's remarks against Wright, natural selection as an answer to "Why is **X** there?" may be a necessary condition for a comprehensive concept of function.[52]

---

[51] Karen Neander, "Functions as Selected Effects: The Conceptual Analyst's Defense," *Philosophy of Science*, 58/2 (1991): 180 and 174.

[52] This reply to Boorse is not an attempt to defend an evolutionary concept of function. Such a defense will be offered in Chapter 7. For now, as a rejoinder to Boorse, it is enough that evolutionary considerations *may* need to be taken seriously when talking about biological functions.

The possible world scenario Boorse uses is the spontaneously generated lion example. Recall that this example is designed to show that if it is possible for a species to emerge in some non-evolutionary generated fashion, then Wright would be forced to accept that the effects produced by such a species or its parts have no functions. The reason why they would have no functions is because neither the species nor their parts came into existence as a result of evolutionary forces.

This criticism could be seen as a compelling counter example to an evolutionary concept of function. The major assumption, however, lurking in the background of Boorse's criticism is that it is grossly counterintuitive to think that non-evolved or spontaneously generated biological entities do not have functions.[53] Yet, Wright could simply reply that intuitions simply do not resolve this issue. Since the findings of science are frequently counterintuitive (e.g., light is both a wave and a particle), it should be no surprise that evolutionary considerations would also reveal counterintuitive insights. So, Wright could reply that his concept of function does account for the function-like activities of spontaneously generated biological entities; that is, such entities do not have genuine functions because they do not (yet) have the relevant Darwinian (i.e., natural selection) causal history.

Now, unfortunately, such a response will not suffice. Since Wright takes himself to be offering a concept of function, he must be willing to defend the view that his concept can withstand possible world scenarios. More cautiously, Wright should claim that his account cannot handle the spontaneously generated creatures or that his account is only designed to handle evolved organisms whose history is deeply tethered to that of the planet Earth. However, since Wright does claim to be defending the former and not the latter, Boorse's criticism against Wright is on the mark—that is, Wright has not offered a necessary condition for what a function is.

Given the qualification made by Wright—that the relevant etiology must be included in the phenomenon under investigation—Boorse's earlier criticism, that Wright's concept of function is not able to range over both organisms and artifacts, is now quite applicable. The reason is that the relevant etiological concept of function for organisms includes natural selection, but natural selection is not part of the concept of function for artifacts. Rather, in the case of artifacts, the intentions of the designer/user represent the appropriate etiology. Wright's qualification reveals that the content of the concept of function for organisms is different than the content of the concept of function for artifacts. Thus, Wright is not able to meet his own adequacy condition of offering a general concept of function that ranges over both organisms and artifacts.[54]

---

[53] McLaughlin argues in this fashion when he claims that "[t]he evolutionary etiological view asserts—*counterintuitively*—that newly advantageous traits have no functions ... [but] there is no *intuitively* plausible reason why the heart of a mule should be denied a function just because the mule turns out to have been spontaneously generated." See McLaughlin, *What Functions Explain*, p. 135 and p. 90 [my addition and italics].

[54] Beth Preston has offered just this conclusion. She notes that, for Wright's account, "In the case of biological organs like the heart, this will be its evolutionary history as mediated by natural selection. In the case of artifacts like the chair, it will be a history of deliberate selection by user or community of users." Given these distinct histories, Preston correctly concludes that "[t]he problem with Wright's analysis is that the two criteria ... pull in opposite

Still, even granting Wright his evolutionary etiological concept of function, Boorse thinks that it is not a sufficient condition for understanding function. Basically, he thinks that a selectionist account would be forced to include many phenomena within a functional perspective that should not be included. Boorse offers the following two examples and the general inference that should be drawn from them:

> A hornet buzzing in a woodshed so frightens a farmer that he repeatedly shrinks from going in and killing it. Nothing in Wright's essay blocks the conclusion that the function of the buzzing, or even of the hornet, is to frighten the farmer. The farmer's fright is a result of the hornet's presence, and the hornet's presence continues because it has this result. Obesity in a man of meager motivation can prevent him from exercising. Although failure to exercise is a result of the obesity, and the obesity continues because of this result, it is unlikely that prevention of exercise is its function. These cases suggest that Wright must say explicitly that the function of **X** is **Z** only when the presence of **X** in a species has resulted from selection pressure deriving from **Z**. But this alone is not enough. An organ **X** once established by selection pressure deriving from its effect **Z** may cease to be functional, as did the appendix, if a change in the rest of the organism or in the environment renders **Z** useless.[55]

Boorse's criticisms in the above two passages amount to three distinct concerns. First, the hornet example, thinks Boorse, tells against Wright's account. Buzzing produces fear, which in turn causes the buzzing to continue. Yet, to think that the function of buzzing is to produce fear seems rather implausible to Boorse. Second, if this first example does not appear conclusive, Boorse thinks his second example suffices to make his point. Whatever the function of obesity might be, no reasonable person thinks that its function is to prevent exercise. Indeed, the obesity example is a case where the use of a functional explanation is entirely inappropriate. Third, Boorse is aware that Wright could qualify his claim to contend with such examples. Wright could say that, for example, the function of **X** is **Z** only when the presence of **X** has resulted from selection pressure deriving from **Z**. Yet, Boorse thinks that such a reply fails because it is possible for **X** to stop its function when either the internal or external environment has changed. To the point, such a move by Wright would not allow for organic entities to stop having functions. Thus, Boorse concludes that Wright has not offered a sufficient condition for what a function is.

Boorse is correct to note that Wright could reply to both of his examples. First, Wright would most likely want to accept that the buzzing sound of the hornet functions to cause fear in the farmer *qua* potential doer of harm. Given that Wright takes seriously natural selection as part of his concept of function, he could reply to Boorse that the token hornet's buzzing functions to cause fear in potential harm doers (of which the farmer is a token) and has evolved to do just this. For example, buzzing may be a product of natural selection as a warning signal for other organisms to stay clear or suffer the pain of a sting. Fear of a hornet attack may very well contribute

---

directions and have proved impossible to weld into harmonious single account of functional ascription-explanation." See Preston, "Why is a Wing Like a Spoon? A Pluralist Theory of Function," p. 218 and p. 219.

[55] Boorse, "Wright on Functions," p. 76.

to the retention of such a feature. Restated, Wright could reply that buzzing is a feature that has and continues to be a boon with respect to the reproductive success of hornets. So long as the farmer remains in the same location as the hornet, the hornet will continue to produce a buzzing sound in order to scare the farmer away from the area. Thus, rather than posing a difficulty to Wright's concept of function, the hornet example actually buttresses Wright's account.

Second, Boorse himself anticipates Wright's reply to his obesity example: obesity does not have the function of preventing exercise, because obesity was not naturally selected to perform such a task. In fact, to the extent that obesity prevents exercise, it is a feature that is deleterious to reproductive success. So, by including natural selection in the discussion, Wright is committed to the idea that X does or brings about Z, because the presence of Z procures a fitness advantage to X's ancestors and X. Boorse acknowledges this reply by Wright, but claims that it leads to the absurd view that Wright cannot allow functions to cease. Yet, as was made clear earlier, Wright does acknowledge that an entity can have a function that ceases, if X stops doing or bringing about Z. Therefore, Boorse has not shown that Wright's account is not sufficient to understand what an organismic function is.[56]

Now that it is clear that Wright does take natural selection seriously as part of the etiology of biological functions, he is able to satisfy the condition of keeping out divine intervention from his account. Recall that his original position of "consequence etiology" left open the possibility that a divine force could have brought about the relevant advantageous consequences for biological functions. His revealed account, however, makes clear that the "force" at work in the case of biological entities is the process of evolution by natural selection. Thus, Wright can claim to have offered a concept of function that is able to resist any sort of theological elements.

*Objection Number 4: The "Common Connection" Criticism*

Boorse's final criticism is that, contrary to Wright's own account, his concept of function does not help to make sense of the possible connection between genuine functions (strong function statements) and accidental functions (weak function statements). The issue here is that in everyday speech people use functional language for entities that really do not have functions. Wright acknowledges this fact by noting that people know that their use of functional language in many instances is really nothing more than a sort of pretending. For example, if a belt buckle deflects an oncoming bullet, people might say that the buckle *functions as* a bullet deflector. In this example, people are aware that the buckle does not really have such a function, but they pretend that it does. Wright makes the point as follows:

> When something does something useful by accident rather than by design, ... we signal the difference by a standard sort of "let's pretend" talk. Instead of using the verb "to be"

---

[56] As it was noted earlier, Boorse could have claimed that Wright is inconsistent in his views. On the one hand, Wright does not allow artifacts to lose their functions. On the other hand, he does allow both artifacts and organisms to lose their functions.

or the verb "to have," and saying the thing in question *has* such and such a function, or saying that *is* its function, we use the expression "function as." We might say the belt buckle *functions as* a bullet shield, or the blowout *functioned as* divine intervention, or the sweep hand *functions as* a dust brush.[57]

Boorse offers the following reply:

> What is puzzling about this explanation is that the idea of usefulness nowhere appears in Wright's analysis ... For Wright the essence of functionality is a certain sort of etiology. But in the "function as" examples he gives, nothing whatever about the etiology of the belt buckle, or the blowout, or the sweep hand is relevant to their useful effects. It remains obscure why in the world we might nevertheless wish to "pretend" that their etiology was of the right sort to justify functional language. If the pretense is made only where a trait has useful effects, that is some argument for a connection between functions and usefulness.[58]

The criticism that Boorse is offering against Wright is that his etiological account of function makes no room for the "pretend" sense of "function" captured in his examples, because his account makes no room for usefulness. That is, the reason that people use functional language in the case of accidental effects (e.g., a belt buckle that accidentally deflects a bullet) is that such effects prove to be useful. Given that Wright's etiological account does not include any sense of "useful," Boorse suggests that Wright would have to argue that such examples reveal that people pretend that they do have an acceptable etiology and it is this pretending that accounts for the use of functional language in such cases. Yet, Boorse replies that it is rather unreasonable to think that people engage in a sort of "pretend thinking" about etiology in the very examples that Boorse provides, because the usefulness of the entities in these examples is not connected to their etiology. Thus, Boorse concludes that Wright's concept of function cannot accommodate the common or everyday pretend use of functional language associated with fortuitous accidental effects.

*A rejoinder to Boorse's objection number 4*  Boorse's fourth criticism of Wright's concept of function is too severe. First, as was made clear in the analysis of Wright's concept of function, he does claim that both artifacts and organic functions are understood in terms of their *advantageous consequences*.[59] On a charitable interpretation, some sense of "useful" or "benefit" is part of Wright's sense of "advantageous consequences." Indeed, as McLaughlin makes the point, "Wright is not able entirely to get by without implicitly appealing to the *benefit* conferred on a system by the function because in all cases that he actually considers, benefit to someone is in fact part of the feedback mechanism by which the function helps to

---

[57] Wright, "Functions," p. 33. This discussion emerges out of Wright's critique of Canfield's concept of function. Wright argues that Canfield's analysis cannot account for the distinction between genuine functions and "pretend" functions. See Wright, "Functions," pp. 31–2 and Canfield, "Teleological Explanations in Biology," *British Journal for the Philosophy of Science*.
[58] Boorse, "Wright on Functions," p. 77.
[59] Wright, "Functions," p. 43.

bring about the function bearer."⁶⁰ At the very least, Boorse should explore why he thinks that Wright's use of "advantageous consequences" does not include the idea of usefulness or benefit. For it is reasonable, at first glance, to think that if **Z** is useful or beneficial to the maintenance of **X**'s existence, then it is an advantage for **X** to have or bring about **Z** in order for **X** to maintain its existence. The reason is that (as McLaughlin hints) "advantage" and "usefulness" include the idea of benefit. Since Boorse offers no analysis concerning the relationship between "advantageous consequences" and "useful," the force of his criticism is weakened.

Moreover, Boorse cannot understand why Wright thinks it is acceptable to use terms such as "pretend" or "function as" when describing those things that really are not functions in Wright's etiological sense. Yet, Wright is clear why such expressions are used:

> It makes perfectly good sense to say the nose *functions as* an eyeglass support; the heart, through its thump, *functions as* a diagnostic aid; the sixth rib *functions as* a pacemaker hook ... This, it seems to me, is precisely the distinction we make when we say, for example, that the sweep-second hand *functions as* a dust brush, while denying that brushing dust is one of the sweep hand's functions. And it is here that we can make sense of the notion of accident in the case of natural functions: it is merely fortuitous that the nose supports eyeglasses; it is a happy chance that the heart throb is diagnostically significant; it would be the merest serendipity if the sixth rib were to be a particularly good pacemaker hook. It is (would be) only accidental that (if) these things turned out to be useful in these ways.⁶¹

As Wright makes clear in the above passage, "function as" signifies that something is not really a function, but rather an accidental feature. When people claim that **X** *functions as* something, Wright is asserting that people use "function" loosely, casually, or figuratively. For Wright thinks that people are aware of an accidental activity from a real function, but employ this "pretend" sense of "function" for lack of a better or more convenient phrase. Indeed, given Wright's own concept of function, it is because these accidents (e.g., sweep-second hand *functions as* a sweep brush) do not have an appropriate etiology that they are really accidents and not true functions. As Wright claims, these beneficial effects are merely fortuitous side effects of genuine functions. Thus, contrary to Boorse's criticism, Wright's allowance for expressions like "pretend" or "function as" do not tell against his own concept of function. In fact, such phrases help to keep genuine advantageous functions distinct from lucky side effects.

Note, however, that Boorse could have criticized Wright for implicitly including useful *qua* beneficial effect in his concept of function. Recall that in his general account of function Wright makes no mention of "useful." Indeed, he criticizes John Canfield's concept of function for the very reason that usefulness is not a necessary condition for what a function is. Wright's justification for rejecting utility as a necessary condition for function is that it is possible for something to have a function even if it is useless. He offers the following assessment:

---

⁶⁰ McLaughlin, *What Functions Explain*, pp. 100–101 [my italics].
⁶¹ Wright, "Functions," pp. 33–4.

My watch has a sweep-second hand, and I occasionally use it to time things to the degree of accuracy it allows: it is useful to me. Now suppose I were to lose interest in reading time to that degree of accuracy. Suppose my life changed radically so that nothing I ever did could require that sort of chronological precision. Would that mean the sweep hand on my particular watch no longer has the function of making seconds easier to read? Clearly not ... [I]f something is designed to do **X**, then doing **X** is its function even if doing **X** is generally useless, silly, or even harmful.[62]

Wright is clear that usefulness is not a necessary condition for a function. Yet, as McLaughlin notes, Wright implicitly includes usefulness in his account. Indeed, Wright's use of "advantageous consequences," which assumes some sense of "benefit," implies some sense of "useful." The point is that Wright is not able to avoid the role of benefit to his concept of function, even though he wishes to keep it out of his analysis. The implication is—much like his criticism against Canfield—that Wright has not offered a necessary condition for what a function is.

To recapitulate briefly, Boorse offers four criticisms against Wright's concept of function. One, Boorse thinks that Wright's concept of function is very close to a tautology. Two, he argues that there are two senses of etiology—one for artifacts and another for organisms—at play in Wright's analysis. These two distinct senses of etiology, thinks Boorse, make it very difficult for Wright to provide a univocal concept of function that ranges over both artifacts and organisms. Three, Boorse claims that Wright's concept of function is neither necessary nor sufficient because Wright insists that the designers of the artifacts must know how their designed artifacts do what they do. Moreover, Wright's account does not allow for nonfunctional parts of artifacts like it does for parts of organisms. Four, Boorse thinks that Wright cannot make sense of the connection between weak and strong function statements, because Wright does not include some concept of usefulness within his concept of function.

Upon close inspection, this analysis revealed that Boorse is partly successful in his overall criticism of Wright's concept of function. First, he revealed that Wright's concept of function is a near tautology. Second, Boorse's charge of equivocation was premature, and unsuccessful to this extent. Third, in the first part of his third criticism, Boorse was not successful in showing that Wright's concept of function is neither necessary nor sufficient for either artifacts or organisms. He was, however, correct to point out that Wright is caught in an inconsistency with respect to whether or not artifacts can become nonfunctional. In the second part, Boorse's critique did reveal that Wright's concept of function is not able to range over both artifacts and organisms, because Wright acknowledges that natural selection is the appropriate causal force behind organisms. Finally, Boorse was not persuasive in his claim that Wright's own etiological analysis cannot account for the distinction between genuine functions and accidental effects. Moreover, this section revealed that Wright has not offered a necessary condition for what a function is, because of his implicit reliance on usefulness to his concept of function.

In the light of Wright's own adequacy conditions, his concept of function is

---

[62] Ibid., p. 31 and p. 32.

1. able to keep distinct genuine functions from accidental effects
2. not able to ignore the sharp distinction between conscious functions and natural functions and is not able to range over both organisms and artifacts
3. able to eliminate the possibility of any divine element from his analysis

Although Boorse's overall criticism of Wright's concept of function is only partially successful, parts of his critique are quite effective in revealing the inadequacy of Wright's analysis. It is now appropriate to turn to Boorse's concept of function and determine whether or not his positive account fares better than Wright's rendition.

## Boorse's Concept of Function

Since Boorse thinks that his concept of function meets all of the adequacy demands required by Wright, his positive account is worth exploring. More to the point, given that his own concept of function is crucial to his concept of health, this section will make clear the details of Boorse's concept of function. Broadly, as was noted at the beginning of this chapter, Boorse thinks that functions are nothing more than those things, which contribute to the goals of a system. As Boorse makes the point, "In every context where functional talk is appropriate, one has also to do with the goals of some goal-directed system ... Any goal pursued or intended by a goal-directed system may serve to generate a function statement. Functions are, purely and simply, contributions to goals."[63] He regards the following formal concept of function, which places much emphasis on goal-directedness, to be similar to his own view:

> To say that an action or a process [X] is directed to the goal [Z] is to say not only that [X] is what is required for [Z], but also that within some range of environmental variation [X] *would have been modified* in whatever way was required for [Z].[64]

For example, mast cells have functions not only because mast cells are required (i.e., contribute to) for immune system defense, but also that within a certain range of environmental changes, mast cells are able to modify their behavior in order to continue to contribute to immune system defense. This additional element concerning goal-directed activities is understood in the function literature as a *regularity condition*—the continued pursuit or achievement of a particular goal(s) in the wake of perturbations. Richard Braithwaite explains the regularity condition in relation to goal-directed systems as follows:

> Coming to a definite end or terminus is not *per se* distinctive of directive activity, for inorganic processes also move towards a natural terminus ... What *is* distinctive is the

---
[63] Boorse, "Wright on Functions," p. 77.
[64] Ibid., p. 78. This version of function, as Boorse notes and hopes to modify, can be found in Gerd Sommerhoff's *Analytical Biology* (Oxford, 1950) [bracketed variables are my addition].

active persistence of directive activity towards its goal, the use of alternative means towards the same end, and the achievement of results in the face of difficulties.[65]

Boorse thinks that there are two difficulties with the above regularity condition element that he hopes to resolve as he moves toward his own concept of function.[66] First, the above version of function would allow for an entity to have a function even when its end-state could not ever be realized. Imagine if there were no allergens at all on the planet Earth as of right now. It is sensible, from Boorse's perspective, to think that the appropriate response would be to claim that mast cells no longer have functions. It is difficult to conceive of how histamine production could help to defend against invaders that are no longer in existence. In the same way, imagine that a cat is waiting to pounce on a mouse at a particular hole. As it turns out, the mouse has vacated this hole. Since there is no actual goal that the cat's mouse-catching behavior can bring to fruition, it is safe to say that the behavior is no longer functional. Yet, Boorse offers the following reply:

> The cat's behavior can, however, fairly be called appropriate to catching a mouse; it is for instance, the kind of behavior that leads to catching a mouse: it is, for instance, the kind of behavior that leads to catching mice when they are there.[67]

The upshot of Boorse's rejoinder to the first problem is that one does not want to say, "[X] is required for [Z]," but that "[X] is able to achieve [Z] so long as [Z] is attainable." If allergens are present such that they can be acted upon by the histamine production of mast cells, then histamine production is the function of mast cells. Along the same lines, if mice are present such that they can be pounced upon by the predatory actions of cats, then the predatory pouncing action of cats is the function of such behavior. Given this modified argument from potentiality, Boorse thinks that the first criticism loses its force.

There is, however, a second more serious problem than the first one noted above that Boorse hopes to dismiss. The concern here is that of multiple functions. It is possible for **X** to exhibit the same behavior for distinct goals such that it is not possible to determine what is the true function of **X**. For example, it could be

---

[65] Richard Braithwaite, "Causal and Teleological Explanations," Ch. 10 of Richard Braithwaite, *Scientific Explanation* (Cambridge, 1964), p. 329. Ernest Nagel offers a similar regularity criterion concerning goal-directed systems when he claims that they "continue to manifest a certain state or property [Z] (or that they exhibit a persistence of development "in the direction" of attaining [Z]) in the face of a relatively extensive class of changes in their external environments or in some of their internal parts—changes which, if not compensated for by internal modification in the system, would result in the disappearance of [Z] (or in an altered direction of development of the system)." See Ernest Nagel, *The Structure of Science* (New York and Burlingame, 1961), p. 411.

[66] Boorse realizes that this preliminary account of the regularity condition for functions has been criticized by Israel Scheffler. So, he hopes to modify this preliminary concept of function to accommodate two of Scheffler's criticisms. Both of these criticisms can be found in Israel Scheffler, "Thoughts on Teleology," *British Journal for the Philosophy of Science*, 9/36 (1959): 265–85.

[67] Boorse, "Wright on Functions," p. 79.

imagined that the cat's pouncing behavior is for catching cream. Indeed, imagine further that the cat has been conditioned in its environment to the point where it takes the requisite steps to acquire a bowl of cream whenever it is present just like the steps it would take to catch a mouse when the mouse is present. The point is that the predatory pouncing behavior is indistinguishable from the cream catching behavior. There is no way to determine if cream catching or mouse catching is the function *qua* goal of the cat's pouncing behavior. Boorse's reply is that "intuitively it seems to make sense to say that mice and not cream are the cat's goal."[68] Boorse justifies this reply in the following way:

> What seems to me required for the possibility that mice are the cat's real goal is something of which the idea of a mouse is only a special case—namely, an internal mechanism which standardly guides mouse-catching but not cream catching. When a process is produced by an internal mechanism which standardly guides pursuit of that goal but not the others.[69]

As can be seen from the above passage, Boorse thinks that the "real function" of the behavior or part(s) of an organism is that which assists in achieving the goal of the particular internal mechanism of the behavior or the part(s). The internal mechanism is that which produces a particular effect for the sake of a particular goal on a standard basis. In this context, "standard" means "on a regular basis" or "on a normal basis." For example, the function of histamines is to assist in the goal of proper immune system response. Now it may be the case that histamines do other things as well. Yet, the internal mechanism for B-cells is that of histamine production. Thus, whatever else histamine production does, its function is to assist in immune system defense. Thus, Boorse *might* be understood to think that a unique or "real" function of an organism's behaviors or its parts is possible to determine.

In fact, contrary to what was concluded in the previous paragraph, Boorse does not seem to think that "the real" function of behaviors of organisms or the parts of organisms can be determined. After the passage noted above, Boorse thinks that his principle of internal mechanism has a specific implication in the case of biological organisms. Specifically, he claims that "[s]ince organisms contain no separate mechanisms that distinguish among the various goals that biological processes achieve, there is no way of finding a unique goal in relation to which traits of organisms have functions."[70] Boorse's point is that a single biological behavior or part can assist to achieve multiple goals. Given this fact, Boorse appears to be suggesting that it is rather arbitrary to single out *the* goal to which an organism or its parts contribute. If choosing a single effect of an organism or its parts is arbitrary, then the determination that the function of an organism or its part is **X** will also be arbitrary. Thus, the ability to determine what *the* function of an organism or its parts is, according to Boorse, not possible.

What, then, is Boorse's concept of function, given his assessment that the function of natural entities cannot be determined definitively? The answer is that

---

[68] Ibid.
[69] Ibid.
[70] Ibid.

Boorse thinks that a *contextualist* concept of function is the correct one. Boorse's own assessment of function statements is quite clear:

> "A function of **X** is **Z**" means that in some *contextually* definite goal-directed system **S**, during some *contextually* definite time interval *t*, the **Z-ing** of **X** falls within some *contextually* circumscribed class of functions being performed by **X** during *t*—that is, causal contribution to a goal **G** of **S**.[71]

Note that there are three context-dependent parts that make-up Boorse's concept of function. First, there is the context-dependent goal-directed system. Second, there is the context-dependent time interval. Third, the activity performed by **X** is one among a limited class of functions that **X** performs. To illustrate, recall that in the badge example the sheriff was able to subdue an approaching desperado with the fortuitous assistance of the reflection of the sun's light off of his star badge into the eyes of the on-coming bandit. Employing Boorse's formula above, the sheriff's badge has a function within the goal-directed "peace-keeping" law enforcement system of which the sheriff is a part. Moreover, that *this* badge has the function of blinding bandits is clear given that it was able to produce this blinding effect just at *the time* of the bandit's advance. Finally, the blinding of the bandit fits within the circumscribed functions of the sheriff's badge—that is, the blinding of aggressive bandits causally contributes to the goal of maintenance of law and order within the city limits. Thus, Boorse thinks that a cogent concept of function is one that is contextual—the contexts include a goal-directed system, a time interval, and a relevant function among a range of functions that brings about the relevant goal(s) of a system.

The above sheriff example might be considered inappropriate due to the fact that Boorse does take seriously the regularity condition. That is, for **X** to be the function of **Z** it must be the case that it brings about **Z** on a regular or standard basis. On the contrary, Boorse thinks that "**X** is performing" is more accurate than "**X** performs." His justification for the progressive use of "performing" as opposed to "performs" is as follows:

> I use the progressive tense rather than "performs" because the latter carries the unwanted implication that the function is performed repeatedly or over an appreciable time. Clearly functions may be performed only once and by accident. The Bible in the soldier's pocket, for example, may perform the function of stopping a bullet only once. Here the system **S** is a soldier plus Bible, and bullet-stopping contributes to its goals by saving his life.[72]

It is clear from the above Bible example that Boorse has relaxed the need for the regularity condition partly to accommodate the need to offer a concept of function that ranges over organisms and artifacts. The sheriff example complements the Bible example to bring about just this point. So long as there is (1) a contextually determined goal-directed system **S**, (2) a contextually determined time interval **t**,

---

[71] Ibid., p. 82 [my italics].
[72] Ibid., p. 80. The tension that emerges between the sheriff example and Bible example for Boorse's concept of function will be addressed later in this chapter.

and (3) some contextually defined class of functions being performed by **X** during time **t**, then **X** will have a function.

Of course, the function of artifacts will change if any combination of contexts changes. For example, imagine that the only time the sheriff makes his badge visible to the public is when he displays it in the presence of the local bartender from whom he wishes to procure a free mug of beer. In such scenarios, where the background conditions have changed, it is not clear the goals of law enforcement are clearly relevant with respect to the function of the sheriff's badge. Indeed, according to Boorse, the function of the sheriff's badge would be something other than for goals associated with law enforcement. As Boorse notes,

> Wright's intentional convention is not part of the meaning of functional talk. It is a generally convenient contextual device reflecting part of the normal background of our discussions of artifacts—namely, the insight of their designers—and would disappear if that background changed.[73]

Thus, contrary to Wright, Boorse claims that the functions of artifacts are not restricted to the intentions of their designers. Rather, the functions of artifacts are contextually determined. As Boorse notes, it may be common that the intentions of designers and the functions of their artifacts are one and the same. Still, according to Boorse, if the contexts in which artifacts find themselves change, then so may the functions of the artifacts.

Now, it is possible to turn to Boorse's assessment of biological entities from the perspective of his contextualist concept of function. With respect to the eating of insects by birds, Boorse notes the following problem and his resolution to biological function statements:

> [The] ambiguity arises partly because biologists see teleology on so many different time scales and levels of organization. At one level, individual organisms are goal-directed systems whose behavior contributes to various goals. By eating insects, say, a bird contributes to its own survival and also (a fortiori) to the survival of the species, but further to the survival of its genes, the equilibrium of the insect population, and so on ... This means that there is no sense in asking which goal **[G]** is *the* goal at which the bird's behavior aims, and respect to which its parts have functions, except in so far as this goal is clear *from the context* of discourse ... At the level of population or species, new goal-directed processes seem to appear—for example, the maintenance of protective coloration—and one can ascend still higher by viewing a whole ecosystem as a teleological unit ... Given this latitude for choice, what has happened is that various subfields of biology have carved out various slices of the teleological pie and interpreted their function statements accordingly.[74]

---

[73] Ibid., p. 83.

[74] Ibid., pp. 83–4 [my italics]. Valerie Hardcastle has argued for a similar contextualist concept of function. See Valerie Hardcastle, "Understanding Functions: A Pragmatic Approach," in Valerie Hardcastle (ed.), *Where Biology Meets Psychology* (Cambridge, 1999), pp. 27–43.

What can be gleaned from the above passage is that Boorse thinks that understanding function statements about biological organisms must be done from a contextualist perspective. His justification is that the practices of the various sub-disciplines within biology focus on particular parts of the biological world, resulting in different function ascriptions to different organisms and their parts. For example, an evolutionary geneticist might argue that the function of the heart is to assist in the passing of genetic material from one generation to another. In contrast, a physiologist might claim that the function of the heart is to pump blood. Drawing from Boorse's concept of function, both specialists have a legitimate claim to the function of the heart; indeed, Boorse is clear that the notion of "the function" is incoherent. Here he must mean that organisms or their parts have multiple functions, which contribute to particular ends, but that the set of contexts determines which functions and ends gain ascendancy in particular explanations and cases.

*Boorse's Concept of Function with Respect to Wright's Adequacy Conditions*

Having offered his contextualist concept of function, Boorse proclaims that he has met the adequacy conditions offered by Wright. Recall that Wright thought that a fruitful concept of function should be able (1) to distinguish accidents from genuine functions, (2) to range over both conscious functions (artifact functions) and natural functions (organism functions), and (3) to eliminate any divine element from the concept of function.

First, Boorse thinks that he has provided a concept of function that ranges over both organisms and artifacts. He says that his analysis, "distinguishes between functions and accidents: all Wright's cases of accidental effects of things which are not their function either fail to contribute to a goal or violate relevance conditions imposed by the context of utterance."[75] Boorse's point is that his analysis is able to distinguish between functions and accidents because the latter either do not contribute to the goals of a system or are not part of the set of functions in the context under consideration.

It is not clear that Boorse has satisfied Wright's first adequacy condition, because Boorse would have to allow certain artifacts to have specific functions, even if they do not. Consider the sheriff's badge example. Imagine that all the witnesses to the duel concur that the badge blinded the bandit gunslinger. That is, within the context of the duel and during the time interval of high noon, the badge's reflection of the sun's rays falls within some circumscribed class of functions being performed by the sheriff's badge, which causally contributes to the success of winning the duel. Under this scenario, Boorse would have to concede that the function of the badge is to blind gunslingers in duels, because it causally contributes to the goal of defeating one's opponent in a duel or to the maintenance of law enforcement.

It is clear that on a given occasion the badge was able to distract the on-coming gunslinger, but distracting gunslingers is not the function of a badge within the system of dueling or law enforcement. The function of a sheriff's badge is to reveal who is in charge of law enforcement and (possibly) who has the legal right to engage in a

---

[75] Boorse, "Wright on Functions," p. 86.

duel with criminals. No doubt, there may be other functions that pertain to a sheriff's badge, but it is highly implausible to think that blinding on-coming gunslingers is part of the set of badge functions in the system of dueling or law enforcement. It is more appropriate to say that the blinding effect produced by the badge is an accident and not a genuine function.

Notice that if the sheriff uses the badge *on a regular* basis to blind gunslingers, then it can acquire this additional function. The difference now is that a *regularity condition* has been added as a necessary condition to the understanding of what a function is. So long as **X** does **Z** on a regular basis, then it becomes possible for **X** to have a function **Z**. It is this lack of a regularity condition in Boorse's analysis that reveals why he is unable to distinguish genuine functions from mere accidents—single fortuitous effects would have to be accepted as functions even though such function attributions are implausible. Boorse should have retained the regularity condition as part of his concept of function.

Indeed, as Boorse makes clear, "Clearly functions may be performed only once and by accident."[76] According to Boorse, he clearly thinks that accidents can be functions. The problem is that if accidents can be functions, then the distinction between genuine functions and mere accidents collapses. Yet, Boorse is clear that he wishes to maintain this distinction. So, Boorse is either caught in a contradiction or he simply cannot satisfy the adequacy condition of keeping genuine functions distinct from accidental effects. In either case, his concept of function runs into difficulties.

Moreover, Boorse's concept of function provides no way to determine which effects do and do not belong to the set of functions that an entity has within a given system. Why would or would not blinding gunslingers be an acceptable function of a badge within the context of dueling or law enforcement? It seems intuitive to think that badges do not have this function of blinding, but relying on intuitions is unsatisfactory—Boorse's intuitions could go in one direction and someone else's intuitions could go another direction. The point is that Boorse needs an account of what can and cannot be allowed in a set of functions for a specific entity in a given context. As it stands, it is possible to construct all sorts of scenarios (like the sheriff's badge example) that allow certain advantageous effects, which are clearly accidental effects, to be genuine functions. The upshot is that Boorse has not provided a concept of function that distinguishes accidents from genuine functions.

Boorse could reply that he agrees that blinding bandits is not the function of a badge, because such an effect is not a function in the context of utterance for dueling. Although the badge does contribute to the goal of either law enforcement or winning duels, it is still an accident in the context of utterance under consideration. The result is that he is still able to distinguish genuine functions from mere accidents. The problem with this reply is that it does not square well with his Bible example. Recall that in this example a Bible in a soldier's pocket stops a bullet from killing the soldier. Boorse concludes from this example that the Bible does have this function in the appropriate context. Yet, it is hard to imagine how a Bible could have such a function within the context of utterance for war. Still, if the Bible can have the

---

[76] Ibid., p. 80.

function of stopping bullets during wartime in a one-time scenario, then Boorse would have to accept that the sheriff's badge has the function of blinding bandits even if this effect occurred only once. Again, Boorse would have to offer an account of why certain causally contributing effects are not part of the set of functions in a particular context.[77] It remains, then, that Boorse's concept of function cannot distinguish real functions from accidental effects.

The above concern is also present in Boorse's discussion of organismic functions. Consider the function of the heart. It is clear that the heart pumps blood and it makes thumping sounds. It is generally regarded that the thumping sounds of the heart are an accidental feature of the function of pumping blood. A persuasive concept of function should be able to accommodate the claim that pumping blood is the function of the heart, but thumping sounds are mere accidents. Yet, Boorse's contextualist account would have to allow for the startling claim that a function of the heart is to make thumping sounds. For example, doctors may very well use the thumping of the heart as a diagnostic measure. Thumping sounds could be initially useful in determining how an individual's pulmonary system is functioning in order to determine if further medical intervention is necessary. That is, the thumping sounds of the heart could contribute to the goal of healing within the context of medicine during the time interval of a doctor checking a patient's heart with a stethoscope. Thus, the thumping of the heart could be viewed as a genuine function as opposed to a mere accidental effect within the context of medical diagnosis.

Boorse could respond that, in the context of medicine, the thumping of the heart *does* have a genuine function because it contributes to the goal of healing within the medical system. Still, this rejoinder is rather implausible. One would have hoped for an account that acknowledges that the thumping of the heart is an accident as opposed to a genuine function. Indeed, the heart example reasonably indicates that it is possible to have an effect that is useful to the goals of a particular system at a certain time interval, but it is merely an accident that it is useful at that particular time interval. Boorse's analysis does not allow for such instances. Thus, it is reasonable to claim that Boorse's account is not able to distinguish genuine functions from mere accidents.

Second, Boorse's concept of function is able to ignore the sharp distinction between conscious functions and natural functions, because this is an implication of his contextualist account. Boorse thinks that natural functions are understood in terms of their goal-directed activities, which do not rely on (conscious) intentions. Rather they are described by different scientific contexts, which focus on different aspects of the natural "teleological pie." Artifact functions, according to Boorse, are understood in terms of the contexts of the intentions of the designer or the intentions of the user. Boorse's account can accommodate both sorts of functions, because they represent different contexts. So, according to Boorse's analysis, this adequacy condition by Wright can be met by his general contextualist concept of

---

[77] Much like the badge example, it is difficult to accept that the function of a Bible during wartime is to stop on-coming bullets. It would be more plausible to suggest that such a one-time event is a fortunate accident.

function—both the function of artifacts and the function of organisms simply fall under different contexts.[78]

Finally, given that Boorse offers a contextualist concept of function, it is reasonable to think that he does not necessarily have to accept a divine intentional designer account within his contextualist concept of function. Recall that Wright is able to satisfy this requirement because, although his account is compatible with a divine intentional designer account, he does not necessarily include such an account in his concept of function. The point is that a concept of function that is compatible with theism is not a problem for Wright because he is only committed to the view that theism is not required to explain functions. Similarly, Boorse could agree that the context of natural theology is compatible with his contextualist concept of function. From this perspective, the heart has the function of pumping blood because this is part of the master plan created by God when he created everything. Alternatively, as Boorse himself holds, biological functions should be understood from the context of the various subfields of biology. Thus, although Boorse's account of function is compatible with a divine intentional designer account, he is able to satisfy the adequacy condition of not necessarily including divine intervention in his account.

This section has revealed that Boorse is not able to satisfy all of Wright's adequacy conditions. Specifically, Boorse's concept of function (1) is not able to distinguish accidents from genuine functions, even though it is (2) able to range over conscious functions (e.g., artifacts) and natural functions (e.g., organs) and (3) able to exclude any theistic element from his concept of function.[79]

## Concluding Thoughts on "Function Talk"

This fourth chapter presented a glimpse into the debate on function. Specifically, in an attempt to understand Boorse's concept of function, Wright's critical analysis of the concept of function and his own positive etiological account was explained. This section assessed the strengths and weaknesses in the concepts of function offered by Wright and Boorse. Wright's concept of function has two strengths: First, it is able to distinguish genuine functions from accidents once it is realized that his etiological account includes natural selection. Second, his account is able to exclude theism as a necessary requirement. However, Wright's concept also has four weaknesses: The first is that his original version appears to be a tautology. Although a modified version could avoid this criticism, it does so at the expense of sacrificing his original account. The second possible weakness is that there is little support for Wright's claim that a virtue of his analysis is that it ranges over conscious functions and natural functions. The difficulty is that his account ranges over both organisms

---

[78] Whether Boorse or Wright is correct about how to understand this adequacy condition depends on how close of connection there is between conscious and natural functions. Recall that it was noted that Wright's insistence that natural and conscious functions are similar is controversial. Ignoring context, Boorse, on the other hand, takes the conventional view that natural functions are entirely distinct from conscious functions.

[79] Keep in mind that Boorse has separated functions from goals. As part of his reply to his critics, Chapter 6 will discuss the role of goals in Boorse's concept of function.

and artifacts, because he reduces both accounts to the common denominator of advantageous consequences. This reduction, however, ignores the fact that artifacts are the result of intelligent thought and rational planning, while biological features are the product of "blind" physiological processes. For his claim to succeed, Wright would have to offer much more than he has in its defense. Thus, to the extent that he has not rigorously defended this claim, Wright is not entirely successful in having his account range over conscious functions and natural functions.[80] Third, Wright is inconsistent as to whether or not organisms and artifacts can lose their functions. Fourth, given certain possible world scenarios and the implicit role of benefit in his analysis, Wright has not provided a necessary condition for function.

Boorse's account has three strengths: First, Boorse's concept of function is able to range over organisms and artifacts. Second, as a result of his contextualist account, he is able to eliminate the necessity of any divine element in his concept of function, although he would agree that a divine intentional designer interpretation of function is compatible with his account. Third, Boorse is able to avoid some of Wright's weaknesses by appealing to the notion of goals. The major weakness of Boorse's concept of function is that it is not able to distinguish genuine functions from mere accidental effects. This difficulty is avoided by Wright's etiological analysis. Part of the issue is that Boorse's concept of function provides no principled way of determining which effects do and do not belong to the set of functions an entity has within a given system or context. The result is that, for both organisms and artifacts, accidents and side effects have to be treated as genuine functions. No doubt, this is a legitimate drawback to Boorse's concept of function.

If one were keeping score, then Boorse's account would appear to be a superior alternative to Wright's account. Yet, this would depend on which of the adequacy conditions one considers most valuable. Putting to one side the charges of inconsistency and tautology against Wright's account, the most valuable adequacy condition could be the one that requires offering a concept of function that distinguishes genuine functions from mere side effects or accidents. Since Boorse cannot meet this requirement, his analysis would be less successful than Wright's account. Alternatively, one might consider a concept of function that is able to range over conscious functions and natural functions as the most valuable achievement. Since Boorse meets this requirement and Wright does not, Boorse might be considered to have a more cogent concept of function than Wright has. The foregoing remarks suggest that a more defensible account of function would attempt to combine their strengths and avoid their weaknesses. Chapter 7 will offer such an account.

Now that Boorse's contextualist concept of function is clear, the way has been paved for a discussion of his functional concept of health and the critical replies to it. It is to the details of Boorse's naturalistic concept of health that will be the focus of the next chapter. Then, Chapter 6 will examine the numerous critical responses to Boorse's concept of health.

---

[80] Again, the details of this debate are beyond the scope of this project. Still, for a defense of a Wrightian-type account, see Preston, "Why is a Wing Like a Spoon? A Pluralist Theory of Function," pp. 244–5.

# Chapter 5

# Boorse's Concept of Health

## Introduction: the Route to Boorse's Concept of Health

The overarching aim of the foregoing three chapters is to provide the background from which Boorse's own concept of health emerges. Chapter 2 presented specific naturalistic concepts of health and Boorse's arguments against them. Chapter 3 offered a critical review of Boorse's dismissal of the idea that the concept of health is normative. Chapter 4 furnished Boorse's contextualist concept of function, which emerged as a response to Wright's etiological concept of function. With these three preliminary chapters in place, it is now possible to turn to Boorse's own concept of health.

There are four parts to this fifth chapter. The first section begins with two separate argument reconstructions designed to makes sense of Boorse's concept of health. In order to understand the details of these two argument reconstructions and how Boorse is using many technical terms, the next section introduces distinctions between mechanism, part-functionalism, and organic functional holism to reveal that Boorse is a part-functionalist. Then, the subsequent section explains four senses of "objectivism"—(1) metaphysical objectivism, (2) methodological objectivism, (3) disciplinary objectivism, and (4) dialectical objectivism—to reveal that Boorse is a combination of (1) and (3). Finally, the fourth section describes the details of how Boorse understands numerous technical aspects (e.g., reference class, normal function, and disease) of his concept of health. Broadly, the goal of this chapter is to offer a rich picture of Boorse's concept of health that will provide a suitable framework from which to evaluate the critical replies to his account in Chapter 6.

*Mechanism, Functionalism, and Objectivism: Some Technical Aspects of Boorse's Naturalistic Concept of Health*

This section offers two argument reconstructions of Boorse's naturalistic concept of health. Recall that Chapter 3 provided a glimpse into Boorse's concept of health. Broadly, the beginning of that chapter made clear that Boorse understands both health and disease in relation to biological function. As Boorse claims,

> The state of an organism is theoretically healthy, i.e., free of *disease*, insofar as its mode of functioning conforms to the natural design of that kind of organism ...[1] If what makes a condition a disease is its deviation from the *natural functional organization* of the species, then in calling tooth decay a disease we are saying that it is not simply in the nature of the species—and we say this because we think of it as mainly due to environmental causes.

---

[1] Christopher Boorse, "On the Distinction Between Disease and Illness," *Philosophy and Public Affairs*, 5/1 (1975): 57 [my italics].

In general, deficiencies in functional efficiency of the body are diseases when they are unnatural, and they may be unnatural either by being atypical or by being attributable mainly to the action of a hostile environment ... *Theoretical health now turns out to be strictly analogous to the mechanical condition of an artifact.* Despite appearances, "perfect mechanical condition" in, say, a 1965 Volkswagen is a descriptive notion. Such an artifact is in *perfect mechanical condition* when it conforms in all respects to the designer's detailed specifications ... Perfect working order is a matter not of the worth of the product but of the conformity of the process to a *fixed design*. In the case of organisms, of course, the *ideal* health must be determined by empirical analysis of the species rather than by the intentions of a designer ...[2] the classification of human states as healthy or diseased is an *objective* matter, to be read off the biological facts of nature without need of value judgments.[3]

In the spirit of philosophical analysis and charity, the discussion to follow will begin with two argument reconstructions of Boorse's claims in the above passage. The reason for this strategy is two-fold. First, it is reasonable to think that Boorse, as a philosopher, is offering an argument in defense of his naturalistic concept of health, as opposed to merely stipulating what he thinks health is. Second, the argument reconstructions provide a way of organizing Boorse's discussion so that it is possible to explain systematically the various aspects of his concept of health. With these two points in mind, the first argument reconstruction, which is called *The Elements of Health*, provides some of the key aspects of Boorse's concept of health. The second argument reconstruction, which is titled *The Concept of Health from Mechanistic Analogy*, focuses on Boorse's analogy between the human body and an automobile. These two arguments are as follows:

*Argument Number 1: The Elements of Health*

P1 If health is the absence of disease, then health is the absence of the conditions that constitute disease.
P2 The conditions that constitute disease are deviations from natural functions.
P3 Deviations from natural functions occur by being atypical or as a result of a hostile environment.
P4. Health is the absence of disease.

\* \* \*

C1 Health is the absence of natural functional deviations that occur by being atypical or as a result of a hostile environment.

*Argument Number 2: The Concept of Health from a Mechanistic Analogy*

P1 If health is the absence of natural functional deviations that occur by being atypical or as a result of a hostile environment, then health can be understood in terms of ideal natural functional efficiency.

---

[2] Ibid., p. 59.
[3] Christopher Boorse, "A Rebuttal on Health," in James M. Humber and Robert F. Almeder (eds), *What is Disease?* (Totowa, 1985), p. 6.

P2 Health is the absence of natural functional deviations that occur by being atypical or as a result of a hostile environment. (= C1)
P3 Health can be understood in terms of ideal natural functional efficiency.
P4 Ideal natural functional efficiency is analogous to the perfect mechanical functional efficiency of an artifact.
P5 Perfect mechanical functional efficiency is an objective condition.

\* \* \*

C2 By analogy, health is an objective condition.

There are many elements to the above two argument reconstructions that require an explanation. The second argument will be examined first. As a start, both "mechanical" and "objective" need to be made clear in the second argument reconstruction. With respect to "mechanical," P5 is the point of focus. In this premise, Boorse claims by analogy that a healthy functioning organism can be understood in terms of a well-functioning automobile.[4] How is this analogy to be understood? Since "mechanism" (which involves an analogy between natural things and machines) has different senses, the machine metaphor needs to be clarified. To this end, E. K. Ledermann has stated that those within the concept of health literature who embrace such machine analogies, like the one put forth by Boorse, also take seriously a *mechanistic* world-view. Ledermann explains "mechanism" as follows:

---

[4] Note that, in his *Treatise of Man*, Descartes offers a similar mechanical picture of the human body and its parts. Specifically, in his attempt to stave off any hint of final causes or vital forces as part of an explanation of human and non-human animal physiology and actions, Descartes provides the following summary judgment: "I should like you to consider, after this, all the functions I have ascribed to this machine—such as digestion of food, the beating of the heart and arteries, the nourishment and growth of limbs, respiration, waking and sleeping, the reception of the sense organs of light, sounds, smells, tastes, heat and other such qualities, the imprinting of ideas of these qualities in the organ of the 'common' sense and the imagination, the retention or stamping of these ideas in the memory, the internal movements of the appetites and passions, and finally the external movement of all the limbs (movements which are so appropriate not only to the actions of objects presented to the senses, but also to the passions and the impressions found in memory, that they imitate perfectly the movements of a real man). I should like you to consider that these functions follow from the mere arrangement of the machine's organs every bit as naturally as the movements of a clock or other automaton follow from the arrangement of its counter weights and wheels." See René Descartes, "Treatise on Man," in John Cottingham, Robert Stoothoff, and Dugald Murdoch (trans/eds), *The Philosophical Writings of Descartes* (Cambridge, 1985), vol. I, p. 108. Of course, I have not done complete justice to Descartes's mechanistic analysis. For example, I have left out the fact that Descartes does think of the mind/soul as a separate entity that acts as a distal cause *qua* controller of many bodily functions (See "Fourth Replies," in John Cottingham, Robert Stoothoff, and Dugald Murdoch (trans/eds), *The Philosophical Writings of Descartes*, vol. II, (Cambridge, 1985), vol. II, p. 161), while the proximate cause of various bodily functions is "[t]he parts of the blood which penetrate as far as the brain serve not only to nourish and sustain its substance, but also and primarily to produce in a certain way fine wind, or rather a very lively and pure flame, which is called the *animal spirits*" (see *Treatise on Man*, p. 100).

The medical scientist who adopts the mechanistic approach ignores the individuality of the patient. The law which he imposes and which determines "every case indifferently from the outside" is discovered as the relationships between parts of the organism. It means that the living being has been divided up, analysed into elements. When the person is ill, the diagnosis consists in identifying the part and the abnormality in the part and in its *function* ... The mechanistic principle is not only applied to the understanding of the healthy and the sick body, the same principle is applied to nutrition ... The body is conceived as a biological machine and food is understood as supplying the energy to enable the machine to work.[5]

In understanding Ledermann's sense of "mechanism" in the above passage, two preliminary points with respect to his use of terms need to be clarified. First, notice that Ledermann uses both "mechanistic" and "function" in the same discussion. This might suggest that the concept of function is similar to the concept of mechanism. Specifically, Ledermann inadvertently may be giving the impression that *mechanism* takes seriously not only the idea that organisms can be reduced to parts, but also the impression that parts of organisms are goal-directed. Historically, however, mechanistic philosophy emerged in opposition to *functional goal-directedness* (i.e., teleology)—the idea that biological entities are by nature moving toward specific end states. Within this historical context, *mechanism* and *teleology* are opposed views. The point is that it is important to keep technical terms associated with machine analogies clear. Indeed, in his discussion of the birth of the "mechanistic world-view" that emerged out of the seventeenth-century Scientific Revolution, Stephen Toulmin offers the following warning:

[A]ny philosophical account of the content of this revolution, and its significance for us today must pay proper attention to the ways in which such words as "machine," "mechanics" and "mechanistic" have been, and are to be, understood in this debate. If we are to do this with confidence, we must take care not to assume that these terms have kept, well defined, fixed meanings throughout the last 350 years.[6]

---

[5] E. K. Ledermann, "Mechanism and Holism in Physical Science," in David Lamb, Teifion Davies, and Marie Roberts (eds), *Explorations in Medicine Volume 1* (Aldershot, 1987), pp. 39 and 40 [my italics]. Norman Malcolm nicely describes mechanism with respect to the human body (using an analogy similar to Descartes and Ledermann) as follows: "The version of mechanism I wish to study assumes a neurophysiological theory which is adequate to explain and predict all movements of human bodies except those caused by outside forces. *The human body is assumed to be as complete a causal system as is a gasoline engine.* Neurological states and processes are conceived to be correlated by general laws with mechanisms that produce movements. Chemical and electrical changes in the nervous tissue of the body are assumed to cause muscle contractions, which in turn cause movements such as blinking, breathing, and puckering of the lips, as well as movements of fingers, limbs, and head." Malcolm's basic point in his description of mechanism is that biological phenomena can be understood entirely through chemical and electrical activities, which can be understood ultimately through the laws of motion in physics. See Norman Malcolm, "The Conceivability of Mechanism," in A. P. Martinich and Ernest Sosa (eds), *Analytic Philosophy: An Anthology* (Oxford, 2001), p. 287 [my italics].

[6] Stephen Toulmin, "From Clocks to Chaos: Humanizing the Mechanistic World-View," in Hermann Haken, Anders Karlqvist, and Uno Svedin (eds), *The Machine as Metaphor and*

In acknowledgment of Toulmin's warning in the above passage (and for the sake of clarity and for the sake of those who are sensitive to this history), it is best to keep "mechanism" and "function" distinct.[7]

The second point is that Ledermann is concerned with part-whole relationships in his description of *mechanism*. Specifically, he thinks that mechanists focus on parts of organisms rather than organisms as a whole. Again, this way of understanding *mechanism* masks a different distinction between part-functionalism and organic functional holism. In order to make sense of Boorse's automobile analogy and the fact that he is a functionalist, it will be necessary to summarize briefly the following technical terms: mechanism, part-functionalism, and organic functional holism. This section will argue that Boorse is best described as a part-functionalist rather than a mechanist or an organic functional holist.

*Mechanism* In his attempt to make sense of René Descartes's use of machine, Dennis Des Chene offers the following general description of mechanism:

> Mechanism is a *method*. It says yes to some modes of explanation and no to others. It promotes the analysis of capacities, and discourages the invocation of irreducible powers. It is also a substantive *doctrine* about bodies and change: bodies have only those properties that follow upon their being extended substances, and perhaps a few additional properties like impenetrability. As a doctrine, it invites us to regard natural things, if complex, as combinations of extended substances interacting only by way of collision.[8]

From the above description, a simple version of mechanism is the view that all natural phenomena are to be understood in terms of (i) a fundamental type of matter (e.g., atoms) (ii) a single set of intrinsic qualities (e.g., electric charge) of the fundamental matter, (iii) a single sort of motion for the fundamental matter (e.g., change in the relative positions of atoms), and (iv) a single uniform way in which the fundamental matter is able to form aggregates (e.g., collision or bonding law).[9]

---

*Tool* (Berlin, 1993), pp. 139–40.

[7] Franz M. Wuketits has offered a nice historical account of how "mechanism" has changed from the atomistic version offered by the ancient Greeks to the contemporary molecular mechanistic version. See Franz M. Wuketits, "Organisms, Vital Forces, and Machines: Classical Controversies and the Contemporary Discussion of 'Reductionism VS. Holism'" in Paul Hoyningen-Huene and F. M. Wuketits, (eds), *Reductionism and Systems Theory in the Life Sciences* (Dordrecht, 1989), pp. 3–28. Note that I am not arguing that mechanistic and functional/teleological explanations are completely incompatible. (Indeed, a Darwinian perspective on teleology could be a way to reconcile these two competing views.) Here, the concern is not to confuse terms that have been thought to be incompatible. For this debate on the incompatibility between these two modes of explanation, see Ned J. Block, "Are Mechanistic and Teleological Explanations of Behavior Incompatible?" *The Philosophical Review*, 21/83 (1971): 109–17.

[8] Dennis Des Chene, *Spirits and Clocks: Machine and Organisms in Descartes* (Ithaca, 2002), p. 14.

[9] A variation on these four points can be found in C. D. Broad, "Mechanism and Emergentism," in Jaegwon Kim and Ernest Sosa (eds), *Metaphysics: An Anthology* (Oxford, 1999), pp. 487–8. No doubt, there are other variations of mechanism that have not been

On this interpretation of mechanism, the idea is that all phenomena can be explained in terms of a basic kind of entity, which has a strict set of fundamental properties. Most importantly for this discussion, an implication of mechanism is that any natural entity can be explained entirely in terms of (i)–(iv) without reference to the system to which it belongs as a whole or to any sort of goal-directed activities of the parts or the system as a whole. In summary, mechanism can be understood as follows:

> Mechanism: A kind of naturalistic explanation that holds that any phenomenon **X** and the set of all of **X**'s constituent parts **P** within a system **S** are to be understood by the structure, arrangement, and properties of a basic entity **B**. In understanding **X** and **B**, there is little or no concern given to **S** as a whole.

Having offered this Cartesian account of mechanism, it is important to note that there are many difficulties with it that make it an implausible position. The first is that the various aggregates formed by the interaction of molecules are the result of distinct types of bonding (e.g., covalent bonding and polar covalent bonding). This fact tells against the view that there exists only one kind of way molecules can form aggregates. Second, if reduction is to be taken seriously, then why does the mechanist stop at the level of atoms? To the point, if the tenets of quantum mechanics are true, then molecules themselves are reducible to quanta (electrons, quarks, etc.), which may either have no distinct intrinsic quality or a stochastic intrinsic nature. Specifically, the foundation of quantum mechanics is that at the level of quanta the laws of classical physics are not applicable. The position and movement of elementary particles cannot be determined in the way macroscopic entities can. Rather, the position and movement of elementary particles can be understood only probabilistically, because the velocity of such phenomena changes unpredictably from one moment to the next. As Brian Greene makes the point, "this inability to know both the positions and velocities of elementary particles implies that the microscopic realm is intrinsically turbulent."[10] Third, assuming the evidence in quantum experiments, there may be no elementary causal law that explains how particles influence each other. As Stuart Glennan observes,

> There is however an obvious limitation to the mechanical theory. Sooner or later the process of decomposition of a system into parts must come to an end. This is the level of fundamental laws. At this point we cannot point to any further or deeper mechanism. Since there is no mechanism, how do we explain the causal connection between events at the level of fundamental physics? The mechanical theory offers us no answers..."[11]

Fourth, some authors argue that emergent properties and the hierarchical nature of the physiology of living organisms have their origin in higher-level physical

---

discussed here. These variations including embracing and rejecting different combinations of (i)–(iv). Still, all of these variations accept the claim that all phenomena, including biological systems, can be understood from the laws of physics—be they associated with Newtonian mechanics, relativity theory, string theory, etc.

[10] Brian Greene, *The Elegant Universe* (New York, 2000), p. 118.
[11] Stuart S. Glennan, "Mechanisms and the Nature of Causation," *Erkenntnis*, 44/1 (1996): 64.

laws that cannot be reduced to lower-level physical laws. Peter Machamer *et al.* defend this anti-reductionistic position when they claim that parts (or mechanisms) of biological entities

> must be understood in their important, vital, or otherwise significant context, and this requires an understanding of the working of the mechanism at multiple levels ... Higher-level entities and activities are thus essential to the intelligibility of those at the lower levels, just as much as those at the lower level are essential for understanding those at the higher level. It is the integration of different levels into productive relations that renders the phenomenon intelligible and thereby explains it.[12]

*Organic functional holism*   As an alternative to the Cartesian-type version of mechanism, organic functional holism is the view that there are certain kinds of natural entities that can be fully understood only with respect to the system to which they belong. Specifically, the organic functional holist rejects elements (i)–(iv) embraced by the mechanist. Moreover, the organic functional holist would argue that an organism and its parts can be understood and explained fully only in terms of *the* function of the organism as a whole. Henry Byerly articulates this holistic view as follows:

> In holistic explanation of a part in terms of a whole, that which does the explaining, the pattern of the whole, must be understood first. The whole is in this sense epistemologically prior to the parts even though the whole may be temporally and causally subsequent to its parts.[13]

For example, the only way to understand and explain fully the various activities associated with an allergic reaction is to understand them within the context of the function of the immune system as a whole and the function of the organism as a whole. A classic organic functional holist is Aristotle. He argues that, in the same way that parts of organisms have functions, organisms as a whole have *a* special or unique function. With respect to determining the function of humans, Aristotle argues as follows:

> Well, perhaps we shall find the best good if we first find the function (*ergon*) of a human being ...[14] just as eye, hand, foot, and, in general, every [bodily] part apparently has its

---

[12] Peter Machamer, Lindley Darden, and Carl F. Craver, "Thinking About Mechanisms," *Philosophy of Science*, 67/1 (2000): 23. Also See Paul Humphreys, "Aspects of Emergence," *Philosophical Topics*, 24/1 (1996): 53–70 and his "How Properties Emerge," *Philosophy of Science*, 64/1 (1997): 1–17, Alexander Rueger, "Physical Emergence, Diachronic and Synchronic," *Synthese*, 124/3 (2000): 297–322, and Niall Shanks and Karl H. Joplin, "Redundant Complexity: A Critical Analysis of Intelligent Design in Biochemistry?" *Philosophy of Science*, 66/2 (1999): 268–82.

[13] Henry Byerly, "Teleology and Evolutionary Theory: Mechanisms and Meaning," *Nature and System*, 1 (1979): 175. See also Herbert A. Simon, "The Architecture of Complexity," *Proceedings of the American Philosophical Society*, 106/6 (1962): 467–82.

[14] Aristotle, *Nicomachean Ethics*, 1097b24–25 (trans. C.D.C. Reeve, *Practices of Reason: Aristotle's Nicomachean Ethics* [Oxford, 1995]).

functions, may we likewise ascribe to a human being some function over and above (*para*) all of theirs?[15]

Aristotle answers the above question in general and specific terms. In general terms, he says:

> Just as every instrument is for the sake of something, the parts of the body are also for the sake of something, that is for the sake of some action (*praxis*), so the whole body must evidently be for the sake of some complex action.[16]

So, generally, the parts of the body and the body as a whole are for the sake of a complex action—that is, the function of the body as a whole is that of a complex action. What is this complex action in the case of humans? In specific terms, Aristotle offers the following answer:

> [A] harpist's function, for example, is to play the harp and a good harpist is to do it well (*eu*). Now we take the human function to be a certain kind of life and take this life to be the activity and actions of the psyche. [Hence] the excellent man's function is to do these finely and well. Each action or activity is completed well when its completion expresses the proper virtue. Therefore, the human good turns out to be an activity of the psyche that expresses virtue.[17]

So, the complex action *qua* the function of the human organism as a whole is the excellent expression of virtue or as he also puts it, "We have found, then, that the human function is the activity of the psyche that expresses reason or is not without reason."[18] Indeed, Aristotle is clear that all activities of the parts of organisms are for the sake of this function (e.g., expressing reason) of the whole organism. So, according to Aristotle, a proper general understanding of the parts of animals will include an understanding of the function of the whole to which they belong.[19] Organic functional holism can be summarized as follows:

> Organic Functional Holism: A kind of naturalistic explanation that holds that any phenomenon **X** and the set of all of **X**'s constituent parts **P** within a system **S** can be understood and explained fully in terms of the function of **S** as a whole.

The major criticism of organic functional holism is that it is impossible (especially in the case of humans) to determine *the* function of an entity like the human organism. Since humans engage in all sorts of activities (e.g., elaborate cooking practices, torture, writing novels, etc.), which are unique or special to our species,

---

[15] Ibid., 1097b31–33.
[16] Aristotle, *Parts of Animals* 645b14–20 (trans. A.L. Peck).
[17] Aristotle, *Nicomachean Ethics*, 1098a13–17 (trans. C.D.C. Reeve).
[18] Ibid., 1098a5–8.
[19] Note that a variation on organic functional holism could be "psyche-soma holism." This latter version of holism attempts to understand organisms in terms of both the physical and the mental. For this latter version of holism, see Ledermann, "Mechanism and Holism in Physical Science," and Joseph Agassi, "Mechanistic and Holistic Models in Psychiatry," *Nature and System*, 3 (1981): 143–52.

it is arbitrary to pick, as Aristotle does, a particular function as *the* function of the human organism. Thus, organic functional holism is not thought to be a plausible account.

*Part-functionalism* As a result of the above difficulties with mechanism and organic functional holism, some scholars have defended a more plausible position, call it *part-functionalism*.[20] On this version of functionalism, the idea that all phenomena can be reduced to a single common denominator is rejected, but it is thought that it is possible to explain parts of systems without attributing functions to the system as a whole. Moreover, the part-functionalist would acknowledge that the causal laws of physics pertain to parts, but would still hold that reducing parts of systems to fundamental elements ignores the hierarchical structure of biological systems and the goal-directed nature of parts.[21]

For example, a part-functionalist could argue that it is possible to discuss how the human heart pumps blood without any reference to the role a heart plays with respect to the function of the human organism as a whole. Basically, the part-functionalist does not necessarily embrace entirely elements (i)–(iv) of mechanism, but endorses the idea that parts may have functions and goals. So, similar to the mechanist and contrary to the organic functional holist, the part-functionalist agrees that in order to understand the parts of a system it is not necessary to know how the parts relate to the function of the system as a whole. In contrast to the mechanist and similar to the organic functional holist, the part-functionalist rejects that parts of a system can be reduced to a fundamental element and accepts that parts of systems have functions that bring about goals. So, part-functionalism is an attempt to steer between the problems present in both mechanism and organic functional holism. Part-functionalism can be summarized as follows:

Part-Functionalism: A kind of naturalistic explanation that holds that any phenomenon **X** and the set of some of **X**'s constituent parts **P** within a system **S** can be understood and explained fully in terms of the functions of **P** and the goals related to **P**'s functions without attributing functions to **S** as a whole.

---

[20] Glennan offers a version of this type of part-functionalism. He says: "A mechanism underlying a behavior is a complex system which produces that behavior by the interaction of a number of parts according to direct causal laws." Note that Glennan labels this definition "market mechanism" as opposed to "mechanism" simpliciter. What Glennan labels "market mechanism," I am calling "part-functionalism." I do this to avoid the possible confusion that may arise from the fact that *mechanism* and *functionalism* have been opposed to one another historically. Moreover, note that Glennan's definition leaves open the possibility that causal laws could be at work at different levels of complexity. See Glennan, "Mechanisms and the Nature of Causation," p. 52.

[21] Samuel Alexander argues for this position in general terms. He says that "the emergence of a new quality from any level of existence means that at that level there comes into being a certain constellation or collocation of the motions belonging to that level, and this collocation possesses a new quality distinctive of the higher complex." See Samuel Alexander, *Space, Time and Deity*, vol. 2 (London, 1927), p. 45.

With respect to the allergy example, a part-functionalist would claim that it is possible to understand how antigen processing cells go about their functions of recognizing allergens and passing them to T helper cells. Moreover, the part-functionalist would claim that such an explanation could be rendered without having to attribute functions to the body as a whole (notably, the part-functionalist acknowledges that not all parts of a system have functions; rather, only those that contribute to the goals of the system have functions). This explains the use of "some" in the above definition. Thus, on this interpretation of part-functionalism, the activities of some parts within a system can be understood and explained fully with respect to the *specific* functions of those parts.

*Boorse as a part-functionalist* The criticisms levied against both mechanism and organic functional holism reveal that they are not very compelling theories.[22] If the above criticisms of mechanism and organic functional holism are on the mark and Boorse's automobile analogy is to be understood from the perspective of either theory, then his account is problematic. For, in general, Boorse would have to justify how it is the case that mechanism or organic functional holism (the versions presented here or some other permutations) can withstand these (or some of these) criticisms. Nowhere in his discussions on the concept of health has Boorse provided any such defense of mechanism or organic functional holism.

Yet, to suggest that Boorse is an adherent of either theory on the basis of his automobile analogy is rather uncharitable. First, the primary reason that Boorse is not a mechanist is that he takes seriously the goal-directedness of the parts of organisms—an element that defenders of mechanism would surely eschew. Moreover, unlike the mechanist, because Boorse acknowledges the goal-directedness of parts of organisms, it follows that he does not embrace the reductionism implicit in mechanism. This point should be quite clear given that Boorse takes seriously functional explanation as an ineliminable part of his concept of health. Thus, it is not appropriate to think that Boorse postulates a mechanistic framework through the use of his automobile analogy.

Second, the following passage reveals that Boorse rejects organic functional holism and explicitly endorses part-functionalism. He says:

> Physiologists obtain their functional doctrines without at any stage having to answer such questions as, What is the function of man? or to explicate "a good man" on the analogy of a "good knife" ... The specifically physiological functions of any component are, I think,

---

[22] Indeed, Ernest Nagel puts the exclamation point on the current implausibility of mechanism as a legitimate explanatory method for understanding biological entities. He says: "No theory can explain the operations of any concretely given system unless a complete set of initial and boundary conditions for the application of the theory is stated in a manner consonant with the specific notions employed in the theory ... we do not know at present the detailed physicochemical composition of any living organism, nor the forces that may be acting between the elements on the lowest level of its hierarchical organization. We are therefore currently unable to state in exclusively physicochemical terms the initial boundary conditions ... Until we can do this, we are in principle precluded from deducing biological laws from mechanistic theory." See Ernest Nagel, *The Structure of Science* (New York, 1961), pp. 442–3.

its species-typical contributions to the typical goals of survival and reproduction ... And the single unifying property of all recognized diseases of plants and animals appears to be this: that they interfere with one or more functions typically performed within members of the species ... The health of an organism consists in the performance by each part of its natural function ... *Functions are not attributed in this context to the whole organism at all, but only to its parts, and the functions of a part are its causal contributions to empirically given goals.*[23]

First, notice that Boorse rejects the idea that the function of man as a whole needs to be determined in order to have a cogent theory of function. Moreover, in contrast to Aristotle, Boorse denies that functional analysis requires determining the overall good of an entity, like the analogy between a good knife and a good human being. This is not surprising given Boorse's rejection of normativism. That is, when defending himself against the normativists, Boorse retreats to a part-function position because he thinks that a whole-function analysis would force him to include what the good of an organism is. Since having to determine what the good of an organism is would put him in the normativist camp, a group with which he does not wish to be associated, he thinks that only a part-function analysis can save him from normativism.

Rather than have to accept the normative aspect of organic functional holism (at least the version proffered by Aristotle), Boorse claims and accepts the view that, with respect to the concept of health, physiologists are only concerned with the functional activities and goals of parts of organisms. This is exactly the position maintained by the part-functionalist,[24] and Boorse makes it clear that he endorses part-functionalism as well. He summarizes his position as follows:

In modern terms, species design is the internal functional organization typical of species members, which (as regards somatic medicine) forms the subject matter of physiology: the interlocking hierarchy of functional processes, at every level from organelle to cell to tissue to organ to gross behavior, by which organisms of a given species maintain and renew their life. The common feature of all conditions called pathological by ordinary medicine seems to be disrupted *part-function at some level of this hierarchy.*[25]

What is to be made of the above passage by Boorse? First, he does acknowledge that there is a hierarchy of functional processes within organisms. Second, it can be inferred from "maintain and renew their life" that survival and reproduction are processes and goals within this hierarchy. This phrase gives the impression that Boorse should be thought of as an organic functional holist, since he does acknowledge higher-level goals within biological systems. The problem, however, is that Boorse goes on to say that pathological states are understood in terms of the disruption of a part-function *within* the hierarchy of biological systems. Nowhere does Boorse suggest that an explanation of a part-function must be understood in terms of its affects on the functions of the system as a whole. This is a reminder that Boorse keeps goals and functions distinct. Even though survival and reproduction

---

[23] Boorse, "On the Distinction Between Disease and Illness," pp. 58–9 [my italics].
[24] Further evidence that Boorse is a part-functionalist will be given toward the end of this chapter, where his account of disease will be discussed.
[25] Boorse, "A Rebuttal on Health," p. 7 [my italics].

are goals of an organism as a whole, they are not functions for Boorse. Thus, his part-functionalist account accepts that parts contribute to the goals of organisms as a whole, but not to the function of organisms as a whole. Thus, it is reasonable to conclude that Boorse is a part-functionalist.[26]

Now that it is clear that Boorse is a part-functionalist, how is his automobile analogy to be understood? Recall that in the beginning of this section, Des Chene's description of mechanism was given. In that quotation, he notes that mechanism "invites us" to accept that complex natural entities can be reduced to simple entities and their qualities. He goes on to say, however, that this invitation is not a requirement. Indeed, he offers the following alternative to mechanism:

> One may simply deny that animals fall within [mechanism's] scope ... [O]ne may compare animals or their organs to machines without adopting a mechanistic philosophy of nature. The machine is useful in comparison because it is familiar, a glass or grid through which to grasp the less familiar. To serve that end, it need not be mechanistically conceived.[27]

Specifically, the answer to the question concerning Boorse's automobile analogy is that he thinks that, in much the same way that it is possible to understand a properly functioning part of an automobile *qua* mechanical device, it is also possible to understand a properly functioning part of an organism. Most importantly, Boorse thinks that if it is possible to determine that a part of a car is working well without trying to figure out how the part affects the function of the car as a whole, then it is also possible to do the same for the parts of an organism. For example, it can be determined whether or not the headlights of a car are performing their function correctly without having to consider the effects on the function of the car as a whole. In general, headlights function properly to the extent that they yield a certain degree of light intensity (within a certain range) to satisfy the designer's goal of improving a driver's ability to drive at night. Analogously, the eyes of a human perform their function properly to the extent that they assist in the production of sight to satisfy the goals of survival and reproduction. In both cases, Boorse would likely claim that the function of the part can be understood without reference to the functions of the systems as a whole (although they do make reference to the goals of the systems). What the machine analogy affords Boorse, as Des Chene suggests generally in the above passage, is the ability to understand complex biological systems in terms of assemblages or aggregates of discrete functional parts. These distinct functional parts (e.g., the eyes) can be understood fully in isolation in terms of their functions and goals—much like the parts (e.g., headlights) of an automobile. Thus, according to Boorse, the machine analogy reveals that health judgments are to be restricted to the parts of a system as opposed to the function of the system as a whole.

In this section, Boorse's use of "mechanical" and "functional" with respect to his concept of health were explained. After distinguishing mechanism from part-functionalism and the latter from organic functional holism, this section made clear that Boorse is best understood as a part-functionalist. Moreover, understanding

---

[26] In Chapter 6, as part of the assessment of his reply to his critics, further justification will be given revealing that Boorse is a part-functionalist.

[27] Des Chene, *Spirits and Clocks: Machine and Organisms in Descartes*, p. 14.

Boorse as a part-functionalist provides a clear understanding of the mechanical analogy represented by P4 of Argument Number 2.

*Understanding Boorse as an Objectivist*

With Boorse's part-functional (non-mechanistic) account of health clarified, it is now possible to turn to his claim that "the classification of human states as healthy or diseased is an *objective* matter, to be read off the biological facts of nature ..." What does Boorse mean when he uses the term "objective"? In the literature, there are at least four senses of "objectivism"—(1) *metaphysical objectivism*, (2) *methodological objectivism*, (3) *disciplinary objectivism*, and (4) *dialectical objectivism*.[28] A brief summary of these different senses of "objectivism" in this section will reveal that Boorse is properly understood (i.e., P5 of Argument Number 2) as both a *metaphysical objectivist* and a *disciplinary objectivist*.

*Metaphysical objectivism* Metaphysical objectivism is the view that there exist phenomena independently (i.e., "in-themselves") of cognizing agents. Another way of stating this is that there is a class of entities (or even a reality itself) that exists irrespective of how anyone thinks, wishes, believes, feels, desires, etc. about it.[29] For example, regardless of whether or not there are cognizing agents to discuss the movement of planets in the universe, it is still the case that, for example, the Earth revolves around the Sun. For an event like the movement of the Earth around the Sun is not at all contingent on the psychology of any observer. Of course, a cognizing agent could be around to report or express some sentiment or judgment about the fact that the Earth rotates around the sun, but any such expression by a cognizing agent is completely distinct from the activities of an entity like the Earth. Metaphysical objectivism can be summarized as follows:

> Metaphysical Objectivism: The doctrine that there come to be and exist phenomena **X** which are not in any way dependent upon the existence of cognizing agents.

With respect to health, metaphysical objectivism is the view that the phenomenon called health comes to be and exists in an organism and/or its parts and does not require the presence of any cognizing agent to affirm its existence.

*Methodological objectivism* Methodological objectivism, is the view that there exists a unique set of standards for representing things "as they really are." Megill succinctly articulates this version of objectivism by stating that "[methodological objectivism] aspires to a knowledge so faithful to reality as to suffer no distortion, and toward which

---

[28] Much of this discussion draws on the works found in Allan Megill (ed.), *Rethinking Objectivity* (Durham, 1994).

[29] Georg W. F. Hegel, in his attempt to explain some of the work of Immanuel Kant, expresses this kind of objectivism as follows: "The thing-in-itself ... expresses the object as it is in abstraction from everything that it is in relation to consciousness, in abstraction from all determinations of feeling and from all determinate thoughts about it." This passage is taken from Ivan Soll's, *An Introduction to Hegel's Metaphysics* (Chicago, 1969), p. 77.

all inquirers of good will are destined to converge."[30] Megill's use of "good will" refers to the allegiance of inquirers to a set of standards usually related to methodological naturalism, which is the view that phenomena are measured in a specific set of ways (e.g., statistical methods) in order that their nature can be properly understood. So, methodological objectivism is the view that methodological naturalism is the correct way to go about understanding the underlying nature of all phenomena. On this interpretation of objectivism, each person should have the same criteria in order to discern the nature of any phenomena, and that as a result of these shared criteria there will be a convergence toward the truth about the phenomena under investigation. For example, so long as inquirers (e.g., nephrologists) are using the same criteria, they will be able to determine a healthy kidney from one that is diseased. Such a determination will reveal the underlying nature of the kidney under observation—that is, the state of the kidney in itself. The formal version of methodological objectivism is as follows:

> Methodological Objectivism: The doctrine that for any phenomenon **X** there exists a unique set of criteria **C** that can be utilized by any capable person **P** to understand the underlying nature of **X**. As an account of health, those individuals who embrace methodological objectivism would claim that a specific set of criteria must be employed by any able person to understand health. For example, assume that the following methodology is the correct way of determining the health status of a patient:
>
> - First decide which organ or body system is likely to be affected by disease.
> - From the signs and symptoms, decide which general category of disease (inflammation, tumor, etc.) is likely to be present.
> - Then, using other factors (age, gender, previous medical history, etc.), compute a diagnosis or small number of possibilities for investigation.
> - Investigation should be performed only if the outcome of each one can be expected to resolve the diagnosis, or influence management if the diagnosis is already known.[31]

According to methodological objectivism, the employment of the above criteria will reveal the true underlying nature of what it means to be a healthy organism—a revelation upon which all interested parties will converge.

*Disciplinary objectivism* The next sense of "objectivism" is disciplinary objectivism. According to Megill, disciplinary objectivism "emphasizes not universal criteria of validity but particular, yet still authoritative, disciplinary criteria. It emphasizes not the eventual convergence of all inquirers of good will but the proximate convergence of accredited inquirers within a given field."[32] The point is that investigators of a given field of inquiry will determine what constitutes an objective claim about certain phenomena. For example, what it means to give an objective account of

---

[30] Megill, "Four Senses of Objectivity," p. 2. Note that Megill uses the label "absolute objectivism" for what I am calling "methodological objectivism."

[31] These are taken from *General and Systematic Pathology*, 2nd edn, ed. J. C. E. Underwood (New York, 1996), p. 10.

[32] Megill, "Four Senses of Objectivity," p. 5.

life and death in physics may be understood in terms of contending with disorder (i.e., entropy). For example, Erwin Schrödinger explains life and death through the concept of entropy. He says:

> Everything that is going on in nature means an increase in entropy of the part of the world where it is going on. Thus a living organism continually increases its entropy—or, as you may say, produces positive entropy—and thus tends to approach the dangerous state of maximum entropy, which is death. It can only keep aloof of it, i.e. alive, by continually drawing from its environment negative entropy ... What an organism feeds upon is negative entropy. Or to put it less paradoxically, the essential thing in metabolism is that the organism succeeds in freeing itself from all the entropy it cannot help producing while alive.[33]

In the field of psychology, however, energy conservation and dissipation may not be included at all in an understanding of life. Rather, the crucial element for determining whether or not an entity is alive in the field of psychology might be whether or not an organism can react to stimuli in a certain way (e.g., behavioral, cognitive, and/or emotional responses).[34] It may be the case that there is "proximate convergence" as to what life means between these two disciplines, but such convergence is not necessary. Nonetheless, both the psychologist and the physicist will be thought of by their peers as offering an objective account of life so long as they adhere to the methodology within their respective fields. This version of objectivism can be expressed in this manner:

> Disciplinary Objectivism: The doctrine that there exists criteria **C** within a given discipline **D** that can be utilized by an accredited person **A** of **D** to understand certain phenomena **X** with the result that **A** will arrive at a "true" understanding of **X** to the extent that **A** has been demonstrated that his analysis is in accord with **C**.

With respect to the concept of health, those who espouse disciplinary objectivism would claim that an objective account of health is possible within a particular field of inquiry. For example, psychology, biology, sociology, etc. could each have its own objective account of health to the extent that the representatives of each of these fields (and sub-fields) offer an account of health that is in line with the tenets of their respective discipline. The result, thinks the disciplinary objectivist, is that there could be a proximate convergence toward a similar account of health as each field independently endeavors to understand what health is. Tristram Engelhardt comes close to capturing what it means to be a disciplinary objectivist. He says the following:

---

[33] Erwin Schrödinger, *What is Life? The Physical Aspect of the Living Cell* (Cambridge, 1944), pp. 71–2.

[34] This is not to suggest that there is a unified understanding of life in psychology. The literature, in fact, seems to suggest the contrary. The point is to offer a plausible contrast between the disciplines of psychology and physics. For a brief account of the history of the field of psychology, see Jaak Panksepp, *Affective Neuroscience* (New York, 1998), pp. 1–23.

The multiple factors in such well-established diseases as coronary artery disease suggest that the disease could be *alternatively construed* as genetic, infectious, metabolic, psychological and social, depending on whether one was a geneticist, an internist, a surgeon, a psychiatrist, or a public health official. The construal would depend upon the particular scientist's appraisal of which etiological variables were most amenable to manipulations. For example, the public health official may decide that the basic variables in coronary artery disease are elements of a lifestyle which includes little exercise, overeating and cigarette smoking. He may then address these social variables and consider such diseases to be ... ways of life.[35]

Given that health is, for Engelhardt, a movement away from disease, he clearly thinks that disease and health can be interpreted differently by different specialists in different fields. Moreover, it is reasonable to infer that Engelhardt's use of "particular scientist" means "particular scientist of a specific sub-discipline within the broader scientific community." Interpretations, then, are "true construals" for Engelhardt to the extent that they are in accord with the established criteria of the discipline from which a specialist makes health judgments, analyzes a particular disease, and investigates the particulars associated with a disease's causal history. Therefore, given his claims in the above passage, it is reasonable to consider Engelhardt as an example of a disciplinary objectivist.

*Dialectical objectivism*  The last version of objectivism is known as dialectical objectivism. Some scholars have argued that the previous senses of "objectivism" give little or no scope for the knowing subject. These scholars claim that metaphysical objectivism excludes the knowing subject altogether. Methodological and disciplinary objectivism greatly constrain the knowing subject as a sort of "passive observer." For example, Megill articulates this concern of the receptive or inactive observing subject in his account of dialectical objectivism as follows: "[D]ialectical objectivity involves a positive attitude toward the subject. The defining feature of dialectical objectivity is the claim that subjectivity is indispensable to the constituting objects. Associated with this feature is a preference for 'doing' over 'viewing.'"[36] Megill goes on to argue that Nietzsche

> contended that unless the historian already has within himself something of what a particular moment of the past offers, he will fail to see what is being given him. In other words, subjectivity is needed for objectivity; or as Nietzsche put it, "objectivity is required, but as a positive quality."[37]

Dialectical objectivism is not easy to understand. If Megill's interpretation is correct, then what does Nietzsche mean by "something of what a particular moment of the past has to offer?" The core idea appears to be that a scrutinizing subject must

---

[35] H. T. Engelhardt, "The Concepts of Health and Disease," in H. T. Engelhardt and S. F. Spicker (eds), *Evaluation and Explanation in the Biomedical Sciences: proceedings of the First Trans-Disciplinary Symposium on Philosophy and Medicine Held at Galveston* (Dordrecht, 1975), p. 133 [my italics].
[36] Megill, "Four Senses of Objectivity," p. 8.
[37] Ibid.

have some understanding of or possess a certain historical (or some other) sensitivity to the phenomenon under investigation in order to provide an authoritative account of the phenomenon. Yet, this subjective requirement appears to be quite inconsistent with the idea that an objective account of **X** is an explanation of representing **X** as it really is. For surely if sensitivity to a particular subject matter includes an observer's idiosyncrasies or biases, then such a sensitivity distorts rather than enhances an understanding of a given subject matter. In reply to this concern of including subjectivity within the concept of objectivity, Megill offers the following:

> At first glance, dialectical objectivity seems antithetical to [methodological] objectivity. But consider Kant, whose *Critique of Pure Reason* offered an account of the understanding, through its imposition of the categories of understanding (unity, plurality, totality, causality, and the like) on the confused manifold of subjective impressions, confers objectivity on those impressions. The account can be taken in two ways. Insofar as one stresses the *universality* of the categories—their sharedness by all rational beings—one will see Kant as a theorist of [methodological] objectivity, an objectivity stripped of everything personal and idiosyncratic. But insofar as one stresses the *active character* of the knowing subject, Kant appears as, despite himself, a theorist of dialectical objectivity. Thus, there is a strange and telling symbiosis between [methodological] objectivity and dialectical objectivity. Indeed, one might even see [methodological] objectivity as a special case of dialectical objectivity, requiring the construction of a particular sort of knowing subject.[38]

The account of dialectical objectivism that Megill has offered above allows for two general interpretations. The first interpretation can be called Nietzschean dialectical objectivism. This is the view that the only way that observers can "actively" make sense of a given phenomenon is that they must bring a certain knowledge or particular kind of sensitivity with respect to the phenomenon under investigation. The second interpretation, call it Kantian dialectical objectivism, is the idea that an objective account of a particular phenomenon requires that all observers possess the same cognitive or rational structures (not personal or idiosyncratic elements of observers) that allow for an "active" understanding of the phenomenon under investigation.[39] Keeping these two senses of "dialectical objectivism" in mind, it is possible to summarize it as follows:

> Dialectical Objectivism: The doctrine that there come to be and exist phenomena **X** that can be understood through either the prior knowledge (or certain sort of sensitivity) of an "active" observer or through the same "active" non-idiosyncratic cognitive structures that all observers share.

With respect to the concept of health, a Nietzschean-type dialectical objectivist would claim that an objective account of health is possible to the extent that the formation of such a concept is the result of the relevant knowledge or particular sensitivity related to the relevant aspects of organisms. Alternatively, a Kantian-type

---

[38] Ibid., p. 10.
[39] It is not clear why Megill thinks that methodological objectivism (what he calls absolute objectivism) is a special case of dialectical objectivism. The former is the view that cognizing agents can access things-in-themselves, but the latter rejects such access.

dialectical objectivist would claim that the concept of health is objective to the extent that the relevant cognitive structures are presently active in knowing subjects when they determine the health of organisms. For example, Robert Aronowitz defends what could be viewed as a Nietzschean-type version of dialectical objectivism. He says:

> Relying on ontological criteria to categorically distinguish psychosomatic diseases from organic diseases results from an overly narrow view of the relationship between culture and disease ... I juxtaposed the different case studies in part to show how changes and choices in the naming and classification of diseases have interacted with changing cultural norms about disease responsibility.[40]

Aronowitz is arguing that an attempt to distinguish physical diseases from psychophysical diseases reflects a lack of sensitivity to the role of culture with respect to disease attribution. Much as Nietzsche thought that an historian must possess a certain "something" inside of himself in order to understand a particular phenomenon at a given time in history, Aronowitz is claiming that, for example, an epidemiologist must have a certain cultural acumen in order to understand a particular disease at a particular time period within a particular culture.

*The four senses of "objectivism" and Boorse's concept of health* To the extent that Boorse is an objectivist, which of the four senses of "objectivism" best captures his use of the term? An answer to this question is connected to Boorse's concept of function. Recall that Boorse thinks that only a contextualist concept of function is possible. His justification is as follows:

> [B]iologists see teleology on so many different time scales and levels of organization. At one level, individual organisms are goal-directed systems whose behavior contributes to various goals. By eating insects, say, a bird contributes to its own survival and also (a fortiori) to the survival of the species, but further to the survival of its genes, the equilibrium of the insect population, and so on ... At the level of population or species, new goal-directed processes seem to appear—for example, the maintenance of protective coloration—and one can ascend still higher by viewing a whole ecosystem as a teleological unit ... Given this latitude for choice, what has happened is that various subfields of biology have carved out various slices of the teleological pie and interpreted their function statements accordingly.[41]

First, the above quotation reveals that Boorse is understood as a disciplinary objectivist. His contextualist concept of function, which is an integral part of his concept of health, is a major part of the justification for putting him in this group of objectivists. Remember that disciplinary objectivism is the view that a thorough understanding of a particular phenomenon is based on criteria employed by an inquirer within a given discipline. So long as experts within a given discipline use the relevant criteria when understanding a given phenomenon, such an account is considered objective *qua* authoritative. Since Boorse thinks that the relevant sub-

---

[40] Robert A. Aronowitz, *Making Sense of Illness: Science, Society, and Disease* (Cambridge, 1998), pp. 176 and 177.
[41] Christopher Boorse, "Wright on Functions," *Philosophical Review*, 85/1 (1976): 83–4.

fields of biology determine goals and functions and that each relevant sub-discipline has a legitimate and authoritative claim to what it considers to be proper functions and goals of organisms and their parts, he is legitimately understood as a disciplinary objectivist.

Second, it is also clear that Boorse is not a methodological objectivist, because he does not think that there is a single procedure from which all trained observers will arrive at the same account. According to Boorse, a geneticist may arrive at quite a different account of health than an ecologist, because they are concerned with different levels of analysis. These different concerns do result in focusing on different functions and goals. For example, on the one hand, a geneticist might argue that the function of *genes* is to ensure their survival in future generations. On the other hand, an ecologist could argue that the function of *organisms* is to ensure a well-balanced ecosystem. If function plays a crucial role in the concepts of health put forth by the geneticist or the ecologist, then these different accounts of function and goal-directedness will result in different concepts of health. Thus, it is clear that Boorse should not be understood as a methodological objectivist.

Third, it is reasonable to think that Boorse is a metaphysical objectivist. When Boorse claims that biologists are able to determine both health and disease states of an organism by "reading off the biological facts of nature," he appears to accept that there exist mind-independent biological phenomena which can be observed. In other words, it is possible to examine biological phenomena out in the world, but such phenomena are not in any way dependent upon observation for their existence. If this interpretation is correct, then it follows that Boorse thinks there come to be and exist phenomena that are not in any way dependent upon the existence of cognizing agents. Thus, Boorse can be considered a metaphysical objectivist.

If it is correct that Boorse is a metaphysical objectivist and a disciplinary objectivist, then it is not entirely clear what sort (if any) of dialectical objectivist he would be. He could be a Kantian-type dialectical objectivist, who takes seriously mind-independent entities and rejects that observers can form concepts that actually make sense of the nature of such entities. For the Kantian-type dialectical objectivist thinks that the application of conceptual/cognitive structures in the representation of things prohibits cognizing agents from actual access to those things. Now, it is true that Boorse does think that different disciplines have authoritative concepts of health that may not coincide. It could be argued that this lack of agreement has its origin in an inability of observers to understand mind-independent entities as they really are. It is this limitation, one could argue, of cognizing agents that accounts for Boorse's contextualist concept of function/health. The difficulty with this interpretation, however, is that Boorse does not hint anywhere in his works that his contextualist analysis is grounded in an allegiance to a Kantian sort of objectivism. Moreover, he does claim that health and disease states of organisms can be determined by "reading off the biological facts of nature." This suggests that observers can form concepts that make sense of the nature of mind independent entities. So, given the dearth of textual evidence and this explicit statement about health and disease states, it is sensible not to consider Boorse a Kantian-type dialectical objectivist.

Maybe, however, Boorse can be interpreted as a Nietzschean-type dialectical objectivist. On such an interpretation, Boorse would have to think that the medical physiologist must have "something" in him (like Nietzsche's sagacious historian) prior to inquiring into the physiology of biological entities. The question is what is this "something" of which the physiologist must be in possession? It is not entirely clear how to answer this question. Definitely, in contrast to Aronowitz, Boorse does not think that the answer is related to a rich understanding of culture because of all the cultural values that would have to be included in such an account. As it was made clear in Chapter 3, Boorse rejects health as a value-laden concept. Thus, if the particular sensitivity required to be a Nietzschean-type dialectical objectivist is a cultural one, then Boorse is surely not this sort of objectivist.

It could be argued that Boorse thinks that the medical physiologists should have a prior appropriate understanding of the concepts of goal-directedness and functionalism and the tool of statistical analysis. It is the incorporation of these concepts and tool into the medical physiologist's understanding of the activities of the parts of organisms that captures Boorse's active observer as a Nietzschean dialectical objectivist. When medical physiologists inquire into the activities of the parts of organisms, they will do so with these prior concepts in mind. The result is that medical physiologists bring a certain degree of subjectivity to an objective understanding. Thus, it could be argued that Boorse is a Nietzschean dialectical objectivist.

The above possibility, however, is already part of the conceptual training most medical physiologists possess. That is, if goal-directedness, functionalism, and/or statistical analysis are the necessary concepts and tools that physiologists must possess prior to understanding correctly the activities of organisms and their parts, then it is not clear how the Nietzschean version of dialectical objectivism is distinct from the disciplinary rendition. For the disciplinary version of objectivism requires that practitioners from various fields have a certain set of concepts and tools in order to inquire into the phenomena relevant to each field. It is with these concepts that practitioners *actively* engage in their inquiries. In the parlance of Megill, Boorse's medical physiologist *qua* subject plays an active role in providing an objective account of health so long as the account includes a prior understanding of the relevant concepts of function, goal-directedness, and the tool of statistical analysis. The consequence is that Boorse could be viewed as a Nietzschean-type dialectical objectivist to the extent that the certain "something" that medical physiologists should have is a thorough understanding of the concepts of function and goal-directedness and a working knowledge of statistical analysis.[42]

Still, the constraints put on disciplinary objectivists, as a result of their adherence to a methodology embraced by their peers, are the sorts of constraints that Nietzschean-type dialectical objectivists would resist. This certain "something" that needs to be present in Nietzschean objectivists is an element that is somewhat unique to them. It is this somewhat unique "something" that captures the subjective element of objectivity. Yet, it is just this sort of unique quality that is not present in disciplinary objectivists, who embraces a methodology endemic to their discipline. The upshot, of course, is that Boorse's concept of health does not include (in any

---

[42] The positive account offered in Chapter 7 will argue that the "something" is a Darwinian perspective.

clear sense) either version of dialectical objectivism. Rather, this is only to say that Boorse is both a metaphysical objectivist and a disciplinary objectivist.

In summary, the preceding sections provided two argument reconstructions to assist in making sense of Boorse's concept of health. These sections also explained Boorse's sense of "mechanical" and "objective." The conclusions to be drawn from this analysis are two-fold. First, Boorse is properly understood as a part-functionalist as opposed to a mechanist or an organic functional holist with respect to his automobile analogy. Second, this section made clear that Boorse is both a metaphysical objectivist and a disciplinary objectivist. Thus far, then, P4 and P5 of Argument Number 2 have been explained. It is now possible to turn to the remaining details of Boorse's concept of health in order to make sense of the rest of Argument Number 1 and Argument Number 2.

*Boorse's Concept of Health: The Final Details*

Boorse labels his naturalistic concept of health as "theoretical,"[43] "biostatistical,"[44] and "functional,"[45] suggesting that these labels are synonymous. Moreover, in Chapter 2, it was made clear that Boorse acknowledges that, although statistical normality is neither a necessary nor a sufficient condition for health, it plays an important role in his concept of health. Thus, in his attempt to include both statistics and function within his concept of health, Boorse offers the following four-part assessment of what health is:

1. The *reference class* is a natural class of organisms of uniform functional design; specifically, an age group of a sex of a species.
2. A *normal function* of a part or process within members of the reference class is a statistically typical contribution by it to their individual survival and reproduction.
3. A *disease* is a type of internal state which is either an impairment of normal functional ability, i.e., a reduction of one or more functional abilities below typical efficiency, or a limitation on functional ability caused by environmental agents.
4. *Health* is the absence of disease.[46]

*The Reference Class* A brief explanation of each of the above statements is in order. First, Boorse is clear that "reference class" refers to an ideal statistical species-type,

---

[43] "Theoretical" is found in Christopher Boorse, "A Rebuttal on Health," and "Health as a Theoretical Concept," *Philosophy of Science*, 44/4 (1977): 542–73.

[44] "Biostatistical" is found in Christopher Boorse, "Concepts of Health," in Donald Van DeVeer and Tom Regan (eds), *Health Care Ethics: An Introduction* (Philadelphia, 1987), pp. 359–93 and "A Rebuttal on Health."

[45] "Functional" is found in all four of the above citations and Boorse's "What a Theory of Mental Health Should Be," *Journal of the Theory of Social Behavior*, 6/1 (1976): 61–84.

[46] Boorse, "A Rebuttal on Health," pp. 7–8. A slightly different version of these same four points can be found in Boorse, "Health as a Theoretical Concept," p. 562 and p. 567. Note

which does not refer to any token of a species-type. This claim helps to make sense of "ideal" in P1, P3, and P4 of Argument Number 2. Boorse explains as follows:

> In general, function statements describe species or population characteristics, not any individual plant or animal ... As a result, the subject matter of comparative physiology is a series of ideal types of organisms: the frog, the hydra, the earthworm, the starfish, the crocodile, the shark, the rhesus monkey, and so on. The idealization is of course statistical, not moral or esthetic or normative in any way. For each textbook provides a composite portrait of what I will call the *species design*, i.e. the typical hierarchy of interlocking functional systems that supports the life of organisms of that type. Each detail of the composite portrait is statistically normal within the species, though the portrait may not exactly resemble any species member ... [T]he field naturalist abstracts from individual differences and from disease by averaging over a sufficiently large sample of the population. The species design that emerges is an empirical ideal which, I suggest, serves as the basis for health judgments in species where we make such judgments.[47]

There are a number of comments that can be made about the above passage. First, the above passage makes clear that it is the statistical sense of "ideal" that Boorse takes seriously. In particular, Boorse brings together "statistical" and "ideal" by claiming that the health judgments of the field naturalist refer to a portrait of ideal functioning of the parts of organisms. This portrait is constructed by the examination of many parts of tokens of a given type of species. The result is a statistical average of what constitutes the normal functioning of, for example, the human thyroid.

The second point to note is that, according to Boorse, the normal functioning of a part, like the human thyroid, does not represent any particular human thyroid. Rather, Boorse endorses the context of the health judgments offered by the field naturalist or comparative physiologist/pathologist. For example, the statistically ideal-functioning thyroid is a composite or portrait that is constructed through the observation of many human functioning thyroids. From such empirical observations, the range of a pathological, normal, or positive functioning thyroid is determined by the comparative physiologist/field naturalist. (Here, again, Boorse's contextualist concept of function is evident.) Figure 5.1, which is taken from Boorse's account, makes clear his functional-biostatistical concept of health.

Starting with the pathological side of the distribution curve above, Boorse defines a *pathological* condition as follows:

> A condition of a part or process in an organism is pathological when the ability of the part or process to perform one or more of its species-typical biological functions falls below some central range of the statistical distribution for that ability in corresponding parts or processes in members of an appropriate reference class of the species.[48]

---

that many scholars have criticized Boorse's understanding of these technical terms. Some of these criticisms will be evaluated in the next chapter.

[47] Boorse, "Health as a Theoretical Concept," p. 557.
[48] Boorse, "Concepts of Health," p. 370.

```
Efficiency of        |  Pathological      ╱‾╲        Positive
part-function        |                   ╱   ╲       health?
                     |                  ╱ Normal╲
                     |_____▓▓_____¦_____
                     |            Statistical distribution
                     |            in reference class
```

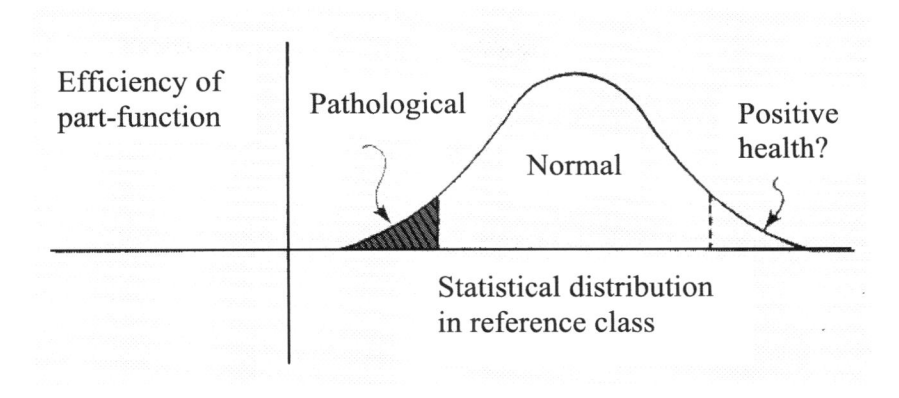

Figure 5.1    Efficiency of the Functioning of the Thyroid[49]

Using the human thyroid will help to explain Boorse's statistical distribution figure above. The thyroid, which is situated in the neck, is a gland that secretes thyroxin. The secretion of this fluid helps to control the body's metabolic processes. The metabolic processes are either sped up or slowed down, according to the amount of thyroxin in the bloodstream. As is clear in the above figure, the inefficient production of thyroxin results in a pathological state of the thyroid. Next, the production at a certain range of efficiency above the pathological level is considered a statistically normal—that is healthy—state of the thyroid.

Moreover, Boorse leaves open the possibility that parts of organisms could perform their function more efficiently than the normal range. Such high-level efficiency would be considered a positive health state. For example, ideal vision in humans is thought to be "20/20," but it is also possible that vision could be better than this norm. Note, however, that Boorse has a question mark in the positive health part of the distribution curve provided above. The reason for this question mark is that Boorse wishes to make clear that his biological sense of function is about efficiency and maximal efficiency as opposed to an excess of function. For example, Boorse would claim that an efficient thyroid is one that produces thyroxin in a normal fashion, and a positive state of the thyroid is when the thyroid produces thyroxin as efficiently as it possibly can. Boorse states his case using the production of acid in the stomach. He says:

> The function of the oxyntic cells of the stomach wall is to secrete acid to aid digestion. But excess stomach acid is ultimately even more dysfunctional than deficiency. The right-hand tail of a function's distribution is maximal physiological efficiency—not maximal quantities of stomach acid or insulin or leukocytes, any of which are, on the contrary, pathological.[50]

---

[49] Note that the figure is taken from Boorse, "A Rebuttal on Health," p. 8, but Boorse does not provide any specific example. The human thyroid is being used to illustrate Boorse's statistical figure.

[50] Ibid.

It is clear that Boorse's sense of "function" includes *how well* an organism or its part(s) progresses and achieves its goal(s). This claim helps make sense of Boorse's use of "efficiency" in P1, P4 and P5 of Argument Number 2. The better a part can bring about its goal than it currently does, the more efficient it can become than it currently is. According to Boorse, "positive health" refers not to the quantity produced by an organism's part(s), but to maximal functional efficiency of the bringing about of particular goal(s) by the part(s). Thus, each of these different states—pathological, normal, and positive—is determined by statistical inferences drawn from the empirical investigations of many of the same parts (e.g., eyes or thyroids) within the same reference class.

Third, Boorse qualifies his account of reference class to focus not only on statistically ideal types, but also to include both age and sex as part of statistically ideal types. As Boorse states:

> [T]he reference class for normality is only a fraction of a species, because medical normality is relative to sex and age (and possibly race). For example, normal males must have prostate glands though most humans (females) do not; normal babies cannot walk even though most humans can. The best reference class for explaining medical judgments of normality may be an age group of a sex of a species.[51]

The thyroid example captures Boorse's age/sex qualification quite nicely. For example, in prenatal development and early development (around six months), the failure of the thyroid gland to produce enough thyroxin results in both poor physical and psychological growth. This deficiency in thyroxin is a condition called *cretinism* and occurs in all degrees of severity. Young children suffering from cretinism are dwarfed and intellectually slow, with thick harsh skin, scanty hair, and large bellies.

In adults, however, a deficiency in the production of thyroxin brings about similar conditions in males and females, but at different age ranges. In general, the thyroid enlarges, the eyes begin to "bulge out," the person becomes nervous and irritable, large appetites with a decrease in weight, attacks of diarrhea, sudden fits of fright, shock, and grief, the skin becomes more brown than usual, and in severe cases depression sets in.[52] All of these symptoms (known as exophthalmic goiter or Graves' disease) occur in women between the ages of 15–30 years old and in men between 30–45 years old. Moreover, usually in only older women, there is also substantial increase in weight, harsh skin, and a loss in hair.[53]

Graves' disease illustrates the point of Boorse's qualification concerning age and sex. A poor production of thyroxin must be assessed differently based on age and sex. In adult males between certain ages, a certain production of thyroxin is normal, but the same production of thyroxin in adult females between certain ages is abnormal.

---

[51] Ibid., pp. 370–71.

[52] Some of these symptoms are discussed in Peter Kopp, "Thyroid Diseases," in Marlene B. Goldman and Maureen C. Hatch, eds, *Women and Health* (San Diego: Academic Press, 2000), pp. 655–73.

[53] Recent research suggests that even paralysis is possible in the case of "hyperthyroidism." See David E. Kelley *et al.*, "Thyrotoxic Periodic Paralysis," *Archives of Internal Medicine*, 149/11 (1989): 2597–600.

The point, according to Boorse, is that not only is the reference class focused on an ideal type of species of "uniform functional design," but also it is further specified in terms of age and sex. Thus, health judgments made by comparative physiologists/field naturalists are the product of statistical inferences that refer to an ideal composite of a species. Such an ideal composite is "restricted by sex and age because of differences in normal physiology between males and females, young and old."[54]

To recapitulate, this section made clear Boorse's use of "reference class," "efficiency," and "ideal type." Specifically, Boorse's explanation of "reference class" captures his qualification of P1–P3 of Argument Number 1 and P1–P3 of Argument Number 2 to include age, sex, and possibly race. Furthermore, Boorse's explication of "efficiency" elucidates P1, P3, and P5 of Argument Number 2. Finally, Boorse's account of "ideal type" helps clarify P1, P3, and P4 of Argument Number 2.

*Normal function* Three parts of Boorse's account of function need to be made clear. First, recall from the previous chapter that Boorse defends a contextualist concept of function. Basically, Boorse argues that a function is a causal contribution to a goal. Moreover, he claims that parts of an organism are goal-directed if and only if the parts are disposed to modify their behavior in the wake of environmental variation to achieve their goals. Finally, Boorse submitted that the parts of organisms contribute to many sorts of goals at the same time (e.g., individual survival, group survival, gene survival, etc.). This fact led Boorse to conclude that many of the sub-disciplines within biology would focus on different sorts of goals. The upshot of this determination, according to Boorse, is that function statements are context-dependent within biology. In the case of medicine, Boorse offers the following justification for choosing physiology as the relevant context/sub-field within biology for health judgments:

[S]ince physiology [is] the sub-field on which somatic medicine relies, medical functional normality [is] presumably relative to the goals physiologists *seem* to assume, viz, individual survival and reproduction.[55]

Thus, it is clear from the above passage that, according to Boorse, physiology *seems* to be the appropriate context/sub-field within biology that is foundational to somatic medicine. It is the goals that physiologists acknowledge—namely, individual survival and reproduction—that *seem* to comprise the meaning of the goal-directed aspect of function statements in somatic medicine.

Second, thus far in the analysis, Boorse's concept of function has been labeled "contextualist." There is one aspect of his contextualist concept of function (noted on the previous page) that needs to be explained. Specifically, Boorse substitutes "disposed" for "being performed." He makes just this modification when he says: "An organism or its part is directed to a goal **G** when *disposed*, throughout a range

---

[54] Boorse, "A Rebuttal on Health," p. 8.
[55] Ibid., p. 9. Note that I have substituted "is" for "was" because Boorse is describing his own view in the past tense. I have changed it to the present tense for smoothness [my italics].

of environmental variation, to modify its behavior in the way required for **G**."[56] So, "being performed" now reads "being disposed to perform." This adjustment by Boorse still makes it the case that he is a contextualist. The difference is that field biologists/medical physiologists, according to Boorse, are concerned about dispositions in their understanding of function. Thus, Boorse also includes a *dispositional* aspect to his contextualist concept of function.

The basic idea of Boorse's sense of "dispositional" is captured in Robert Cummins's dispositional account of function. Cummins says the following:

> [I]f something functions as a pump in a system $s$, or if the function of something in a system $s$ is to pump, then it must be capable of pumping in $s$. Thus function-ascribing statements imply disposition statements; to attribute a function to something is, in part, to attribute a disposition to it. If the function of $x$ in $s$ is to $f$, then $x$ has a disposition to $f$ in $s$.[57]

For example, human lungs have a function because they perform a particular activity within the respiratory system. As long as environmental forces within a certain range of intensity do not destroy the actual activities of the lungs, the dispositional trait of the lungs remains. To illustrate further, the function of the lungs is to eliminate carbon dioxide (produced by cells) from the body and exchange it for oxygen because that is what the lungs do. According to the dispositional view, the actual activity of assisting in gas exchange includes a corresponding disposition to assist in gas exchange. What this means is that lungs are disposed to exchange carbon dioxide with oxygen. So long as the lungs actually assist in the performance of these relevant gas exchanges, they have a disposition *qua* function to perform such activities. If, however, a token set of lungs is filled with excess water or smoke, then gas exchange becomes greatly limited or impossible. Also, if acute asthma, emphysema, or bronchitis is present, then the flow of air is considerably reduced. The result is that respiratory muscles must work much harder than they usually do, making gas exchange greatly limited or impossible. In such extreme cases, the disposition to bring about gas exchange in lungs is destroyed as a result of the inability of the lungs actually to engage in the activity of gas exchange. A dispositional concept of function can be summarized as follows:

> Dispositional Concept of Function: **X** is a function in a system **S** only if **X** is disposed to do **Y** in **S**. **X** is disposed to do **Y** in **S** if and only if **X** actually does **Y** in **S** when the conditions within **S** make it the case that **X** can actually do **Y**.

Again, Boorse's contextualist concept of health includes this dispositional element noted above. Indeed, Boorse is clear that normal function ability is "defined *dispositionally*, as the readiness of *an internal part* to perform all its normal functions on typical occasions with at least typical efficiency."[58] So, for Boorse,

---

[56] Boorse, "A Rebuttal on Health," p. 9.

[57] Robert Cummins, "Functional Analysis," in Elliott Sober (ed.), *Conceptual Issues in Evolutionary Biology*, 2nd. edn (Cambridge, 1994), p. 61. This essay was originally published in *Journal of Philosophy*, 72 (1975): 741–64.

[58] Boorse, "A Rebuttal on Health," p. 8 [my italics].

a part of an organism is healthy to the extent that the part is disposed to perform its function. This function *qua* disposition is determined by the actual activities of the part that is being studied. Thus, according to Boorse, the medical physiologist embraces this dispositional-part-function concept of function in his study of the parts of organisms.

Third, Boorse suggests that "normal function" is understood in terms of statistical inferences drawn by physiologists in their empirical investigations of the activities of parts and processes. For example, there is a certain way that thyroxin is produced by the thyroid that constitutes the normal functioning of the thyroid. This normal way of producing thyroxin (as well as the pathological or positive) is determined by the physiologist through his study of many thyroids within a particular age/sex group of a specific reference class. Importantly, Boorse makes the following qualification:

> [T]he lower limit of normal functional ability—the line between normal and pathological—is arbitrary. Although statisticians often use of 95 percent central range, no reason for such a choice applies here. The concept of a pathological state has vague boundaries—though the vast majority of disease processes involve functional deficits by any reasonable standard.[59]

Boorse is quite clear in the above passage that determining where pathology ends and normal begins is arbitrary. Boorse is making two points here, a minor point and a major point. First, as it was made clear in Chapter 2, statistical normality is understood to be that range within 2.5 percent on either side of a distribution curve. In that discussion, it was made clear with the albumin example (the liver-synthesized protein that regulates blood pressure) that such a distribution does not always capture what is normal. Boorse's minor point is that the traditional 95 percent range may be quite irrelevant in cases like albumin production. Thus, Boorse thinks that the 95 percent range is not always a relevant standard.

More importantly, Boorse is suggesting that there is enough variation within populations such that it is not possible to determine precisely where pathological states of entities end and normal states of entities begin. The dividing line between pathological and normal, claims Boorse, is simply sort of a *reasonable* guess on the part of the physiologist. Still, Boorse is quick to note that such ambiguity is not present in most cases. It is only at "the border" between pathology and normal where this uncertainty is present. Thus, Boorse concedes that there is a degree of imprecision in determining whether or not a certain level of functional efficiency (at "the border" between pathology and normal) of an organism's part(s) is in either a normal or pathological state.

To summarize, this section made clear Boorse's account of function that was developed in Chapter 4. It is now clear that Boorse argues for a dispositional concept of function. Moreover, Boorse explains his use of "normal functional ability" in terms of statistical normality, conceding that there is a degree of arbitrariness in determining where pathology ends and health begins. Finally, these aspects of Boorse's concept of natural function help to make sense of P2 and P3 of Argument Number 1 and P1–P5 of Argument Number 2.

---

[59] Boorse, "Concepts of Health," p. 371.

*Disease* Since it is the case that Boorse thinks that health is the absence of disease, a brief account of how he understands "disease" is in order. Moreover, Boorse's way of handling the concept of disease will help make sense of the argument reconstructions provided at the beginning of this chapter. To begin, there is a broad sense of "disease" and a narrow sense of "disease" which Boorse discusses.[60] In the broad sense, disease classification ranges over defects (e.g., cleft palate), disorders, abnormalities, injuries, lesions, illnesses, and handicaps.[61] In the narrow sense, disease classification excludes many of the above conditions as diseases, although there is no agreed upon account of what the narrow sense of "disease" is.[62] In response to this vexing problem, Boorse offers the following resolution:

> [We can abstract from all problems of disease classification and definition by using a more general term; pathological. All the conditions in the [AMA's Standard Nomenclature of Diseases and Operation] are correctly described as pathological, or medically abnormal, however classified or subdivided. I suggest that the distinction between normal and pathological conditions is the basic theoretical concept of Western medicine. A bodily state or process is disease, disorder, injury, lesion, defect, sickness, or illness only if it is abnormal in the sense of pathological; in other words, these are all specific kinds of pathological conditions.[63]

As it is clear from the above account, Boorse thinks that disease in the broad sense can be fundamentally understood through the concept of pathology. Recall that from the discussion on "reference class" above, Boorse thinks that a pathological state is a condition of a part or process in an organism, only if the part or process performs its activities below the species-typical performance of such activities. So, when Boorse claims that health is the absence of disease, what he means is that health is the absence of pathological states. These final words from Boorse provide his considered view on the concept of health as the absence of pathological conditions and the upshot of such a view:

---

[60] Ibid., p. 362.

[61] See the AMA's *Standard Nomenclature of Diseases and Operations*, 4th edn, eds Richard J. Plunkett and Aladine C. Hayden (New York, 1951). Boorse notes the following categories employed by the AMA under what he calls the broad sense of "disease": (1) Diseases due to genetic and prenatal influence (e.g., webbed fingers), (2) Disease or infections due to a lower plant or animal parasite (e.g., malaria), (3) Diseases due to intoxication (e.g., opium poisoning), (4) Diseases due to trauma or physical agent (e.g., bone fractures) (5) Diseases secondary to circulatory disturbance (e.g., gangrene), (6) Diseases secondary to disturbance of innervation or of psychic control (e.g., muscular paralysis), (7) Diseases due to or consisting of static mechanical abnormality (e.g., varicose veins), (8) Diseases due to disorder or metabolism, growth, and nutrition (e.g., scurvy), (9) New growths (e.g., all tumors), (10) Diseases due to unknown or uncertain cause with the structural reaction manifest (e.g., liver cirrhosis) and (10) Diseases due to unknown or uncertain cause with the functional reaction alone manifest (e.g., epilepsy). See Boorse, "Concepts of Health," pp. 362–3.

[62] For more on this point about the difficulties of disease classification, see R. E. Kendell, *The Concept of Disease and Its Implications for Psychiatry* (Edinburgh, 1975) and Lawrie Reznek, *The Nature of Disease* (London, 1987).

[63] Boorse, "Concepts of Health," pp. 364–5.

Local part-dysfunctions need not have any gross effects on disability or deformity or distress. A small skin lesion or intestinal polyp is pathological because it involves local dysfunction or nonfunction of parts (i.e., cells and tissues). But such local pathology often leaves gross abilities or the organism unscathed. Liver cells, to be normal, must perform a host of metabolic functions because that is what liver cells collectively contribute to survival and reproduction. But a large number of liver cells can be pathological without clinically detectable effects or appreciable risk of such effects. Finally, pathology is occasionally desirable just because biological functions are occasionally undesirable. Reproduction, for example, is a quintessential biological function; but there is no reason why everyone should want to reproduce at every opportunity. A woman who has her tubes tied after five children deliberately acquires a pathological condition in the interest of values she prefers to normality.[64]

There are three points to note from the above passage. First, Boorse's attempt to make sense of the concept of disease is accomplished by returning to his concept of function and his concept of statistical normality. As he notes in the above quotation, local dysfunction is understood in terms of pathology, which, in turn, is understood in terms of species-specific statistical normality.[65] Second, upon making clear that the concept of health is understood in terms of the absence of pathological conditions, Boorse reminds the reader that he is only concerned about part-dysfunction. Boorse is underscoring that his contextualist dispositional concept of function is based on his allegiance to part-functionalism. Finally, Boorse offers a gentle reminder that part-dysfunction is a value-free concept, but that one can either value or disvalue a pathological state of a part-function, depending upon one's circumstances and interests. Thus, with respect to the discussion of normativism in Chapter 3, Boorse still considers himself a non-normativist.

In summary, Boorse's concept of disease is understood in terms of the absence of pathological conditions. It follows, according to Boorse, that health is the absence of pathological conditions. This account of disease clarifies Boorse's sense of "disease" in P1, P2 and P4 in Argument Number 1. So, Boorse's concept of health can be summarized as follows:

Boorse's Naturalistic Concept of Health: Health is the absence of pathological conditions of parts of organisms, a condition that is understood as an ideal dispositional-functional state of parts of organisms of a particular species, gender, and age group.

---

[64] Ibid., pp. 371–2.

[65] Given that Boorse rejects the statistical concept of health as a necessary condition (see Chapter 2), it may seem like a contradiction for him to endorse it in his own positive account. This is a reasonable criticism. Minimally, Boorse should explain why he thinks that drawing on statistical considerations is an acceptable part of his concept of health, but is not subject to the necessary and sufficient conditions analysis he uses in his criticisms of the statistical concept of health. Possibly, Boorse could reply that the inclusion of statistical norms is part of his contextualist concept of function that he thinks is part of pathology. That is, statistical normality is included in his concept of health because it is required from the contextualist perspective of understanding the function of parts within biological systems. It is this contextualist perspective, and not meeting necessary and sufficient conditions, that explains why Boorse might think that he is not caught in a contradiction. Clearly, more information from Boorse would be needed to resolve this concern.

## Conclusion

Much has been accomplished in the chapter. The first part of the chapter presented two argument reconstructions of Boorse's concept of health that revealed many technical terms, including "mechanical," "objective," "function," "disease," "reference class," and "normal." Fittingly, the second part of this chapter, upon explaining the subtle differences between mechanism, part-functionalism, and organic functional holism, made clear that Boorse is best described as a part-functionalist. Then, after distinguishing four senses of "objectivism," the next section argued that Boorse is best understood as a combination of a metaphysical objectivist and a disciplinary objectivist. Then, the third part of the chapter elucidated the technical terms of Boorse's concept of health. Briefly, Boorse understands "normal" in an ideal statistical sense, and he makes clear that his contextualist concept of function is properly understood as a dispositional concept of function. Moreover, by "reference class" Boorse means that functional explanations are to be understood in terms of the age, sex, (possibly) race, and class (i.e., species) to which an organism and its parts belong. Finally, Boorse's concept of disease is understood in terms of his concept of pathological. The upshot is that Boorse thinks that the concept of health is a value-free statistical/part-functional/dispositional concept, which is understood in terms of the absence of pathological conditions specific to a particular reference class.

# Chapter 6
# Boorse and His Critics

**Introduction: Boorse's Defense against His Critics**

The previous chapter explained the details of Boorse's naturalistic concept of health. Briefly, Boorse thinks health is an ideal dispositional-functional state of parts of organisms of a particular species, gender, and age group. Importantly, he maintains that this account is value-free and complements the theoretical framework embraced by medical pathologists. Boorse's analysis has come under attack by critics from many different directions. For example, some argue that his account includes faulty reasoning, is not in fact objective and value-free, neglects to consider seriously environment factors of biological systems, and is at odds with the practice of medicine. Boorse, however, thinks that his reply to his critics reveals that his naturalistic concept of health "best explains medical disease judgments and our reactions to them."[1] This chapter will determine the extent to which Boorse is successful in this claim.

This chapter discusses four general categories of criticism against Boorse's naturalistic concept of health.[2] These include the charges of (1) circular reasoning, (2) covert normativism, (3) bad biology, and (4) bad medicine. Each section will begin with a presentation of each criticism, followed immediately by Boorse's rejoinder to each criticism, and then an assessment of Boorse's rejoinder. This will permit a full examination of each criticism. The upshot of this analysis is that there are serious difficulties with Boorse's concept of health. Nonetheless, Chapter 7 will argue that there is a way to salvage important elements of Boorse's account and, at the same time, avoid the pitfalls that render his analysis problematic.

*The Charge of Circularity*

The first criticism launched against Boorse's naturalistic concept of health is that his reasoning is circular or question begging. There are two distinct charges of circularity levied against Boorse. The first focuses on his claim that disease is an *internal state*, and the second emphasizes his use of *normality* in understanding health and disease states.

---

[1] Christopher Boorse, "A Rebuttal on Health," in James M. Humber and Robert F. Almeder (eds), *What is Disease?* (Totowa, 1985), p. 6.

[2] These four categories of criticism are acknowledged by Boorse. See ibid.

126  In Defense of an Evolutionary Concept of Health

*Charge of Circularity Number 1*

J. B. Scadding offers the first charge of circularity against Boorse's concept of health. He says:

> [Boorse's] identification of disease with an "internal state" is confusing. This state is presumably regarded as the explanation of the phenomena constituting a disease; but at the same time, it is itself implied from these phenomena.[3]

Scadding's criticism can be understood through the following example:

**X→** The internal state of a cancer victim is a state of uncontrollable cell reproduction.
**Y→** The phenomenon that constitutes the disease of cancer is uncontrollable cell reproduction.

Using the above example, Scadding claims that Boorse thinks that **X** is the explanation for **Y**. The problem, according to Scadding, is that **X** provides no independent support for **Y**, because the internal state of cancer and the phenomenon that constitutes cancer are one and the same condition. A cause can explain an event only if they are distinct events. But internal state **X** implies phenomenon **Y**, since both imply uncontrollable cell reproduction. Thus, Boorse's account of disease is circular or question begging, according to Scadding, since he has not provided in his explanation of disease any independent support for thinking that internal state **X** causes phenomenon **Y**.

*Boorse's reply to Scadding*  Boorse offers the following reply to Scadding:

> I do not claim that all diagnoses are explanatory rather than descriptive; I have said almost nothing about the form of disease explanation. And disease as an "internal state" is consistent with Scadding's "sum of abnormal phenomena" if none of these phenomena is external to the organism.[4]

There are two parts to Boorse's reply to Scadding. First, Boorse notes above that he has not discussed the form of disease explanation. He suggests that it is uncharitable of Scadding to ascribe a particular form of disease explanation to him. Yet, if Boorse thinks that a disease is constituted by a particular internal state, he must also think that an explanation of a given disease should include (at least in part) the internal state by which it is constituted. Indeed, Boorse analyzes the presence of a diseased internal state in terms of impairment of function or limitation of function. Cancer is the impairment of function of cell reproduction. It is the presence of such dysfunctional cells that brings about the internal state.

This is the reply Boorse should have given to Scadding. That is, according to Boorse, the internal state is not identified with the presence of a disease. This is

---

[3]  J. B. Scadding, "Health and Disease: What Can Medicine Do for Philosophy?" *Journal of Medical Ethics*, 14/3 (1988): 123.
[4]  Boorse, "A Rebuttal on Health," pp. 16–17.

where Scadding's criticism goes wrong. Rather, Boorse thinks that impairment or limitation of the function of **X** renders **X** diseased. So, the internal state will be whatever results from the limitation or impairment of **X**. Cancer is a disease involving cell dysfunction. The internal state of a cancerous body is the presence of rapid and uncontrollable cell growth. It is this reply that avoids the charge of circularity; that is, contrary to Scadding's criticism, Boorse identifies disease with dysfunction, not with the phenomena that constitute disease. Thus, although Boorse does not directly address Scadding's criticism, it is clear that he does have the resources to deflect his charge of circularity.

Second, Boorse notes that his account of "internal state" is similar to Scadding's "sum of abnormal phenomena," so long as external factors (i.e., external environmental phenomena) are excluded. This claim by Boorse is persuasive. For Scadding defines disease as "the sum of the abnormal phenomena displayed by a group of living organisms in association with a specified common characteristic or set of characteristics by which they differ from the norm of their species in such a way as to place them at a biological disadvantage."[5] Similarly, Boorse claims that disease is (in part) "a type of internal state which is ... an impairment of normal functional ability ..."[6] Boorse's point is that the details of Scadding's account are captured in his "impairment of normal functional ability." Since Boorse thinks that the concepts of health and disease are species specific (recall this point from Chapter 5), he is correct to claim that his and Scadding's account are similar.[7]

*Charge of Circularity Number 2*

William Bechtel offers the second charge of circularity as follows:

> Boorse appeals to a standard of normality to distinguish healthy from diseased functioning. First, however, he gives the impression of trying to explain what normal is. He cites a statement from [Daly] King that appears to define normal in terms of the design of the organism: "The normal ... is objectively, and properly, to be defined as that which functions in accordance with its design." This, however, will not work, because it puts Boorse in the same predicament as Kass, needing criteria for determining what something's design is. As I noted ... within an evolutionary framework, one cannot equate the design of something with its internal essence, because the organism is changing under selection pressures. But Boorse thinks he has a way out. He says "a function ... is nothing but a standard causal contribution to a goal actually pursued by the organism." These goals, in turn, can be ascertained empirically, "without considering the value of pursuing them." This is accomplished by studying the normal behavior of the organism, with normal taken in the statistical sense. Boorse has rather clearly moved in a circle now, for normal is

---

[5] Scadding, "Health and Disease: What Can Medicine Do for Philosophy?," p. 123.
[6] Boorse, "A Rebuttal on Health," p. 7.
[7] Note that Boorse also thinks that disease can come about from environmental factors (e.g., bacteria or viruses) that cause part-dysfunction, but this point is not the focus of this exchange between him and Scadding. Indeed, they both set it aside for the sake of understanding disease in terms of "internal state."

being used to define functioning according to design, which was to explicate the notion of normal.[8]

In order to make sense of Bechtel's criticism of Boorse, it is necessary to summarize briefly his concern about C. Daly King's notion of "normal" and Leon R. Kass's idea of "well working."[9] As Bechtel notes, Daly King's concept of normal is tied to an unexplained notion of design. Without a clear and general account of the design of an organism (or of the species to which it belongs), it is very difficult to make sense of an organism functioning well or normally. Thus, Bechtel thinks that Daly King's use of "design" sheds little or no light on his use of "normal."

Bechtel also argues that Kass has offered no criteria for determining the design of an organism. Critical to Kass's naturalistic concept of health is his understanding of function in terms of "well-working," which

> will vary from species to species ... Yet it is at the whole animal that one should finally look for the measure of well-working ... Thus, it is ultimately to the workings of the whole animal that we must turn to discover its healthiness. What, for example, is a healthy squirrel? ... [T]he healthy squirrel is a bushy-tailed fellow who looks and acts like a squirrel; who leaps through the trees with great daring; who gathers, buries, and covers but later uncovers and recovers his acorns ... To sum up: Health is a natural standard or norm—not a moral norm, not a "value" as opposed to a "fact," not an obligation, but a state of being that reveals itself in activity as a standard bodily excellence or fitness, relative to each species and to some extent to individuals, recognizable if not definable, and to some extent attainable. If you prefer a more simple formulation, I would say that health is "the well-working of the organism as a whole," or again, "an activity of the living body in accordance with its specific excellences."[10]

Bechtel's concern is that Kass appears to think that there are specific kinds of activities and behaviors in which squirrels engage and these activities and behaviors can be empirically determined. The problem, notes Bechtel, is that once a Darwinian world-view is embraced, it becomes clear that new behaviors and activities (and genetic changes as well) of organisms manifest themselves out of the complex interaction between organisms and the niche(s) they occupy. Thus, Bechtel is suggesting that Kass's assumption that there exists a finite and closed set of activities and behaviors of organisms is false.

Now, Bechtel is well aware that Boorse realizes the force of the above objection. But Boorse's attempted resolution, according to Bechtel, results in circular reasoning, since Boorse's relevant technical terms, "function" and "normal," are explained by each other. In order to determine that **X** is a function, one has to determine whether or not **X** is a normal behavior. Yet, Boorse (according to Bechtel) thinks that normal behavior is determined by how the design functions. The problem is that function *qua*

---

[8] William Bechtel, "A Naturalistic Concept of Health," in James M. Humber and Robert F. Almeder (eds), *Biomedical Ethics Reviews 1985* (Clifton, 1985), p. 143 [bracketed addition mine].

[9] Bechtel is referring to C. Daly King, "The Meaning of Normal," *Yale Journal of Biology and Medicine*, 17 (1945): 493–501 and Leon R. Kass, "Regarding the End of Medicine and the Pursuit of Health," *The Public Interest*, 40 (1975): 11–42.

[10] Kass, "Regarding the End of Medicine and the Pursuit of Health," pp. 27–8.

causal contribution to a goal is determined by normal behavior, but normal behavior is determined by function. Thus, Bechtel thinks that Boorse uses his definition of "function" to explain "normal" and vice-versa, rendering his argument circular.

*Boorse's reply to Bechtel* Boorse addresses directly Bechtel's charge of circularity as follows:

> If I understand this criticism, it may rest on some confusion of medical and statistical normality. I called C. Daly King's statement an "admirable explanation of clinical normality." I should have said "medical," not "clinical," since my basic analysis really aims at the pathologist's, not the clinician's, concept of disease. But I see no circle. What I proposed was to explicate medical normality as statistical normality of function (or more accurately, statistical nonsubnormality of function). *Medical normality, as King said, is functioning according to design. But species design is, in fact, simply those functions statistically typical in species members.* Given a focus on functions, medical normality and statistical (nonsub)normality are the same thing. But one must add the function concept to the statistical-normality concept to get medical normality, so the two kinds of normality differ. If any circle remains here, then perhaps the [Daly] King quote is not as admirable as I thought. In any case ... my careful version of the basic analysis, neither cites Daly King nor uses the term "species design" on any definition.[11]

The first part of Boorse's reply is that he thinks that he may have misled Bechtel into thinking he was offering an account of medical normality from the perspective of a clinician's understanding of disease. Boorse goes on to explain that he thinks that medical normality is to be understood in terms of the perspective of the pathologist's (not the clinician's) concept of disease. This perspective of the pathologist, according to Boorse, emphasizes statistical normality. Indeed, Boorse thinks that medical normality and statistical normality are one and the same concept from the perspective of the pathologist.

The second part of Boorse's reply is his justification for thinking that medical normality and statistical normality are identical from the perspective of pathologist *qua* physiologist. It is at this point that Boorse introduces his notion of function. Recall that Boorse thinks that a contextualist theory of function is correct. To this extent, the context of the pathologist *qua* physiologist is to figure what, on average, are the goals of parts of a biological system. According to Boorse, if a part, which usually brings about a certain goal(s), does not perform its function within a certain range of efficiency, it is thought to be statistically subnormal. It is the presence of such functional subnormality, according to Boorse, that leads the pathologist to render the judgment that such inefficient functioning is a sign of disease.

Now, Boorse thinks that his account is not circular. Since he stipulates that species design is nothing more than "the functions statistically typical in species," he thinks that he has evaded the charge of circularity. This reply, however, does not address adequately Bechtel's charge of circularity. First, Boorse's attempt to equate medical normality to statistical normality, as a way of distinguishing medical normality from clinical normality, is irrelevant to the issue. Bechtel is not concerned

---

[11] Boorse, "A Rebuttal on Health," pp. 17–18 [my italics].

about making sure that Boorse has explained adequately why medical normality is distinct from clinical normality. Rather, Bechtel's concern is that Boorse is using a definition of "normal," which includes the concept of function according to design, to explain "normal." Again, reminiscent of Scadding's concern, Bechtel is claiming that Boorse *defines* "function according to design" in terms of "normal." Since both "function according to design" and "normal" are defined in terms of one another, *independent* support must be offered in order to *explain* either one of these concepts. Bechtel's challenge is that Boorse has not provided such support.

Note that Boorse tags a disclaimer at the end of his reply to Bechtel. He says that if his reply still smacks of circularity, then his "careful version" of statistical normality and function (which excludes Daly King's ideas and the idea of "species design") is not circular. Boorse inserts this disclaimer because part of his reply to Bechtel in the above passage is to state that "species design is, in fact, simply those functions statistically typical in species members." The concern is that Boorse has substituted "statistically typical" for "normal." This maneuver, however, will not do. Bechtel could simply reply that the charge of circularity remains despite the substitution of terms. For "statistically typical" and "normal" are synonymous terms for Boorse such that species design is both defined and explained by "statistically typical" *qua* "normal." Thus, the charge of circularity remains.

Given that the charge of circularity is a legitimate concern, however, it is possible that Boorse's "careful version" does avoid this difficulty. Recall that Boorse states his "final definition" of function and disease as follows:

1. The *reference* class is a natural class of organisms of uniform functional design; specifically, an age group of a sex of a species.
2. A *normal function* of a part or process within members of the reference class is a statistically typical contribution by it to their individual survival and reproduction.
3. A disease is a type of internal state which is either an impairment of normal functional ability, i.e. a reduction of one or more functional abilities below typical efficiency, or a limitation on functional ability by environmental agents.

It is true that Boorse does not mention either Daly King or "species design" in the above account. Recall that Bechtel's concern is that Boorse appears to give an *explanation* of "normal" by way of his *definition* of "normal." In the above careful version, Boorse notes that "normal function" is to be understood as the statistically typical activity of a part or process within a specific reference class that assists in the survival and reproduction of an individual belonging to the reference class. Reasonably, Boorse's addition of "survival and reproduction" resolves the problem of circularity. Normal is *defined* in terms of statistically typical activities, but normal is now *explained* in terms of how such activities ensure survival and reproduction. More carefully, since Boorse is a part-functionalist, normal is explained by the goals and activities of specific parts within the body. Nevertheless, Boorse has provided independent support for his notion of "normal" that is neither circular nor question begging. The reason is that "normal" refers to the actual activities of parts of biological systems. Thus, Boorse has addressed adequately the charge of circularity submitted by Bechtel.

In summation, both Scadding and Bechtel charge Boorse with circular reasoning. They both claim that Boorse's attempt to explain certain technical terms (e.g., normal, function, and species design) is unpersuasive because he does not provide independent support for the explanation of these terms. Rather, they claim that he uses the definition of particular terms as part of the explanation of those same terms. In response, Boorse rejects Scadding's charge of circularity because he claims that he is not providing an explanation. Moreover, Boorse replies to Bechtel by acknowledging the criticism and suggesting that he has the resources to thwart it. Finally, this section revealed that Boorse's reply to Scadding is correct in the light of his definition of disease. Moreover, this section argued that Boorse's initial reply to Bechtel is wanting, but suggested that Boorse is correct to think that he has provided the kind of independent support to block Bechtel's charge of circularity.

*The Charge of Covert Normativism*

There are five distinct "covert normativism" criticisms of Boorse's naturalistic concept of health. The first one is offered by K. W. M. Fulford, who argues that Boorse slides from descriptive terms to normative terms in his account of disease. The second criticism is R. M. Hare's claim that Boorse ignores the fact that cultural norms are part of the concept of health. The third criticism is offered by Tristram Engelhardt, who argues that Boorse's choice of reproduction and survival as the goals of species reflects a value/normative judgment. The fourth criticism, which is put forth by Miller Brown, is that Boorse's claim that his concept of health is non-normative is mistaken because the science of biology is value-laden. The fifth criticism is due to George Agich, who argues that Boorse's naturalistic concept of health is value-laden, because science in general is unavoidably value-laden. A close examination of each of these criticisms and Boorse's reply to them will reveal that Boorse is mostly successful in his reply to criticisms 1–4, but his reply to criticism 5 is not entirely persuasive.

*Covert Normativism Number 1*

In the form of a dialogue between two philosophers, Fulford's opponent of Boorse argues that Boorse frequently moves from descriptive language to normative language. For example, Fulford notes that "Boorse's *claim* notwithstanding, he continues to use both 'dysfunction' and 'disease', and the ideas expressed by these terms, evaluatively."[12] For the sake of this discussion, the following examples, according to Fulford, capture Boorse's slide form the descriptive to the evaluative:

1. Boorse defines disease as a "deviation from natural functional organization." Then, Boorse goes on to substitute "deficiency" for "deviation" when he refers to disease.

---

[12] K. W. M. Fulford, *Moral Theory and Medical Practice* (New York, 1989), p. 37.

2. Boorse moves from "the affects of the external physical and cultural environment" to "hostile" or "injurious" environment.
3. Boorse moves from "**X** is an obstruction" to "**X** is an interference."
4. Boorse moves from "hindering" to "disrupting."
5. Boorse moves from "variations in behavior" to "incompetent" behavior.

*Boorse's reply to Fulford*   Boorse replies generally and to each of Fulford's five points above as follows:

> Admittedly, my rhetorical seas rose a bit high in the last passage, but Fulford's charge seems to me unfounded. Some terms that he calls normative need not be so ... where my terms are normative, they can easily be replaced by nonnormative ones; the evaluative rhetoric is eliminable without loss. Fulford misses this because ... he pays no attention to my empirical view of functions based on ... goal-directedness ... The function of a physiological process is its contribution to physiological goals.
>
> Reply to 1 → By "deficiency" of function, then, I mean simply less function, less contribution to the goals, than average. This is an arithmetic, not an evaluative, concept.[13]
>
> Reply to 2 → I am not sure that "hostile" is evaluative at all. Surely it and its synonyms ("aggressive") are common enough in biology. A hostile person, like an enemy, is someone who is trying to harm you. In physiology, harm is lowered functional efficiency in serving physiological goals.
>
> Reply to 3 and 4 and 5 → "Interference" is used even in physics, and many sciences talk of "disrupting" an equilibrium. To interfere with or disrupt a functional process is, for me, to lower its degree of achievement of physiological goals empirically given ... If the goals aren't achieved at all, the functioning is incompetent. So it seems to me that the terms Fulford complains of, insofar as they are evaluative, are easily eliminable.[14]

Boorse's general reply to Fulford underlies each of his specific replies. Basically, Boorse concedes that he was speaking casually when he moved from descriptive terms to normative terms. Still, Boorse insists that non-normative terms can be re-substituted for the normative terms without doing any damage to his account. His justification for this re-substitution is that his use of terms like "hostile" and "incompetent" refer to the way a part of an organism is functioning. If the heart functions below what is normal for its species, then it is incompetent *qua* diseased *qua* pathological. If bee stings cause breathing difficulties, then the bee sting is hostile to the extent that breathing has been compromised below normal functional efficiency. The point is that, although Fulford is right to point out Boorse's somewhat casual use of language, Boorse does have the resources to deflect this concern. Thus, Fulford's attempt to show that Boorse's concept of health is laden with many kinds of values is not successful.

---

[13] C. Boorse, "A Rebuttal on Health," pp. 20–21.
[14] All of these passages are from Boorse, "A Rebuttal on Health," pp. 20–21.

*Covert Normativism Number 2*

R. M. Hare offers what he takes to be a serious criticism against Boorse's non-normative concept of health. Using both the condition of baldness and a hypothetical genetic engineering example, Hare argues that the effects of a condition on a person's psychology and the person's response to that condition (and not survival and reproduction) are ineliminable to the concept of health. In summary, Hare claims that baldness is a disease, not because it hinders survival or reproductive success, but simply for the reason that "people do not *like* to be called bald."[15] Hare then asks the reader to imagine a genetic engineer who is able to create an organism that can prevent hair growth without the organism itself spreading throughout the body. He further asks the reader to imagine that this organism is sold on the market as a form of hair remover for women's legs. Upon offering this scenario, Hare addresses the concern of whether or not the induced loss of hair (in those women who use this product) is a disease.[16] He answers in the following way to those who think that such a hair loss condition is a disease:

> I suspect that, if we did [call it a disease], we should put quotation marks round the word, and would hesitate to say that the skins of the ladies who used it were not healthy. Doctors would probably not concern themselves with this condition if it were thought harmless.[17]

The point about the two examples, according to Hare, is that in one instance hair loss from baldness is thought to be a disease, but hair loss from the genetically engineered microorganism is not really considered a disease. Hare goes on to claim that the upshot of these examples is that they

> may be an indication that the differentia between pathological and non-pathological conditions is the badness of the effects of the condition, and not its interference with survival and reproduction, nor with natural function. For in neither example is there interference with survival and reproduction; and in both there is interference with natural function in the ordinary sense of that expression. It is the fact that ladies want to get rid of their hair, but balding men want to keep theirs, that makes the difference ... There seems, then, to be missing from Boorse's definition of "disease" as cited, and thus "healthy," an element which he does include in his definition of "illness": the evaluative element.[18]

Hare is quite clear that he thinks that values are ineluctably part of the concept of health, and Boorse is simply not acknowledging this point. In fact, Hare thinks that the differing intuitions about his baldness example and genetic engineering thought experiment support his position that both cases must be understood within a normative framework. Indeed, Hare concludes, "we seem to classify conditions as diseases if and only if they are bad things for the patient, in general."[19]

---

[15] R. M. Hare, "Health," *Journal of Medical Ethics*, 12/4 (1986): 178.
[16] Ibid.
[17] Ibid. [bracketed addition mine].
[18] Ibid.
[19] Ibid.

*Boorse's reply to Hare* There are three parts to Boorse's reply to Hare. First, Boorse claims that if there is no other effect than leg-hair loss in the genetic engineering case, then he is not sure what a pathologist would say. Alternatively, if it turns out that the falling of the leg-hairs is the result of damaged cells (caused by the genetically engineered organism), such a condition would be a disease. It just happens to be the case, Boorse argues, that this particular pathology "is a kind of convenient pathology, much as oviduct blockage is for some women."[20] Boorse's point is that the health status of a part of an organism is distinct from whether or not it is of value. He notes, for example, that women who do not wish to get pregnant and come to have oviduct blockage may very well welcome the pathological state.[21] The point here is that the value one places on a biological physical condition **X** is neither necessary nor sufficient for determining the health status of **X**. Thus, Boorse's conclusion, contrary to Hare, is that health and disease are not normative concepts.

Second, Boorse argues that baldness is a generic term that masks different conditions. For example, if baldness (a loss of scalp hair known as alopecia) is due to the malfunctioning of the pituitary gland or the thyroid, then the baldness is not pathological, but the pituitary gland or thyroid is. Alternatively, Boorse notes that common male-pattern baldness (androgenic alopecia) afflicts most men to some degree (statistical average) such that it would not be a disease. If, however, the baldness is excessive or premature, then it would be a disease (due to dysfunction). Notice that this reply fits in well with Boorse's claim that the concept of health is limited with respect to species, age, and gender. In the light of these variations in baldness, Boorse concludes, "I would wish to be sure of pathologists' determination to call any sort of baldness pathological before I rested the normativity of health and disease to this example."[22]

The third part of Boorse's reply to Hare is connected to human evolution. He argues that his naturalistic concept of health could predict how these two examples could be understood. With respect to leg hair, Boorse claims that body hair is a vestigial organ (much like the appendix), but face and scalp hair are not. His justification is that "[s]ince, in our evolution from earlier primates, hair has almost vanished from the rest of the body but not the head, that is some proof that it retained a function there. There is no generally accepted view of what that function is or was. One possibility is that the head hair has a protective or insulating function."[23]

The first two parts of Boorse's reply to Hare are quite reasonable. First, as Boorse suggests, the idea that disease is understood necessarily and/or sufficiently through the values people express about conditions they have is distinct from the actual function or dysfunction of the part. Moreover, the actions of doctors may not have a direct bearing on determining whether or not a particular condition is pathological. Contrary to Hare, it does not follow that if a doctor does not treat a patient for a particular condition, then that condition is not pathological. Thus, Hare's use of his two examples does not produce the outcome he would have hoped.

---

[20] Boorse, "A Rebuttal on Health," p. 70.
[21] Note that Boorse offers much the same reply to Hare's version of normativism as he did to Marmor's account discussed in Chapter 3.
[22] Boorse, "A Rebuttal on Health," p. 70.
[23] Ibid., p. 71.

Moreover, Boorse's distinctions of the different sorts of baldness help to understand how a pathologist might assess a particular case from a part-functionalist perspective. Rightly, Boorse notes that baldness is a generic term. The condition of baldness is manifest in many ways. As Boorse notes, it is an empirical question as to what function or dysfunction produces a particular case of baldness. Thus, there is no reason to turn to values, when a particular case of baldness is unknown.

Boorse's third reply to Hare is surprising. In Chapter 2, he argued against an evolutionary account of health. Moreover, in Chapter 4, his contextualist part-function account, which is the concept of function he thinks is embraced by pathologists, makes no mention of evolution. The point is not that Boorse has understood the function of hair incorrectly from an evolutionary perspective—indeed, his account is quite plausible. Rather, the point is that his attempt to include evolution in his reply to Hare is inconsistent with his rejection of it.[24]

Moreover, evolutionary concepts of function are etiological accounts. Recall, however, that Boorse went to great lengths to distance himself from Wright's etiological concept of function. The problem is that if Boorse takes evolutionary functions seriously, then he must also accept an etiological account of function. Since Boorse is clear that he does not wish to accept an evolutionary account of function, he cannot help himself to it as part of his reply to Hare. Thus, this reply by Boorse is not persuasive. The further suggestion is that, since the previous two parts of his reply to Hare are on the mark and the fact that he is caught in a contradiction, it is best that he eliminate this third part of his reply to Hare.

*Covert Normativism Number 3*

The next charge of covert normativism is offered by Engelhardt, who argues that Boorse imposes "the survival of species as an overriding good."[25] This criticism also includes a subsidiary charge of appeal to authority against Boorse by William Stempsey that is appropriate to Engelhardt's primary criticism. To start, Engelhardt offers the following argument:

> [O]ne can escape value judgments in ... defining disease and health only if one either defines disease as merely atypical function, which is clearly unsatisfactory, or accepts species survival as the goal (i.e., so that all judgments about disease and health simply presuppose this and no further value judgments). Otherwise, what counts as disease counts so not because of the designs of nature but because of our goals and expectations.[26]

---

[24] Importantly, Boorse's part-functionalism is not incompatible with evolutionary theory. For example, hair on the head could be viewed as promoting evolutionary goals. This account fits with Boorse's insistence that he does not want to attribute functions to organisms as a whole, but only to their parts. Yet, Boorse cannot make this argument given his explicit rejection of evolution. If readers are unconvinced by this criticism, then they should hold their judgment until later on in the chapter. Specifically, the section on "Bad Biology" argues that Boorse is caught in a contradiction with respect to how he thinks evolution fits into his analysis.

[25] H. Tristram Engelhardt, "Ideology and Etiology," *Journal of Medicine and Philosophy*, 1/3 (1976): 265.

[26] Ibid., p. 264.

Engelhardt criticizes Boorse's choice of species survival as the goal for organisms because it goes against the medical establishment's mantra of care for "the plight of individual persons." It may be the case that medical physiologists focus on the goals of survival and reproduction, but those who provide medical care for patients are concerned about the well-being of their patients. Engelhardt describes a case of sickle sell anemia. In summary, he notes that a medical physiologist might claim that those who have sickle cell anemia are not diseased and are not in need of medical care, because of the long-term survival advantages to the heterozygote condition. A medical doctor, however, might very well consider sickle cell anemia a disease, because of the suffering from certain side effects and the patient's request for medical assistance.[27] Engelhardt's general point is that Boorse makes a normative choice when he picks species survival over the choices of individual patients.

*Boorse's reply to Engelhardt*  In reply, Boorse offers the following:

> First ... it is incorrect that biological functions aim at species survival: units of selection are the genes of individuals, and therefore biological functions work to preserve the individual and his close kin. Secondly, the definition above incorporates no value judgments it only states what health (i.e., medical normality) *is*, namely biologically normal part-function. The normal-pathological distinction is a reasonable foundation for medical practice because biological normality is almost always in the interest of the patient. Where this presumption fails ... other values take precedence over health. Although the value of health is usually important, it is also limited ...[28]

First, in his reply to Engelhardt, Boorse makes it quite clear that biological functions do not range over the survival of species, but genes of individual organisms. From this claim he goes on to infer that the unit of selection is the individual organism and its close kin. This is an important move for Boorse if he is to offer a concept of health that respects the functioning parts of individual organisms. For many would think that it is quite counter intuitive that a proposed concept of health could only make sense of the health of species, but not the health of individuals (or species' health at the expense of individual health). Indeed, Boorse thinks that this reply, contrary to Engelhardt's claim, allows for his concept of health to range over individual organisms.

Second, as it was argued earlier in this chapter and in Chapter 5, Boorse is a part-functionalist and the above passage confirms this interpretation. The reason why Engelhardt's criticism fails, according to Boorse, is that he fails to take notice of the fact that parts of organisms can be understood simply in terms of the purely descriptive notion of medical normality. Basically, Boorse is claiming that Engelhardt has set up a "straw man" argument. That is, Engelhardt, thinks Boorse, has misrepresented his argument to make it easier to criticize. The upshot is that Engelhardt is attacking an argument that does not belong to Boorse. Thus, Engelhardt has simply interpreted

---

[27] Ibid., p. 264.
[28] Boorse, "A Rebuttal on Health," p. 24. This same quotation can be found in Boorse, "Concepts of Health," in Donald VanDeVeer and Tom Regan (eds), *Health Care Ethics: An Introduction* (Philadelphia, 1987), p. 372.

Boorse's concept of function/health incorrectly. If this is correct, then Engelhardt's criticism loses its force.

Boorse's move from the gene as the unit of selection to the individual organism and its kin as the units if selection is very controversial. Specifically, within the philosophy of biology, there is much debate as to what is the unit of selection. Some scholars have argued that individual organisms are the unit of selection, but others argue that genes are the unit of selection. Still, others argue that the group or species can be the unit of selection, while others recommend that a plurality of these selection models should be used to represent the process of natural selection. Boorse stipulates that Engelhardt's claim in favor of group/species selection is false, but he subsumes genic selectionism under individual selectionism. The problem is that some genic selectionists think that individual organisms are merely vehicles in which genes can go about replicating themselves. Thus, they conclude that the unit of selection is the gene, not the individual organism. On this view, individual selectionism and genic selectionism are opposing accounts of what is the unit of selection. The point is that Boorse needs to offer arguments in favor of why genic selectionism and individual selectionism are compatible positions, but that species/groups selection is ruled out. He has not done so in any of his works.[29] Although Engelhardt's species/group selectionist account of evolution may be false, Boorse has offered neither an argument against Engelhardt's position nor a defense of his allegiance to individual selectionism. As it stands, his reply to Engelhardt is unpersuasive.

Moreover, the second part of Engelhardt's concern may render Boorse's concept of health problematic. Even if Boorse is only a part-functionalist,[30] he still appears to value part-functions over the choices of individual patients. Such a choice, Engelhardt could claim, runs against common practice in medicine. Boorse's reply to this point is that, most of the time, his non-normative concept of health coincides with the values underlying the choices made by individuals. Thus, Boorse thinks that

---

[29] Note that the unit of selection debate is far subtler than the general picture I have presented here. Nonetheless, the classic genic selectionist is Richard Dawkins, *The Selfish Gene* (New York, 1976); David Hull, "Individuality and Selection" *Annual Review of Ecology and Systematics*, 11 (1980): 311–32, stands as the exemplar of the individual selectionist camp; defenders of the possibility of group selection are Elliot Sober and David Sloan Wilson, *Unto Others The Evolution and Psychology of Unselfish Behavior* (Cambridge, 1998); and John Maynard Smith, "How to Model Evolution," in John Dupré (ed.), *The Latest on the Best: Essays on Optimality and Evolution* (Cambridge, 1987), pp. 119–31, has defended the plurality of models position. Note that Chapter 7 will offer a brief defense of the individual as the unit of selection to fill this gap in Boorse's analysis.

[30] Boorse is correct to make clear that Engelhardt has constructed an inaccurate version of his account. Boorse is a part-functionalist and he thinks that this is the appropriate account of function for understanding health. Still, in fairness to Engelhardt, Boorse does not give an extensive defense of his allegiance to part-functionalism in his article, "On the Distinction Between Disease and Illness," *Philosophy and Public Affairs*, 5/1 (1975): 49–68. It is to this article that Engelhardt is replying. Nonetheless, on p. 58 of this article, Boorse makes clear that he is a part-functionalist. So, it is clear that Engelhardt missed this point in Boorse's discussion.

there is no genuine tension between his value-free concept of health and the values that may accompany patient choices.

Notably, in his above reply to Engelhardt, Boorse makes a qualification about individual medical choices. He states that in those cases where a patient (i.e., a part of a patient) is not considered to be unhealthy and the patient still chooses medical treatment, the values of that patient should take precedence.[31] Yet, Boorse is clear (much like his claims in the normative discussions in Chapter 3) that the values patients may have with respect to the physical states of their body parts are completely distinct from the description of those parts. If it is the case that sickle cell anemia patients and their doctors wish to treat this condition (knowing that future generations may suffer from such a decision), then Boorse does not have a problem with such a decision. This would simply be one of those cases in which patients and their doctors decided to act against the medical notion of pathology.[32] Thus, because Boorse thinks that suffering is neither necessary nor sufficient for pathology (see Chapter 3), he does not think that his account is disturbed by Engelhardt's criticism.

The linchpin of Boorse's argument above is the justification he gives in defense of why it is the case that medical physiologists think that health is the absence of disease *qua* pathology. An earlier section of this chapter noted that Boorse thought that normal part-function in terms of medical normality *seems or appears* to be the accepted position of medical physiologists/pathologists (see section on normal function). Boorse goes on to say with respect to his concepts of health and disease that he is "content ... to live or die by the considered usage of the pathologists."[33] The problem is that Boorse's use of "seems" is rather weak. The move from "seems" to "is" is clearly too fast without further justification. Restated, why should anyone think that medical physiologists do, in fact, understand function in the way that Boorse claims they do? The concern is that Boorse's contextualist concept of function/health is more of a stipulated or assumed position rather than one that is rigorously defended. A stronger case than what Boorse provides is required if he is going to (as he does above) claim that disease *is* understood in terms of biological part-dysfunction. Thus, as it stands, Boorse has not provided a very persuasive reply to Engelhardt.

Of course, Boorse need only provide some evidence of those pathologists who do defend his part-functionalist account. This information, at the very least, would reveal that Boorse is not simply being dogmatic in his approach, but is following

---

[31] This qualification by Boorse is a complicated point. Would he want to allow every moral and social context to take precedence over healthy physiology? For example, it is not clear that a patient should be entitled to insurance coverage for purely elective cosmetic plastic surgery. Boorse is likely thinking of cases in which a patient is physiologically healthy, but suffering. Possible examples include the need for an epidural during pregnancy or gene therapy for certain sickle-cell anemia patients. However, Boorse does not offer any boundary conditions as to which medical treatments should and should not take precedence over physical health. Boorse would need to offer additional details to make this qualification clear.

[32] In the evolutionary account of health that will be offered in the next chapter, this sickle cell anemia case will be examined more carefully than the brief discussion here.

[33] Boorse, "A Rebuttal on Health," p. 53.

a particular disciplinary approach. For example, one of the key figures in the early history of pathology, Rudolf Virchow, defends a part-functionalist account. He says:

> In my view, the disease entity is *an altered body part*, or expressed in first principles, an altered cell or aggregate of cells, whether tissue or organ. In this sense, I am a thoroughgoing ontologist, and I have always regarded it as a merit to have brought the old and essentially justifiable requirement that disease should be a living entity, and lead a parasitic existence, into harmony with genuine scientific knowledge.[34]

Given the above passage, Boorse could argue that, much like Virchow and other similar pathologists, it is part-functionalism that is relevant to the concept of health. Boorse could claim that his disciplinary objectivism has its origin in the discipline of pathology that was pioneered by the views of Virchow. Indeed, since Boorse does not think that a definitive concept of function is forthcoming, he could claim that the Virchowian piece of the teleological pie is what is relevant to his concept of health. Again, at the very least, Boorse is defending a disciplinary objectivism concept of function that is well defined within the history of pathology.

Still, one could argue that, although Boorse could draw on the history of pathology in defense of his part-functionalism, he still has not offered genuine support for such a view. Recently, William Stempsey has launched just this criticism against Boorse. He explains as follows:

> Most pathologists are not philosophically trained. They study the morphological characteristics of disease, not disease itself. When they speak of disease, they are actually speaking of morphology that they attempt to correlate with a patient's phenomenological experience of sickness. Pathologists generally do not study the concept of disease. Concepts like disease and death are philosophical concepts. Pathologists generally are not philosophers. Hence, defining the concept of disease according to the way pathologists use the term relies on what Robert Veatch has called the "fallacy of generalization of expertise." It would be more plausible to look at the considered usage of those who are trained in both medicine and philosophy.[35]

Stempsey is arguing, much like Veatch,[36] that Boorse is relying on the expertise of pathologists, who do not have the skills of conceptual analysis. According to Stempsey, Boorse is claiming that, since some expert pathologist (like Virchow) asserts that part-functionalism is correct, it must be the case that part-functionalism is correct. This move by Boorse, claims Stempsey, amounts to nothing more than an appeal to authority, rather than a genuine argument in defense of non-normative part-functionalism.

---

[34] Rudlof Virchow, "One Hundred Years of General Pathology," in L. J. Rather, trans., *Disease, Life, and Man: Selected Essays of Rudolf Virchow* (Stanford, 1958), p. 192 [my italics]. This quotation is taken from William E. Stempsey, "A Pathological View of Disease," *Theoretical Medicine*, 21/4 (2000): 323.

[35] Stempsey, "A Pathological View of Disease," p. 322.

[36] Robert M. Veatch, "Generalization of Expertise: Scientific Expertise and Value Judgments," *Hastings Center Studies*, 1 (1973): 29–40.

Stempsey's criticism needs to be clarified and expanded, because, in general, it is not clear that appealing to authority is necessarily problematic. Given the complexity of the world, no single person can come to know more than a small percentage of all there is to know. Thus, relying on the expertise of others may be a necessity. Of course, there are legitimate and illegitimate appeals to authority. Usually, an appeal to authority is legitimate if the following two conditions obtain:

1. The person to whom an appeal is made is an authority in the subject being discussed.
2. There is general agreement among experts concerning the matter being discussed.[37]

The fallacy of appeal to authority occurs when either one or both of the above conditions fails to obtain. In Boorse's case, both conditions fail to obtain, claims Stempsey. First, although a particular pathologist may be an expert in *the practice* of his field, he is not necessarily an expert in the conceptual and theoretical elements of his practice. The point is that Stempsey insists that appealing to a "bench scientist" about the concept of disease is a mistake. Rather, it is the philosopher or medical practitioner to whom one must appeal for expert advice about the concept of disease. If Stempsey is correct, and given the above criteria, it follows that the first condition does not obtain. Thus, according to Stempsey, Boorse has committed the fallacy of appeal to authority.

Second, it turns out that there is no general agreement, even within pathology, about the scope of the claims made by pathologists. For example, Rubin and Farber claim that "pathology has been defined as the medical science that deals with *all aspects* of disease, but with special reference to the essential nature, the causes, and the development of abnormal conditions."[38] Moreover, in their preface, Ramzi S. Cotran, Vinay Kumar, and Stanley L. Robbins define pathology as follows:

> Translated literally, pathology is the study (*logos*) of suffering (*pathos*). As a science, pathology focuses on the structural and functional consequences of injurious stimuli on cells, tissues, and organs and ultimately the consequences on the entire organism.[39]

Interestingly, both Christian Nezelof and Thomas A. Seemayer offer a similar account to the one above:

> Since the beginning of time, people have wished to know more about the causes of the evils and afflictions that befall them. The answer to these basic queries have evolved with time and reflect the main philosophical, religious, and scientific concepts, as well as the technical possibilities of the day ... Pathology, from the Greek *pathos*, meaning "suffering" and *logos*, meaning "word," the discipline that deals with the causes and mechanisms of

---

[37] This discussion is drawn from James Stuart and Donald Scherer, *Logical Thinking: An Introduction to Logic*, 2nd edn (New York, 1997).

[38] Emanuel Rubin and John L. Farber, *Pathology* (Philadelphia, 1988), p. ix.

[39] Ramzi S. Cotran, Vinay Kumar and Stanley L. Robbins, *Robbins Pathologic Basis for Disease*, 4th edn (Philadelphia, 1989), p. 1.

human diseases, originated from the above mentioned fundamental physical concerns, and hence can be considered to be as old as medicine itself.[40]

The first quotation from Rubin and Farber includes "all" in the description of the range of phenomena with which the science of pathology concerns itself with respect to disease. This means that the functions of organisms as a whole would be included in such a range. Cotran, Kumar, and Robbins claim that the *entire* organism is included within the pathologist's understanding of disease. This means that, contrary to Virchow and Boorse, pathology (according to some experts) includes any functions an organism as a whole might have. These passages from other pathologists *qua* experts reveal a rather different account of pathology than that of Boorse and Virchow. These differences suggest that there is no general agreement amongst experts within pathology on the scope of their field with respect to disease. Thus, the second condition of the appeal to authority does not obtain. It further follows, according to Stempsey, that Boorse has committed the fallacy of appeal to authority.[41]

Stempsey's criticism that Boorse has committed the fallacy of appeal to authority is rather uncharitable. First, it is not clear that Boorse's reliance on pathology is the product of relying on "bench pathologists." To the contrary, Boorse's contextualist concept of function/health is the result of quite a detailed critique of Wright's concept of function (see Chapter 4). Boorse came to the conclusion that a unique concept of function is not possible only after examining the function debate. It is at this point that Boorse turned to the field of biology. Conceding that different sub-disciplines in biology carve up the "teleological pie" in different ways, Boorse argued that part-functionalism is appropriate to a naturalistic concept of health. The move to part-functionalism is the product of rigorous debate with philosophers on the concept of function. The point is that Boorse's reliance on the sub-field of pathology is not the result of simply drawing on the works of pathologists who are part-functionalists.

---

[40] Christian Nezelof and Thomas A. Seemayer, "A History of Pathology: An Overview," in Ivan Damjanov and James Linder (eds), *Anderson's Pathology*, 10th edn, vol. 1 (St. Louis, 1996), p. 1.

[41] Although Stempsey does mention the pathologists quoted here, he does not specify any pathologist who explicitly claims that the field of pathology is or should be concerned with the functions or functioning of organisms as a whole. Yet, it appears implicit in his analysis that the pathologists quoted in this discussion do include the functions or functioning of organisms as a whole when they use phrases like "all aspects of disease" and "consequences on the entire organism." These passages, however, are not as explicit as one might like to reveal a possible tension in pathology concerning whether or not its practices range over only the functional parts of an organism or the functions or functioning of an organism as a whole. To make the tension more explicit, Stempsey could have mentioned that Kurt Goldstein's holistic claim about disease comes close to capturing the tension. Goldstein claims that "[d]isease appears when an organism is changed in such a way that, though in its proper, "normal" milieu, it suffers catastrophic reaction. This manifests itself not only in specific disturbances of performance, corresponding to the locus of the defect, but in quite general disturbances because, as we have seen, disordered behavior in any field coincides always with more or less disordered behavior of the whole organism." See Kurt Goldstein, *The Organism, A Holistic Approach to Biology Derived from Pathological Data in Man* (Boston, 1963), p. 432.

Therefore, Boorse's critical debate with philosophers of function leaves open the possibility that the first condition of the appeal to authority obtains, because philosophers of function could be viewed as the appropriate experts for a naturalistic *qua* functional *concept* of health and disease.

With respect to the second condition of the appeal to authority fallacy, Stempsey's criticism reveals a lack of charity on his part. Basically, Stempsey is requiring that Boorse should have examined his concept of disease within the framework of the different conceptions of disease in the history of pathology. Since it is clear that there is no clear-cut consensus on the scope of disease within pathology, Boorse cannot simply assume that there is. It is this assumption by Boorse, argues Stempsey, that does not allow condition two to obtain. It follows, thinks Stempsey, that Boorse has simply appealed to authority.

The difficulty with Stempsey's criticism is that it ignores Boorse's entire discussion on normativism and mental health. Recall that in Chapter 3, Boorse evaluates the different normative concepts of health and argues why he considers them problematic. With respect to the claims made by some of the pathologists noted above, Boorse could simply locate them within one of the normative concepts of health against which he has already argued. Since these pathologists claim that the field of pathology ranges over *all* aspects of disease, many of the norms associated with cultural, moral, and aesthetic values would be relevant. Yet, Boorse has argued why these various norms should not be included in the concept of health (see Chapter 3). Thus, by challenging the many normative concepts of health, Boorse has indirectly addressed the normative dimensions present in the claims made by some of the pathologists noted above. Therefore, contrary to Stempsey, Boorse does not simply assume a version of pathology at the expense of ignoring others versions. Rather, upon having dismissed the major normative concepts of health and the idea that a single concept of function is possible, Boorse suggests that it is reasonable to accept a non-normative part-dysfunction concept of health.

Moreover, Boorse has argued that suffering is not a legitimate part of a naturalistic concept of health, because of the controversial nature of mental health. Although Boorse's concept of mental health is beyond the scope of this project, it should be noted that Boorse does defend a functionalist theory of mind in his attempt to make sense of mental health. He notes, however, that his account assumes mental causation, which he concedes is a rather contentious issue.[42] Again, if Stempsey is going to argue that psychology *qua* suffering is part of the concept of health, then he needs to address directly Boorse's efforts in the topic of mental health.

It further follows that the second condition of the appeal to authority is not directly relevant to Boorse's account. Since Boorse does address the difficulty of various normative concepts of health, he has (indirectly) addressed the issue of whether or not there is controversy with respect to the field of pathology. Of course, it is true that Boorse should have made clear that pathologists who embrace normativism run into the same difficulties as other normativists do. The point, however, is that Boorse has cleared the way (through his analysis of normativism and functionalism) so that

---

[42] See Boorse, "What a Theory of Mental Health Should Be," *Journal of the Theory of Social Behavior*, 6/1 (1976): 61–84.

he can embrace a concept of disease/pathology that is not the result of appealing to authority. Thus, it is reasonable to conclude that Boorse does not appeal to authority in the way Stempsey suggests.[43]

Recall that the point of this discussion is to determine whether or not Boorse has successfully replied to Engelhardt's concern. There is still a difficulty with Boorse's reply in that he has not demonstrated why the field of pathology/medical physiology should be authoritative for understanding the concepts of disease and health; that is why it should take precedence over other accounts. Engelhardt argues that Boorse's description of disease as atypical dysfunction is "unsatisfactory" as follows:

> The term *clinical problem* underscores the fact that an attempt to give a neutralist, purely descriptive, account of disease fails. Diseases stand out for us as problems to be solved, all else equal ... [A] disease is a disease because it is disvalued—in a particular way. It is a clinical problem ... Whether it is athlete's foot, tuberculosis, a deformed nose, or unwanted pregnancy, disease or clinical problems are not good things to have.[44]

Engelhardt thinks that the meaning of "disease" is determined by the doctor-patient relationship in medical practice. That is, the psychology of a patient is sufficient to proclaim a bodily conditioned diseased. Boorse offers the following reply:

> Engelhardt seems to hold that clinical problems are diseases, and unwanted pregnancy is a disease or clinical problem; therefore, unwanted pregnancy is a disease. But it isn't, despite having been thoroughly medicalized in every other way ... Medicine could have easily christened [unwanted pregnancy] with some bogus disease name like "dysgravida," or "gestation adjustment disorder," or "organismic hypernumerosis." But medicine did not, and that is because doctors, in general, know what is a disease and what isn't, even if they have trouble reducing their knowledge to a tight definition.[45]

Boorse's objection above is similar to the one he offered in his reply to the Marmor-type normativist in Chapter 3. To reiterate, Boorse is making clear that a patient's psychological state with respect to physical condition **X** does not necessarily suggest anything about **X** itself. For example, it is true that women (in general) suffer a great deal during the birthing process. It does not follow that such a process is unhealthy or bad because of the suffering.[46] It is these sorts of examples, which Boorse uses

---

[43] With respect to conceptual analysis, the second condition of the fallacy of appeal to authority may be unreasonable. For example, there is little consensus in philosophy about how the concept of health is to be understood. Conceptual analysis, at least in philosophy, may assist in getting clear on what the problem is on a given topic, but it is not clear that a definitive resolution to the problem would be forthcoming. Thus, it is not at all clear why philosophers (or medical professionals) would be "experts" on Stempsey's account.

[44] Tristram H. Engelhardt, *The Foundations of Bioethics* (New York, 1986), pp. 174 and 175.

[45] Boorse, "A Rebuttal on Health," p. 27.

[46] Of course, Boorse's claim that doctors know what is and is not a disease is unmotivated. He did not need to include this claim to make his point. Also, Engelhardt has restricted his discussion only to the doctor–patient relationship. This comes off as a bit anachronistic. Clearly, his account fails to take into consideration that doctors and patients today operate in a wider context that includes health plans, insurance companies, and all sorts of laws and regulations governing the practice of medicine.

against criticisms like that of Engelhardt, that make it clear that (at the very least) the psychological state of an individual is not sufficient for determining the health status of a part of an individual. So, Boorse has persuasively argued against Engelhardt's insistence that normativity is covertly part of his concept of health. Thus, upon further inspection, Boorse has provided a cogent reply to Engelhardt.

*Covert Normativism Number 4*

The fourth criticism offered by W. Miller Brown pushes Boorse further on conceding that norms are part of his concept of health. Miller Brown states the following:

> How are we to determine those highest-level goals of organisms which lower processes function to achieve? ... It may be true that what interests the physiologist is what promotes individual survival and reproduction. But Boorse's account was designed to show that the concept of disease is non-normative. At best, what he has shown is that *given* such a choice of highest-level goals, "function statements will be value-free ..." But such "empirical matters" are significant only in terms of the goals chosen. What assurance do we have that these *are* the goals of the system whose "species design" we have determined?[47]

Miller Brown is claiming, much like Engelhardt and others,[48] that Boorse has not offered an account of why it is the case that one area of the teleological pie should be preferred over another. Moreover, Miller Brown thinks that Boorse's attempt to argue for a value-free concept of health is weakened on the grounds that the physiologist's choice of goals is a value. This choice of survival and reproduction, argues Miller Brown, is a value that is part of the concept of disease.

*Boorse's reply to Miller Brown* Boorse offers the following riposte to Miller Brown:

> My answer ... is that there is no choice here—that is simply what disease is, as the concept is best reconstructed from medical classifications. The real normative choice is medicine's commitment to combat disease ... Unquestionably medical practice rests on a normative choice to combat disease. But that does not show that the meaning of "disease" rests on a normative choice unless one assumes that the meaning of "disease" is fixed by medical practice. And this is just what writers like Engelhardt, Agich, and Miller Brown assume.[49]

Boorse's reply to Miller Brown ignores his own discussion on function, which anticipates Miller Brown's objection. (All that he has done in his reply is stipulate that disease is what medical taxonomists claim it is. Such a response appears to support Stempsey's appeal to authority criticism.) To reiterate, Boorse claims that a naturalistic concept of health is grounded in the concept of function. As it

---

[47] W. Miller Brown, "On Defining 'Disease'", *Journal of Medicine and Philosophy*, 10 (1985): 315 and 316.

[48] See George J. Agich, "Disease and Value: A Rejection of the Value-Neutrality Thesis," *Theoretical Medicine*, 4/1 (1983): 27–41.

[49] Boorse, "A Rebuttal on Health," p. 25.

turns out, argues Boorse, the concept of function can only be contextually defined. This means that there is some degree of legitimacy to different concepts of health, depending upon the goals chosen by a particular kind of biologist in a specific subfield. In Boorse's own words, "Given this latitude of choice, what has happened is that various subfields of biology have carved out various slices of the teleological pie and interpreted their function statements accordingly."[50] The point is that goals of systems are contextually determined because, according to Boorse, there is no universal concept of function available. So, based on Boorse's own contextualist account of function, he would be forced to reply to Miller Brown that there is no assurance that the goals of parts of organisms *really are* the goals embraced by pathologists and physiologists.

Although the above concession would put Boorse in a position where he would have to accept that there are choices/values on which goals to focus, he still could claim that part-functionalism is the relevant concept of function for the physiologist or pathologist. The point is that Boorse should have conceded to Miller Brown that there is a choice of goals, depending upon a given practitioner's area of specialization.[51] Still, such a concession would not put Boorse in a position to concede that values are part of the concepts of health and disease. From the fact that a scientist makes a value judgment in studying phenomenon X rather than Y, it does not follow that this value is part of the concept of X. For example, if a geologist decides to study crystals instead of minerals, the value that the geologist places in crystals is not thereby part of the concept of crystal. In the same way, the fact that pathologists value the function of parts of organisms (i.e., part-functions) as opposed to, say, the function of ecosystems, it does not follow that the value they place in the function of parts of organisms is part of the concept of part-function. The point is that Boorse can concede to Miller Brown that there are choices and values about which part of the teleological pie is worthy of study, but make clear that such choices and values are not necessarily part of the concepts that comprise the various parts of the pie. Thus, although Boorse's reply to Miller Brown is not entirely persuasive, it is evident that such a criticism does not cause any serious damage to his analysis.

*Covert Normativism Number 5*

George Agich furnishes the final charge of covert normativism. Agich argues that Boorse's concept of health cannot be value-free, because science is not value-free. Thus, according to Agich, since Boorse does rely heavily on the practice of science, his concept of health is value-laden.

---

[50] Christopher Boorse, "Wright on Functions," *Philosophical Review*, 85/1 (1976): 84.
[51] Indeed, Boorse acknowledges just this point in defense of his contextualist part-functionalist account against Larry Wright. Moreover, Boorse notes that different biologists could carve up the teleological pie in different ways. But this constraint on who gets to carve up the pie does not follow from his account. His contextualist concept of function allows for all kinds of specialists in different disciplines to offer all sorts of different contexts from which to understand functions.

In general, the debate about values in science is a battle between *constructivists* and *descriptivists* about the nature of concept/judgment formation. Constructivists argue that science is value-laden, because it is not possible simply to provide a non-interpretive concept of a phenomenon through human non-cognitive and cognitive systems. Rather, constructivists think that objects are constituted or constructed through the use of value-laden non-cognitive and cognitive systems. Helen Longino articulates this constructivist view of science as a deeply value-laden enterprise as follows:

> The idea of a value-free science presupposes that the object of inquiry is given in and by nature, whereas contextual analysis shows that such objects are constituted in part by social needs and interests that become encoded in the assumptions of research programs. Instead of remaining passive with respect to data and what the data suggest, we can, therefore, acknowledge our ability to affect the course of knowledge and fashion or favor research programs that are consistent with the values and commitments we express in the rest of our lives. From this perspective the idea of a value-free science is not just empty but pernicious.[52]

Longino argues that epistemic values and non-epistemic values (e.g., social, personal, religious, and/or political values) associated with particular research plans comprise the practice of science. Her justification is that an object under investigation is not simply taken in by human perceptual and cognitive systems. Rather, she claims that these systems take part in *constructing*—not simply describing—the object under investigation. At bottom, Longino denies that it is possible to offer a purely descriptive account of an object, because the perceptual and cognitive systems involved in such descriptions are imbued with all kinds of personal, professional, social, political, religious, and epistemic values. Since, according to Longino, human perceptual and cognitive systems are value-laden and actually construct objects that are under investigation, it follows that all such constructions are value-laden.[53]

In sharp contrast, descriptivists claim that science follows a fixed set of rules and concepts in its attempt to offer knowledge about the workings of the external world. These rules and concepts may be valued, but such value does not enter into the characterization of objects under investigation. A classic descriptivist is Henri Poincaré. With respect to ethical values and science, he offers the following judgment:

> Ethics and science have their own domains, which touch but do not interpenetrate. The one shows us to what goal we should aspire, the other, given the goal, teaches us how

---

[52] Helen E. Longino, *Science as Social Knowledge* (New Jersey, 1990), p. 191.

[53] Stephen Jay Gould offers much the same assessment of science as Longino does. He says: "Science, since people must do it, is a socially embedded activity. It progresses by hunch, vision, and intuition. Much of its change through time does not record a closer approach to absolute truth, but the alternative cultural contexts that influence it so strongly. Facts are not pure and unsullied bits of information; culture also influences what we see and how we see it." See Stephen Jay Gould, *The Mismeasure of Man* (New York, 1981), pp. 21–2.

to attain it. So they never conflict since they never meet. There can be no more immoral science than there can be scientific morals.[54]

More prosaically than Poincaré, Hugh Lacey articulates the descriptivist's value-free image of science as follows:

> The world, "the facts of nature," the spatio-temporal totality, is fully characterizable and explicable in terms of "its underlying order"—its underlying structures, processes and laws. All objects belonging to the underlying order can be fully characterized in quantitative terms; all interactions are lawful; and laws (not necessarily deterministic) are expressible in mathematical equations. *Such objects are not constructed as objects of value. Qua* objects of the underlying order, they are part of no meaningful order, they have no natural ends, no developmental potentials, and no essential relatedness to human life and practices. Values—and objects, *qua* objects of value—are not represented as emergent from the underlying world ... The aim of science is to represent this world of pure "fact," the underlying order of the world, independently of any relationship it might bear contingently to human practices and experiences. Such representations are posited in theories which, in order to be faithful to the object of inquiry, must deploy only categories devoid of evaluative content or implications.[55]

Lacey's depiction of science as value-free is quite clear. First, there is an underlying value-free (i.e., "pure") structure of reality. Second, the methodology of science can access and characterize this reality without the intrusion of values associated with the personal or social domains of life. Specifically, science simply employs mathematics to reveal the true structure of reality and its laws. Thus, because science is concerned with the use of quantitative measurements (e.g., statistics,) the descriptivist concludes that science is value-free.

With descriptivism and constructivism clearly explained, it is possible to turn to Agich's concern. Basically, Agich argues that Boorse's "descriptivist" value-free concept of health is value-laden because science in general is value-laden. Agich's justification for biomedical science being value-laden is that the language of disease is embedded in both the science of understanding pathological conditions *and* the medical goal of elimination of pathological states in order to secure patient freedom.[56] Thus, Agich concludes the following about Boorse's defense of a value-free science:

---

[54] Henri Poincaré, *The Value of Science* (New York, 1920/1958), p. 12. This same point about science in terms of means and ends is discussed by Michael Scriven, "The Exact Role of Value Judgments in Science," in Kenneth F. Schaffner and Robert S. Cohen (eds), *PSA 1972* (Dordrecht-Holland, 1974), pp. 219–47.

[55] Hugh Lacey, *Is Science Value-Free?* (London, 1999), pp. 2–3.

[56] George J. Agich, "Disease and Value: A Rejection of the Value-Neutrality Thesis," pp. 36–7. For a similar account, see Edmund L. Erde, "Philosophical Considerations Regarding Defining 'Health', 'Disease', etc., and Their Bearing on Medical Practice," *Ethics and Science in Medicine*, 6 (1979): 42–3 and Tristram H. Engelhardt, "Human Well-Being and Medicine: Some Basic Value Judgments in the Biomedical Sciences," in Tristram H. Engelhardt and Daniel Callahan (eds), *Science, Ethics, and Medicine* (New York, 1976), pp. 120–39.

This approach is based on an unacceptably simplistic view of science as value-free. In these terms, medicine appears value-laden and is often criticized for that reason. Work in philosophy of medicine, however, has helped question this view and aided in the recognition that science, too, is a practice laden with particular value as well as conceptual commitments.[57]

Agich's point in the above passage is that medicine, unlike science, has been criticized for being value-laden. The problem with this view, claims Agich, is that science is as value-laden as medicine. No doubt, it is clear that Agich thinks that any attempt to divorce science from medicine with respect to both epistemic and non-epistemic values is misguided. In order to make sense of Agich's claims above, an account of what he means by "particular value" and "conceptual values" needs to be made clear.

First, what is the *particular* value of science? There are at least two distinct senses of "particular value." The first sense refers to particular values that are not associated with knowledge acquisition. For example, particular values of science could include social norms (e.g., improving technology), personal norms (e.g., science as a justification for monogamy), religious norms (e.g., science as justification for forbidding the teaching of evolution), or political norms (e.g., the use of science as justification for the advancement of military practices).

The second sense of "particular value" refers to *the* single end of doing science. Although he does not necessarily endorse the following claim, Peter Caws notes that, traditionally, "Science is the explanation of nature on its own terms."[58] Morris R. Cohen and Ernest Nagel elaborate on this "explanation of nature" in terms of *truth*. They offer the following summary judgment:

If we look at all the sciences not only as they differ among each other but also as each changes and grows in the course of time, we find that the constant and universal feature of science is its general method, which consists in the persistent search for truth ...[59]

As Cohen and Nagel note, the constant and universal feature of science is the pursuit of truth. Whether or not science can arrive at such an end point is debatable, but it is clear that truth is the overarching value or "particular value" that distinguishes science from many other activities. Thus, the particular value to which Agich refers would be science's pursuit of understanding/knowing the natural world as it is; that is, the pursuit and achievement of truth or a particular social, political, personal, etc. value.

Agich's "conceptual values" (also known as epistemic or cognitive values) refer to a set of rules or standards that underlie the practice of science. Edward O. Wilson hints at these standards (which he thinks should be valued) in his advice to the pubescent scientist:

Throw everything you can at the subject, as long as the procedures can be duplicated by others. Consider repeated observation of a physical event under varying circumstances,

---

[57] Ibid., p. 39 (end note 3).
[58] Peter Caws, *The Philosophy of Science* (Princeton, 1965), p. 287.
[59] Morris R. Cohen and Ernest Nagel, *An Introduction to Logic and Scientific Method* (New York, 1934), p. 192.

experiments in differing modes and styles, correlation of supposed causes and effects, statistical analyses to reject null hypotheses (those raised to deliberately threaten the conclusion), logical argument, and attention to detail and consistency with the results published by others.[60]

Wilson's advice to the young scientist is a reminder that there is a set of rules (that should be valued) which form the methodology of knowledge acquisition. These epistemic values[61] usually include, though are not limited to, the following:

(1) Explanatory/Unifying Power—A theory that unifies phenomena in a wide range and variety of domains is superior to one that does not.[62]
(2) Simplicity/Parsimony—A theory that postulates fewer entities or processes is preferable to one that posits more.[63]
(3) Fecundity/Predictive Power—A theory that is able to provide knowledge beyond its targeted explananda is superior over one that does not.[64]
(4) Replicability—Theories and the results of theories that are the product of experiments and tests, which can be replicated by others, are favored over those that cannot be replicated.[65]

---

[60] Edward O. Wilson, *Consilience: The Unity of Knowledge* (New York, 1998), pp. 58–9. This reminder by Wilson of the importance *qua* value of following agreed upon rules is not at all new. Aristotle also called on the need for an agreed upon set of rules for understanding natural phenomena: "[I]t is clear that in the investigation of nature, or natural science, as in every other, there must first of all be certain defined rules by which the acceptability of the method of exposition may be tested, apart from whether the statements made represent the truth or not." See Aristotle, *Parts of Animals*, A. L. Peck, trans. (Cambridge, 1937), 639a13–15.

[61] Note that these values represent only a sample of epistemic values. For example curiosity, intuition, falsifiability, and other so-called epistemic values have been left out. Also, there is no consensus on a unique set of epistemic values. For an excellent discussion on this topic, see Lacey, *Is Science Value-Free?*

[62] For example, the rejection of the geological theory of continental drift in favor of plate tectonics brought together previously unrelated fields (e.g., study of volcanoes and the study of the sea floor) within what is now geological science. See Naomi Oreskes and Homer Le Grand (eds), *Plate Tectonics: An Insider's History of the Modern Theory of the Earth* (Boulder, 2001).

[63] For example, Copernicus's attempt to explain retrograde motion did not require the use of any *major* epicycles as did Ptolemy's account. Since Copernicus postulated a fewer number of entities (i.e., epicycles), than Ptolemy did, his account is favored over Ptolemy's (everything else equal) based on simplicity or parsimony. See Thomas H. Kuhn, *The Copernican Revolution* (Cambridge, 1957).

[64] The theory of evolution/natural selection not only helps to explain biological organisms, but it also provided unexpected knowledge in paleontology, systematics, embryology, physics, and geography. See Michael Ruse, *Mystery of Mysteries: Is Evolution a Social Construction?* (Cambridge, 1999).

[65] Many of the experiments performed on the genetics of *Drosophila melanogaster* in Thomas Morgan's "fly room" were designed to confirm the hypotheses resulting from other experiments. See chapter sixteen of John A. Moore's *Science as a Way of Knowing: The Foundations of Modern Biology* (Cambridge, 1993), pp. 328–59 and Peter Lawrence, *The Making of a Fly: the Genetics of Animal Design* (Oxford, 1992).

(5) Internal Consistency—The parts of theories that are connected together without contradiction are favored over those that have internal contradictions.[66]

(6) Impartiality/Neutrality—A theory that is successful as a result of rigorously employing only epistemic values is superior to one that does not.[67]

In summary, when Agich claims that the practice of science includes particular values and conceptual values, he is referring to (1) non-epistemic values (e.g., social, political, personal, etc. values), (2) the overriding value of knowledge and truth, and (3) epistemic values that assist in the pursuit of knowledge and truth. Moreover, much like Longino's version of constructivism, Agich likely thinks that concept formation is value-laden in terms of the value-laden nature of human cognitive and non-cognitive systems and the value-laden nature of the goals and projects that humans pursue. This explains why Agich considers Boorse's description of science as "simplistic." (Using the language introduced in Chapter 3, Agich is a mixed normativist.) So, according to Agich, scientific concepts necessarily include all three sorts of values.

*Boorse's reply to Agich*   Boorse replies to Agich as follows:

> If health and disease are only as value-laden as astrophysics and inorganic chemistry, I am content. I admit having no sympathy for the view that scientific concepts or knowledge is evaluative. Obviously, we do science, as we do everything, for evaluative reasons. But I do not see why our motives for information gathering must infect the information gathered, injecting values into science, mathematics, and the Bell telephone directory. However, I leave defending the value-freedom of physics to physicists and philosophers thereof. If [my concept of health] shows that health in medicine is as objective as physics, it achieves everything I ever dreamt of for it.[68]

There are two parts to Boorse's reply to Agich. The first is his standard reply, but the second is rather unanticipated. First, much like his reply in Chapter 3 to mixed normativism, Boorse is unrepentant in defending a non-normativist position. Indeed, similar to his rejoinder to some of the other charges of covert normativism in this section, Boorse rejects the idea that norms are part of scientific concepts. Primarily, Boorse is claiming that being motivated by or with respect to **X** does not necessarily make it the case that the concept of **X** includes the norms that underlie such motivation. Notice that Boorse's reply to Agich is similar to the assessment

---

[66] As part of his discussion of the relationship between science and religion, Robert Root-Bernstein reveals the internal inconsistencies of those who claim that creationism is a legitimate theory (like those in science) of the origin of biological entities. See Robert Root-Bernstein, "On Defining A Scientific Theory: Creationism Considered," in Ashley Montagu (ed.), *Science and Creationism* (Oxford, 1984), pp. 64–94.

[67] In his analysis of the various theories of evolution from the time of Charles Darwin's grandfather (Erasmus Darwin) up through present day geneticists (e.g., Geoffrey Parker), Michael Ruse shows the steady transition from the inclusion of both non-epistemic and epistemic values in theories of evolution to the inclusion of only/mostly epistemic values in theories of evolution. See Ruse, *Mystery of Mysteries: Is Evolution a Social Construction?*

[68] Boorse, "A Rebuttal on Health," p. 56.

made by Poincaré at the beginning of this discussion. Poincaré's point is that, although there are values, desires, and interests with respect to the end(s) pursued by science, the means to achieve those ends are value-neutral. For example, if the end of medical science is to achieve a society in which most of its members are healthy, then even if it is the case that values are part of this end, it does not follow that the means to this end are value-laden. As Boorse notes through the use of his automobile analogy, "'perfect mechanical condition' in, say, a 1965 Volkswagen is a descriptive notion."[69] Thus, much like Poincaré, Boorse is a descriptivist in the sense presented by Lacey.

To some extent, Boorse's reply to Agich is not satisfactory. Admittedly, Agich makes a very strong claim by insisting that all three types of values are part of scientific concepts. It needs only to be shown that Agich's argument fails if any one of the value-types—especially the non-epistemic values—is not part of scientific concepts. Indeed, Michael Ruse goes to great lengths to show that the transitions in the history of biology reveal a move away from non-epistemic norms to epistemic norms. Ruse's findings are revealing. He says:

> [T]he history of evolutionism, from the middle of the eighteenth century to the end of the twentieth, is one of ever-greater manifestation and adherence to the epistemic norms ... Moving forward to this century, we see yet greater attempts to make evolutionary theorizing epistemically rigorous ... we can truly say that the epistemic norms play a major role in the structure of evolutionary theorizing and that their satisfaction is significantly above what it was in earlier times.[70]

If Ruse's claims above are on the mark, it could be the case that at some future date only epistemic norms would be part of biological concepts.[71] Thus, more generally, it might be possible to show that non-epistemic norms can be eliminated from scientific concepts by the diligent efforts of scientists themselves. The upshot of this possibility would render Agich's (and Longino's) argument unsound. So, it is possible (though not certain) that Boorse could have a persuasive reply to Agich.

Moreover, both Poincaré and Boorse make a legitimate claim that the values attached to particular ends do not necessarily attach themselves to the means to those ends. Formally, even if scientist **S** employs method **M** as means to bring about end **Y**, because **S** attaches a set of values **V** to **Y**, then it does not follow that **V** is part of the concept of **Y** given that **S** Employs **M** to bring about **Y**. For example, if providing the true concept of health is the end being pursued *qua* valued by medical science, both Boorse and Poincaré argue that the means to achieving that end do not include the values attached to such an end. The reason for this claim is that both authors think that the method **M** that brings about **Y** is what forms the concept of **Y**, not the set of values **V** for **Y**. Thus, the concept of health could not only exclude non-epistemic norms, but it could also exclude norms attached to the end(s) pursued

---

[69] Boorse, "On the Distinction Between Disease and Illness," p. 59.

[70] Ruse, *Mystery of Mysteries: Is Evolution a Social Construction?*, p. 237.

[71] Ruse goes on to note that non-epistemic values that help foster the ends of science should be understood as meta-values. These meta-values, notes Ruse, are values *"about* science, rather than *within* science." Ibid., p. 75.

by science. The further effect of this point is that two of the three types of norms that Agich considers ineliminable to the concept of health, namely non-epistemic values and the value of truth, could possibly be eliminated.

Still, it is possible to render Agich's argument in a disjunctive way rather than in his conjunctive approach. On this interpretation, even if it is the case that non-epistemic values and values attached to the goals of science are not necessarily part of scientific concepts,[72] it does not follow that epistemic values are not part of scientific concepts. If this were Agich's argument, then he could claim that Boorse's rejoinder is, at the very least, premature since it still needs to be determined whether or not scientific concepts are value-laden.

Indeed, Boorse's second point in his reply to Agich is that he acknowledges this disjunctive interpretation. Specifically, Boorse submits that if it is the case that there are norms that are part of the concepts in astrophysics and inorganic chemistry, then he concedes that his concept of health would also include such norms. It is somewhat surprising that Boorse would make this concession, given that he has defended the non-normativist position throughout his reply to his critics. But recall from Chapter 2 that Boorse is not really concerned with epistemic norms, but non-epistemic norms. So, even if it turned out to be the case that his concept of health includes epistemic norms, such a finding would neither reveal that he has conceded much nor that it renders a fatal blow to his analysis.

First, keeping in mind Boorse's inclusion of statistics in his naturalistic concept of health, it is clear that he does take metrical values seriously. Of course, in the debate between normativists and naturalists, the real issue is whether or not non-metrical values (e.g., moral norms) are included in the concept of health. No doubt, if accepting metrical values is what it means to be normativists, then Boorse would affably agree that he is a normativist. So, claiming that Boorse is a normativist because he accepts the use of metrical values within his concept of health is not a major part of the debate between normativists and naturalists.

Second, since Boorse does embrace science, he does think that it is truth about health that is the overarching goal. If this is correct, then he must think that statistics is a means to achieving this end. Thus, statistics has instrumental value (i.e., it is a useful means) with respect to bringing about truth. Specifically, Boorse's concept of health includes some of the instrumental values associated with statistics. These values include the epistemic values of explanatory power, simplicity, fecundity, replicability, internal consistency, and impartiality. Note that these values are not part of the goal of truth, but are part of the means to bring about truth. Such values would be part of any descriptive account, since such values are part of providing a good/acceptable scientific account. Ruse's comments on this point about epistemic values are instructive:

---

[72] Again, the history of biology tells against Boorse's non-normative stance. That is, it is clear that both epistemic and non-epistemic values were deeply connected to biological concepts from Charles Darwin to contemporary biologists like Richard Lewontin. See David J. Depew and Bruce Weber, *Darwinism Evolving: System Dynamics and The Genealogy of Natural Selection* (Cambridge, 1995) and Richard C. Lewontin, *Biology as Ideology: The Doctrine of DNA* (New York, 1992).

[O]bjectivists are surely right. There is a set or body of norms or values or constraints that guides scientists in their theorizing and observing: predictive accuracy, internal coherence, external consistency with the rest of science, unificatory power (consilience), predictive fertility, and to some degree simplicity or elegance. Satisfying this set of demands is the mark of good science—the kind of science one expects from a professional ... [These values] are above the vagaries of societal change or whim or fashion. In this sense, they are pointing toward truths about the real world: objectivity.[73]

The point is that, although Boorse could claim that the values attached to bringing about *the end* state of truth are not part of a descriptive concept of health, it is not clear that he could make this claim about the values attached to *the means* of bringing about a descriptive concept of health. Thus, much like it would be for the astrophysicist, the inorganic chemist, or the evolutionary biologist, epistemic values that are for the sake of truth are part of scientific concepts, including Boorse's concept of health. The upshot is that Agich could, at the very least, claim that Boorse should concede that he embraces epistemic norms. Unfortunately for Agich, such a concession is a minor one for Boorse within the normativism debate.

Finally, it may seem obvious that Boorse's concept of health includes only non-moral/social values. Since he embraces the practices of science, which employs mathematics to make sense of phenomena, there would appear to be no justification to think that Boorse would accept moral/social values into his concept of health. For the most part this is correct, but there is one major qualification that needs to be noted. Specifically, the use of metaphors in science suggests that cultural values (which may include moral values) may be part of scientific concepts. Ruse makes the point as follows with respect to evolutionary biology:

Although cultural values may have declined in evolutionary biology, in our evolutionizing today we still rely very heavily on many, many elements from our culture and that of our forefathers. A list comes to mind: struggle for existence, natural selection, sexual selection, adaptive landscape, dynamic equilibrium, arms race, and much more. These do not even start to include the more controversial and arguable notions, like selfish genes ... My point is that there is still something deeply cultural about evolutionary biology, even at its most mature or professional or praiseworthy level. Through the language, ideas, the pictures, the models, above all the metaphors that evolutionary biology uses, culture comes rushing right back in ... From the tree of life to evolutionary stable strategies, we have culturally rooted metaphors: an idea from one domain, that of culture, is taken and applied to another domain, that of organisms ... I would certainly agree that cultural values can seep back into science because of the use of cultural metaphors. It is difficult to think of evolutionary trees without getting progressionist, precisely because trees in our culture are associated with upward striving.[74]

---

[73] Ruse, *Mystery of Mysteries: Is Evolution a Social Construction?*, p. 236.

[74] Ibid., p. 239. Note that this account by Ruse is controversial. Many scientific terms are drawn from ordinary language, but given a more precise scientific connotation (e.g., "force," "gravity"). These terms have normative connotations in ordinary language that are no longer directly relevant in physics. Similarly, the biologist tries to give a value-free precise definition of terms like "selfish" and "altruistic." Ruse is aware of this concern and tries to handle it by making a distinction between *values* and *metavalues*. This distinction will be explained momentarily.

The above passage from Ruse suggests that cultural values are a deep part of the science of evolutionary biology. Ruse concedes that the role of cultural values has diminished considerably in the past few centuries, but that they are still quite prevalent.[75] Indeed, Susan Sontag argues just this point in her assessment of how cancer is described:

> The controlling metaphors in descriptions of cancer are, in fact, drawn not from economics but from the language of warfare: every physician and every attentive patient is familiar with, if perhaps inured to, this military terminology. Thus, cancer cells do not simply multiply; they are "invasive."[76]

Assuming that Ruse's depiction of the history of biology is on the mark and Sontag's claims above are accurate, it appears that cultural values are an integral part of the practices of science. Given that Boorse is wedded to the scientific enterprise, it follows that he should embrace cultural metaphors *qua* cultural values as part of his concept of health.

Of course, Boorse could simply reply that the history described by Ruse suggests that metaphors can and have been (in theory and practice) eliminated or greatly marginalized in the actual descriptions offered by contemporary scientists. As Jerry Fodor claims, "When you actually start to do science, the metaphors drop out and the statistics takes over."[77] Thus, Boorse could claim that it is possible to ignore cultural values by way of the actual descriptive statistical activities of scientists. The problem, however, is that Boorse himself employs the cultural metaphor of an automobile in his attempt to make sense of the human body (This metaphor/analogy was discussed in Chapter 4.) In modern Western society, the automobile is a prized machine because of its usefulness, appearance of precision, and its disclosure of social and economic status. So, even if Boorse's automobile metaphor does not reveal that he embraces moral values, it *might* suggest that he tacitly endorses certain cultural values associated with the wonders of the automobile (not necessarily the ones suggested here, but some set). Thus, it could be argued that Boorse's naturalistic concept of health does include cultural values.

No doubt, Boorse would object to the idea that his concept of health includes cultural values. This supposed problem between naturalism and values can be resolved by making a distinction between *values* and *metavalues*. The former refers to the values of science associated with epistemic values. These values include (though not limited to) explanatory power, simplicity, fecundity, replicability, internal consistency, and impartiality. It is the allegiance to these values by scientists

---

[75] Many years after *The Structure of Scientific Revolutions*, Thomas Kuhn described the relationship between metaphors and science as follows: "Metaphor plays an essential role in establishing links between scientific language and the world. Those links are not, however, given once and for all. Theory change, in particular, is accompanied by change in some of the relevant metaphors and in the corresponding parts of the network of similarities through which terms attach to nature." See Thomas Kuhn, "Metaphor in Science," in Andrew Ortony (ed.), *Metaphor and Thought*, 2nd edn (Cambridge, 1993), pp. 533–42.

[76] Susan Sontag, *Illness as Metaphor* (New York, 1978), p. 64.

[77] Jerry Fodor, "Peacocking," *London Review of Books*, 18 April 1996, p. 20.

that justifies their claim to objectivity. The latter refers to values that support epistemic values. That is, metavalues are values about science, rather than values that are within science. When scientists employ a metaphor/analogy from one area to help make scientific sense of a particular phenomenon, they do so with the goal of furthering epistemic values. So, when Boorse uses the automobile metaphor, he values this metaphor because he thinks it can help make sense of the human body without compromising explanatory power, simplicity, replicability, etc. That is, the automobile metaphor allows the scientist to see a similarity between automobiles and humans (and their respective parts) from which to sharpen theories and descriptions about what it means to be a healthy human. Again, Ruse makes the point about the importance of metaphors to science:

> [E]ven if metaphor could in theory be eliminated, no sensible scientist would ever think seriously of making such a move ... Most crucially, one would at once lose one of the most important of the epistemic values, namely, predictive fertility. Metaphors, as it is sometimes said, are absolutely vital for their "positive heuristic" as they push one into new fields and new forms of thinking ... Without metaphors—which are vehicles for seeing similarities in otherwise dissimilar things—one would lose a value so essential that in its absence science would simply grind to a halt.[78]

As Ruse makes clear, metaphors in science are an integral part of sustaining epistemic values in the pursuit of understanding, explaining, predicting, and describing phenomena. The upshot of this point is that it would be a mistake for Boorse not to include in some fashion the importance of metaphors to his concept of health.

Moreover, it does not follow that Boorse has to include cultural values within his concept of health on the grounds that he acknowledges the importance of metaphors to science. The reason is that, although epistemic values are part of scientific concepts, it does not follow that metavalues are part of scientific concepts. The fact that **X** (metavalues) supports **Y** (epistemic values), it does not follow that **X** (metavalues) is part of **Y** (epistemic values). For example, assume that an epidemiologist thinks that the best way to understand viral infections is by using war metaphors (e.g., "attack," "defense," "invasion," etc.). It does not follow from the fact that war metaphors are used in many social settings (e.g., sports) that the value society attaches to the use of such metaphors is part of the concept of virus. The reason is that the cogency of a particular metaphor as an explanatory tool in science is judged by the epistemic values of empirical success. If the war metaphor is useful in understanding and possibly eliminating a particular virus, then the usefulness of the metaphor is determined by the epistemic standards within science. Yet again, Ruse substantiates this point as follows:

> Through the metaphors of culture, predictions are made possible. But then the science produced can and must be judged simply by the epistemic standard of empirical success. However socially or culturally congenial one may find the science, if it does not succeed in the fiery pit of experience, it can and should be rejected.[79]

---

[78] Ruse, *Mystery of Mysteries: Is Evolution a Social Construction?*, p. 241.
[79] Ibid., p. 246.

Ruse's point is that cultural metaphors may give the impression that a particular theory, description, or explanation is true, because the accompanying metaphors have a familiarity through their cultural uses. Still, according to Ruse, the success of a theory, description, or explanation will be judged by the epistemic values within science. If the theory withstands scientific scrutiny, then the metaphor is retained because of its support of epistemic values. Conversely, if a theory, description, or explanation is abandoned because it does not meet the rigors imposed by epistemic values, then the metaphor is discarded. Thus, rather than seeing cultural values as part of Boorse's concept of health, they should properly be seen as values that support and espouse epistemic values, which are part of Boorse's concept of health.

The conclusion of this analysis is that the second part of Agich's claim, that science includes values, is partially on the mark. Boorse is a covert normativist to the extent that he does embrace epistemic values. Indeed, Boorse's challenge that he is willing to accept those values that are part of astrophysics and inorganic chemistry has been met. Specifically, Boorse's concept of health necessarily includes epistemic values.

In this section, some of the major objections to Boorse's non-normative concept of health were presented. First, Fulford argued that norms are present in Boorse's concept of health as a result of his slide form normative to non-normative terms. Second, Hare insisted that the concept of health is value-laden based on the badness of the effects of a physical condition on a person. Third, Engelhardt defended the view that Boorse's concept of disease is unsatisfactory, because the norms that encompass the doctor-patient relationship are covertly present. Fourth, Miller Brown pronounced Boorse's concept of health is normative to the extent that choices have to be made as to which goals in a system merit privilege. Fifth, Agich argued that since science is value-laden and Boorse embraces the practices of science, his scientific concept of health is also normative. Along with Boorse's reply to these criticisms, this section offered a rejoinder to each of Boorse's replies. The results of this analysis are that Boorse is successful in his replies to Fulford, Hare, and Engelhardt, somewhat successful in his reply to Miller Brown, and partially successful in his reply to Agich. More generally, with respect to the issue of normativism, it is clear that Boorse's concept of health has not suffered much damage.

*The Charge of Bad Biology*

There are three criticisms levied against Boorse's understanding of biological entities in the light of evolutionary/Darwinian accounts of *species design*. The first criticism is introduced by Engelhardt (and reinforced by Win J. van der Steen and P. J. Thung), who claims that Boorse relies on an antiquated understanding of biology that emphasizes uniformity rather than variation within and across species. The second criticism is put forth by Wim J. van der Steen and P. J. Thung. These authors claim that Boorse's construction of an "ideal species type" runs counter to contemporary accounts of biological classification. The third criticism is put forth by Engelhardt and Jerome Wakefield. These authors argue that, since Boorse thinks that an evolutionary concept of function is correct, he cannot make sense of the present functions of organisms. The upshot of these criticisms is that Boorse's concept of health, which relies on a poor account of the biological concepts of species, disease, and function, is untenable.

*Bad Biology Number 1*

To begin, Engelhardt offers his criticism as follows:

> Views such as Boorse's tend to gloss over the important role of intraspecies variability, while at the same time imposing the survival of species as an overriding good. Given an evolutionary biology and variability within a species (not to mention the variability of environments and therefore variability as to what will be functional or dysfunctional), there is no absolute standard with regard to which one can identify an organism as healthy ... *There is simply no single natural design* ... Rather, there are variations, including aging and even special debilities, which may play their role in the overall survival of a particular species. What will count as successful function in one environment may count as disease in another ...[80] There may not be a single design, but rather a number of designs. When such is the case, one cannot speak straightforwardly of either species design or species typicality ...[81]

In the above passage, Engelhardt claims that Boorse thinks that species design is a fixed notion. The result of this error, thinks Engelhardt, is that Boorse does not have an accurate understanding of biological bodies that are the product of evolutionary adaptation. In what is to follow, an explanation of these points by Engelhardt will be provided, followed by Boorse's reply, and an assessment of Boorse's reply.

In philosophical terms, Engelhardt claims that Boorse accepts the idea that tokens of a species type not only share, at least, some identical properties in common, but that there exists a unique immutable species-type. The problem with accepting this fixed notion of species and properties, argues Engelhardt, is that there are no identical characteristics shared by biological tokens. Van der Steen and Thung (hereafter VT) echo Engelhardt's criticism when they claim that taxonomists "nowadays emphatically reject the typological way of thinking ... Philosophers concentrating on taxonomy share their opinion."[82]

Engelhardt's reason for rejecting natural kind species-design is that there is enough variation in each biological entity from the "genetic lottery" that no two tokens of a type will share any identical property. Restated, a Darwinian view of organisms rejects the notion of fixed natural properties (i.e., the rejection of universals or real essences). Rather, an evolutionary perspective on biological entities emphasizes variation in natural design such that there is a family resemblance amongst token entities, but no "real" ideal type of resemblance.[83] Thus, Engelhardt and VT conclude

---

[80] Engelhardt, "Ideology and Etiology," p. 264.
[81] Engelhardt, *The Foundations of Bioethics*, p. 168.
[82] Wim J. van der Steen and P. J. Thung, *Faces of Medicine: A Philosophical Study* (Dordrecht, 1988), p. 88. Note that VT are referring to the philosopher of biology, David Hull and his article, "The Effect of Essentialism on Taxonomy: Two Thousand Years of Stasis," *British Journal of the Philosophy of Science*, 15/60 (1965): 314–26.
[83] See L. Van Valen, "Morphological Variation and the Width of Ecological Niche," *American Naturalist*, 99/3 (1965): 377–90 and Kenneth J. Halama and David N. Reznick,

that Boorse's concept of health, which relies on a fixed notion of species design, is unserviceable to the concept of health in the light of a Darwinian world-view.

*Boorse's reply to Engelhardt (and VT)*   In response to both Engelhardt's and VT's charge of incorporating obsolete biology into his concept of health, Boorse reminds these critics of his view about species design. Specifically, he notes that they have ignored his resistance to Aristotelian essentialism[84] and his account of "empirical ideal." With respect to the latter, Boorse reminds these authors of what he said:

> It would be a mistake to think that this notion of a species design is inconsistent with evolutionary biology, which emphasizes constant variation. The typical result of evolution is precisely a trait's becoming established in a species, only rarely showing major variations under individual inheritance and environment. On all but evolutionary time scales, biological designs have a massive constancy vigorously maintained by *normalizing selection*. It is this short-term constancy on which the theory and practice of medicine rely.[85]

As Boorse correctly notes, he is sensitive to the evolutionary underpinnings of biological entities. When he uses the term "fixed design," he means a design that is *stable* in the short-run as a result of selection pressure. Indeed, Boorse does not endorse in any of his written work the sort of typological thinking that Engelhardt and VT claim he does endorse.

In fact, Boorse's use of "stabilizing condition" further supports his allegiance to (at least some) concepts in evolutionary biology. Specifically, "natural selection" usually refers to three distinct sorts of selection processes: (1) directional, (2) stabilizing, and (3) disruptive. To clarify these different senses of "natural selection," beak size will be the character trait used. Also, assume that half-inch and two-inch beak sizes represent extremes. First, "directional section" refers to cases in which there is selection pressure in favor of certain beak sizes. For example, if evidence reveals that one-inch beaks are more successful (i.e., increase in production of offspring) than two-inch beaks, and that there is a trend toward smaller beak sizes, then (so long as the differences are heritable) natural selection is said to be directional.[86]

Second, "stabilizing selection" refers to cases in which there is selection pressure in favor of a particular beak size (e.g., one-inch). For example, imagine that whenever a given bird population deviates from the one-inch beak size, there is a tendency to return the population to this one-inch beak size. In this scenario, natural selection

---

"Adaptation, Optimality, and the Meaning of Phenotypic Variation in Natural Populations," in Steven Hecht Orzack and Elliott Sober (eds), *Adaptationism and Optimality* (Cambridge, 2001), pp. 242–72.

[84]   Christopher Boorse, "Health as a Theoretical Concept," *Philosophy of Science*, 44/4 (1977): 554.

[85]   Ibid., p. 557 [my italics].

[86]   As a result of intense fishing for large pink salmon in British Columbia since the 1950s, there has been directional selection in favor of small-sized salmon. See W. E. Ricker, "Changes in the Average Size and Average Age of Pacific Salmon," *Canadian Journal of Fisheries and Aquatic Science*, 38 (1981), 1636–56.

works against change, and keeps the population's beak-size constant through time.[87] Evidence suggests that stabilizing selection is more common than either directional selection or disruptive selection.[88]

Third, "disruptive selection" refers to cases in which selection favors the extreme beak sizes as opposed to intermediate sizes. In such cases, the intermediate beak size is not able to flourish in the wake of harsh environmental conditions. Rather, the half-inch and two-inch beak sizes diverge and proliferate.[89]

With these different senses of "natural selection" clarified, Boorse's account can be elucidated. Much like the case in which the one-inch beak-size is stabilized in a population of birds when there is a certain degree of disruption, Boorse is claiming that this is how physiological features (in general) in organisms ought to be understood. He notes that major changes do occur on geologic time scales, but that in the short run stabilizing selection (as opposed to directional or disruptive selection) is the proper way to understand the state of functional traits of organisms. Thus, it is now clear that by "constancy" Boorse is referring to the process of stabilizing selection.

As it stands, then, Engelhardt and VT have attacked a straw person version of Boorse's actual position. Indeed, it this trivializing of Boorse's position that leads him to conclude that these authors "seem too concerned with my efforts to show continuity between ancient and modern disease concepts, and too little with my efforts to distinguish them."[90] Thus, Boorse is correct to dismiss this first criticism offered by Engelhardt and VT.

*Bad Biology Number 2*

VT offer the second critical point made against Boorse's use of biology. They argue that Boorse has completely underemphasized the importance of environmental factors that contribute to what it means to be a normal or abnormal biological entity. This lack of concern for environmental factors leads them to consider Boorse's biology too simplistic or elementary. The details of their criticism are as follows:

> Boorse's conception of design becomes inadequate even within physiology, his favorite discipline, as one leaves the realm of elementary textbooks of medical physiology. The physiological functions change with the environment, *so there are no reference values simpliciter*. Reference-values will have to be *context-dependent*. They are sensible only if they are related to the environment besides age and sex. Blood cell counts change with

---

[87] Stabilizing selection is apparent in the weight of human babies. Data reveals that infants weighing eight pounds at birth have a higher survival rate than lighter or heavier children. See L. Ulizzi and L. Terrenato, "Natural Selection Associated with Birth Rate," *Annals of Human Genetics*, 56 (1992): 113–18.

[88] This point is made by Mark Ridley, *Evolution*, 2nd edn (Cambridge, 1996), p. 75. Much of this discussion on the different senses of "natural selection" owes to Ridley's efforts.

[89] This actually occurred in the beak size of finches on the Galapagos Islands in the wake of El Niño. Also, experimental research on fruit flies has revealed the actuality of disruptive selection. See both Jonathan Weiner, *The Beak of the Finch* (New York, 1994) and J. M. Thoday and J. B. Gibson, "Isolation by Disruptive Selection," *Nature*, 193 (1962): 1164–6.

[90] Boorse, "A Rebuttal on Health," p. 40.

altitude, metabolic rates with temperature, and so on. Clinical diagnosis in fact makes allowances for such items. Many conditions, which are pathological according to Boorse's definition, may be biologically normal in some, and abnormal in other environments. Plain biology would not justify their being classified as diseases in our nomenclatures.

Boorse apparently wants to use idealizations representing optimal designs in hypothetical environments without pathogens and harsh physical conditions. Such environments are not very "biological." They represent ideals one would like to realize. Boorse's idealizations are nonsense in the context of biology.[91]

The point that VT make in the above passage is that, by abstracting away from the particular details of organisms in their environments, Boorse's account cannot accommodate the fact that organisms (or their parts) can only be deemed healthy or diseased based on how they actually function in their local environments. It is Boorse's lack of attention to environmental considerations, argue VT, that makes his biology "bad biology."

*Boorse's reply to VT* To address the above criticism adequately, recall that Boorse's ideal-type is a portrait constructed out of actual token parts of organisms observed by pathologists. That is, the portrait of a functioning part (e.g., kidneys) on Boorse's functional concept of health is a statistical generalization of how token parts (e.g., token kidneys) actually function. In defense of his account, Boorse turns to the work of Ernst Mayr:

> All organisms and organic phenomena are composed of unique features and can be described collectively only in statistical terms. Individuals ... form populations of which we can determine only the arithmetic mean and the statistics of variation. Averages are merely statistical abstractions ... The ultimate conclusions of the population thinker and of the typologist are precisely opposite. For the typologist, the type (*eidos*) is real and the variation an illusion, while for the populationist the type (average) is an abstraction and only the variation is real. No two ways of looking at nature could be more different.[92]

Given the above account from Mayr, Boorse concludes that his understanding of species design is consonant with the idea that a species is "a variable population of unique individuals for whom a statistical abstraction of normal functioning defines health."[93]

Boorse's reply to VT is not very satisfying. Specifically, neither he nor Mayr address carefully the role of the environment in their account. The issue at hand is whether or not environmental considerations are lost in such statistical abstractions. If the role of the environment is eliminated as result of statistical abstraction, then both Boorse and Mayr (and biologists in general) may be at fault. Alternatively, if the role of the environment is included in such statistical abstractions, then the criticism of VT loses much of its force. Unfortunately, Boorse does not offer any

---

[91] van der Steen and Thung, *Faces of Medicine: A Philosophical Study*, p. 90 [italics in original].

[92] See Ernst Mayr, "Typological Versus Population Thinking," in Ernst Mayr, *Evolution and the Diversity of Life* (Cambridge, 1976), pp. 27 and 28.

[93] Boorse, "A Rebuttal on Health," p. 40.

other support for his position. To this extent, Boorse has not given a powerful reply to this second criticism offered by VT.

Still, assume that a statistical concept of health does include a role for the environment. Is Boorse's reply then satisfactory? The answer would be no. The reason is that VT argue that an environment is a constantly changing domain. The fact that statistical analysis could acknowledge the environment as part of its abstraction is unhelpful because the abstracted environment would not capture the actual dynamics of a genuine environment in constant flux. For Boorse to offer a serious rejoinder to VT, he would need to address this point in one of two ways. He could argue that a statistical concept of health does capture a fluctuating environment in its abstraction from token environments. Alternatively, he could argue against a constantly changing environment of the sort envisioned by VT. Unfortunately, Boorse offers no such reply in either direction. Thus, Boorse has no offered a persuasive reply to VT.

*Bad Biology Number 3*

A few authors have argued that Boorse's concept of function, as it relates to his concept of disease, is problematic because the former relies on evolutionary biology, which obscures an understanding of the latter. Engelhardt states his concern as follows:

> One cannot simply turn to the results of evolution to determine what a disease is. We are the product of blind, selective forces, which, if they have been successful, have adapted us to environments in which we no longer live. Since what is species typical may represent an adaptation to environments in which we no longer live, it may not afford us the same degree of adaptation as that provided by some species-atypical trait.[94]

Wakefield makes a similar claim as Engelhardt, but he endorses the importance of evolution. He says that Boorse was

> right to [think] that there must be an evolutionary foundation to our judgments of disorder ... However, the biological disadvantage approach mistakenly uses deceased longevity and fertility in the present environment as the criterion for mechanism dysfunction. The fact that the organism's mechanisms were originally selected because they increased longevity and fertility in a past environment does not imply that some mechanism is malfunctioning when longevity and fertility decrease in the present environment. Thus, despite its evolutionary roots, the biological disadvantage definition actually fails to require a dysfunction and thus is subject to counterexamples.[95]

*Boorse's reply to Engelhardt and Wakefield* Both Engelhardt and Wakefield think that Boorse's recruitment of evolutionary theory to his concept of health is misguided.

---

[94] Engelhardt, *The Foundations of Bioethics*, p. 169. Variations on this same criticism are offered by Martin Bunzl, "Discussion: Comment on 'Health as a Theoretical Concept'," *Philosophy of Science*, 47/1 (1980): 116–18 and William K. Goosens, "Values, Health, and Medicine," *Philosophy of Science*, 47/1 (1980): 100–115.

[95] Jerome C. Wakefield, "The Concept of Mental Disorder: On the Boundary Between Biological Facts and Social Values," *American Psychologist*, 47/3 (1992): 379.

Boorse's reply to each author is now in order. First, in reply to Engelhardt, Boorse notes that he is not necessarily wedded to an evolutionary or etiological concept of function. In an attempt to remind Engelhardt that he has argued against an etiological concept of function (of which an evolutionary concept of function is a version), he notes how his concept of function is distinct from Wright's concept of function:

> Regarding function, a contrast between Wright's view and mine is that I require a function to be an actual contribution to a goal, whereas Wright says that something can "have" a function that it no longer performs.[96]

The details of Boorse's reply to Wright will not be rehashed here (see Chapter 4). The important point to remember is that Boorse rejects the etiological account of function defended by Wright. Rather, as Boorse claims above, it is the current/actual functions of parts of organisms that are important in determining whether or not such parts are healthy or diseased. The point is that Boorse is quite clear that he does not defend an evolutionary concept of function. Indeed, Boorse makes just this point as follows:

> For biologists, the standard abilities of organisms are adaptations to their environments ... The notion cannot be "Darwinian fitness," or pure reproductive success. Parents hardly become healthier with each successive child, nor would anyone maintain that the healthiest traits are the ones that promote large families.[97]

Thus, Boorse thinks that Engelhardt's criticism is off the mark.

No doubt, Boorse is correct to point out that Engelhardt has overlooked his analysis of Wright's concept of function (much of the literature fails in this regard as well) and his own resistance to evolution. The problem with Boorse's reply is that even if he does not accept an evolutionary concept of function, he does endorse a dispositional concept of function. Recall from Chapter 4 that Boorse claims that "[a]n organism or its part is directed to a goal **G** when *disposed*, throughout a range of environmental variation, to modify its behavior in the way required for **G**."[98] Being disposed to achieve or bring about **G** does not necessarily require that the parts of an organism be *actually* bringing about **G** at time t. Thus, Boorse does not want to claim (as he does in reply to Engelhardt) that functions are limited to actual goal-directed behavior. Nonetheless, Boorse is clear that he rejects an etiological/evolutionary concept of function.

Now, in his reply to Wakefield, Boorse claims the following:

> I do see a species as extending over time as well as space, so for me some of the past affects what is species-typical ... Human beings suffer many difficulties rooted in the fact that our physiology ... evolved to fit a different way of life, such as primitive hunter-gatherer society.[99]

---

[96] Boorse, "A Rebuttal on Health," p. 66.
[97] Boorse, "Health as a Theoretical Concept," p. 548.
[98] Ibid., p. 9.
[99] Boorse, "A Rebuttal on Health," p. 66.

Boorse's reply to Wakefield reveals a problem that has been hinted at throughout this analysis; namely that Boorse is caught in a contradiction as a result of his concept of function. In the above passage, Boorse is clear that he wants his concept of function to respect the fact that functions (at least some) are a product of a certain Darwinian history. This point is also clear (in his reply to Engelhardt and VT) when Boorse claims that he defends a stabilizing selection interpretation of natural selection. Yet, it is just this sort of Wrightian etiological account that he was at pains to reject in his reply to Engelhardt. So, sometimes Boorse agrees that his concept of function includes an etiological/evolutionary dimension, but at other times he is adamant that his concept of function does not include an etiological/evolutionary dimension. Clearly, Boorse is not consistent with respect to his concept of function. The result is that not only is Boorse's reply to Wakefield unpersuasive, but it also reveals that he has not provided a persuasive concept of function. Indeed, Boorse's biology is bad, because he does not make clear what exactly is his considered view with respect to his concept of function.

This section on Boorse's "bad biology" reveals that following three points. First, Boorse offers a persuasive reply to Engelhardt and VT's charge that he does not have a clear understanding of what an evolved species is. Second, it was made clear that Boorse's reply to VT's claim that he cannot accommodate real environments in flux is not very persuasive. Third, in reply to Engelhardt and Wakefield, Boorse inconsistently endorses and rejects survival and reproduction as part of his concept of function. This inconsistency suggests that his concept of function is not entirely persuasive.

*The Charge of Bad Medicine*

In this final set of objections, critics argue against how Boorse understands the field of medicine. Margolis and Miller Brown balk at Boorse's claim that there really is genuine theory in medicine. In contrast, Germund Hesslow concedes that there is genuine theory in the biomedical sciences and Boorse's concepts of health and disease are most likely correct in this arena. He goes on to argue, however, that such theoretical concepts of health and disease defended by Boorse are irrelevant to clinical decision-making.

*Bad Medicine Number 1*

In an attempt to make sense of health and disease, Margolis argues the following about medicine:

> [It] is primarily an art and, dependently, a science: it is primarily an institutionalized service concerned with the care and cure of the ill and the control of disease, in facilitating which certain purely descriptive and causal inquiries are pursued ... [S]ince medicine in general must subserve, however conservatively, the determinate ideology and ulterior goals of given societies, the actual conception of diseases cannot but reflect the state

of the technology, the social expectations, the division of labor, and the environmental conditions of those populations.[100]

In the spirit of Margolis's claims above, Miller Brown makes a similar assessment. He concedes that "it is theory, not practice which Boorse seeks to analyse,"[101] but he goes on to argue as follows:

> Medicine is largely a practical activity since it is concerned with diagnosis and treatment of illness, usually as a matter of medical crisis; and, as such, it is more akin to a technology ... As a practical discipline, medicine and its concepts of "disease" and "health" are bound up with medical practice and the interests of doctors and patients as well as with the advances of science. And it is this fact which adds to the complexity and variety that confounds efforts to find simple definitions ... There can be, then, only in a derivative sense a theoretical medicine, and accordingly it makes little sense to argue that "disease" is a theoretical concept of medicine...[102]

The criticism offered by Miller Brown (and noted by Margolis) is straightforward. He thinks that Boorse's naturalistic *qua* theoretical concepts of health and disease are misguided, because they are not appropriate to the ends of medicine. It is the diagnosis *and* treatment of an ill patient, argues Miller Brown, over which the concept of health and disease must extend. Once these ends are understood as the ends of medicine, then appropriate concepts of health and disease can be proffered. In effect, Miller Brown and Margolis are claiming that Boorse's theoretical concepts of health and disease may be appropriate to the field of biology, but they are simplistic in the medical arena. Their justification is that Boorse's concepts of health and disease do not acknowledge the doctor-patient relationship and the social background as the reason for such concepts. Thus, Margolis and Miller Brown conclude that Boorse has over-simplified the concepts of health and disease.

*Boorse's reply to Margolis and Miller Brown*  Boorse offers the following blunt reply to both Margolis and Miller Brown:

> This objection seems to me of that rare variety which can be answered in one word: "pathology." Pathology, one of the "basic sciences" studied in the first or second year of medical school, is the scientific study of disease. It is based on anatomy, physiology, biochemistry, genetics, and other biological sciences, but is distinctively medical in being wholly devoted to disease ... Since it certainly uses the term "disease," it is the venue of a scientific, theoretical, medical disease concept unless either pathology is not science, or not theoretical, or not medicine. To call it unscientific would be odd, since, of the various demarcation tests philosophers of science have proposed, pathology seems to pass every one that biology passes.[103]

---

[100] Joseph Margolis, "The Concept of Disease," *Journal of Medicine and Philosophy*, 1/3 (1976): 242 and 252 [bracketed additions mine].
[101] Brown "On Defining 'Disease'," p. 315.
[102] Ibid., p. 326.
[103] Boorse, "A Rebuttal on Health," p. 52.

Believing that he has established that pathology is a science, Boorse adds the following reply to Miller Brown:

> I don't know why one must in this way read pathology out of medicine ... Does [Miller Brown] realize that there is an actual discipline called "pathology" that counts as one of the basic sciences, is housed almost entirely in medical schools, and so is, one would think, part of medicine and a suitable venue for medical theory? ... Even if one declares pathology part of biology, it is still a scientific discipline concerned with disease ... Thus, whether pathology is biology or medicine, [my concept of health] can claim that it furnishes medicine with a basic scientific concept of disease as a scaffold on which medicine, and society at large, can build clinical and social disease concepts.[104]

Boorse's reply to Margolis and Miller Brown is clear. It has three parts. First, Boorse claims that his theoretical concepts of health and disease are ineliminable aspects of medicine. His justification is that pathology, which is the study of disease, is an integral part of the early stages of medical training. It is this elementary training that lays the foundation for the rest of medical training. Thus, according to Boorse, for Margolis and Miller Brown to claim that medicine does not include a theoretical foundation distinct from social and clinical norms is simply false.

Second, Boorse claims that the field of pathology satisfies all the criteria given by philosophers of science of what a science is. It can be inferred that Boorse is referring to some combination of the epistemic values noted in the previous section. Thus, **X** is a science if and only if **X** adheres to epistemic values. Since, according to Boorse, pathology does adhere to epistemic values, it follows that pathology is a genuine science. Therefore, Boorse concludes that Miller Brown is wrong to consider pathology unscientific.

Third, Boorse points out in the second quotation that it is unclear why Miller Brown (and indirectly Margolis) is so adamant about excluding his theoretical concepts of health and disease from medicine. Boorse points out that his theoretical account can been seen as a foundation or framework from which Miller Brown's patient-centered concepts of health and disease can be understood. Thus, rather than being a simplistic view of medicine, Boorse is arguing that his account provides a necessary foundation to complement the clinical and social dimensions of medicine noted by Margolis and Miller Brown.

Boorse's overall reply to Margolis and Miller Brown is persuasive for the following reasons. It is the case that medical training takes pathology as one of its foundations. Indeed, the pathologists Christian Nezelof and Thomas Seemayer concur with Damjanov and Linder when they claim that "pathology is one of the basic medical sciences and is vital to the understanding of disease and hence its appropriate treatment."[105] Rodney Markin and James Linder claim that "[t]he practice of pathology produces vast amounts of *data*, which are communicated to physicians and others. As these individuals process the data, it becomes information that guides clinical decisions. The data and their availability influence greatly the

---

[104] Ibid., pp. 52 and 53 [bracketed addition mine].

[105] C. Nezelof and T. A. Seemayer, "A History of Pathology: An Overview," in Ivan Damjanov and James Linder (eds), *Anderson's Pathology*, p. 1.

decisions made in the care of the patient."[106] Nezelof and Seemayer make it clear that pathology is foundational in medicine and that treatment of diseases requires the study of pathology. Moreover, Markin and Linder add that this foundation of pathology does guide clinical decisions. The point is that pathology does include theoretical concepts, which produce information that is used by doctors for treatment. The autopsy pathologists, Bruce McManus and Shelina Babul, make just this point when they advise that "[t]he need to understand the distinction between immediate, proximate, and remote causes of death, mechanisms of death, and the manner of death should be stressed to medical students at key points in their educational programs. The confusion of cause of death with mechanism of death is frequent."[107] Thus, Boorse is correct that pathology *qua* scientific study of disease is one of the foundations of medicine that employs theoretical concepts.[108]

The second part of Boorse's reply to Miller Brown is a fair generalization, but it must be made clear that there are some sub-disciplines in pathology that are more scientific than other sub-disciplines. For example, surgical pathology does not appear to be as rigorous a sub-discipline as other sub-disciplines in pathology with respect to replicability of its findings (Recall that replicability of findings is a fundamental epistemic value to the practice of science.). Pathologists Richard Cote and Clive Taylor offer the following confession about the sub-discipline of surgical pathology:

> Surgical pathology is an inherently subjective discipline. Although "standard" histologic criteria can be described for virtually all diagnoses, in fact overlap among different entities and dissimilarities among the same entity can be enormous. This is compounded by the subjective evaluation by the individual pathologist, each of whom varies in skill, training, experience, patience, and local habits ... In the clinical laboratory, intralaboratory variation can be minimized through a variety of quality assurance programs. However, these programs are less easily applied to surgical pathology.
>
> Unlike many precise assays and numerical results (with normal reference ranges) that emanate from the clinical laboratory, the surgical pathology report itself also invites clinical misrepresentation, not only because of its inherent subjectivity (alluded to above),

---

[106] Rodney S. Markin and James Linder, "Informatics," in Ivan Damjanov and James Linder (eds), *Anderson's Pathology*, p. 110.

[107] Bruce M. McManus and Shelina Babul, "The Autopsy," in Ivan Damjanov and James Linder (eds), *Anderson's Pathology*, p. 25.

[108] Jeremy R. Jass, a professor of pathology, echoes this point. He claims that the anatomical aspect of pathology "is based on use of the microscope to examine wafer thin sections ... to achieve a diagnosis on behalf of a living patient. A diagnosis is reached rather in the same way that an art expert distinguishes a genuine Rembrandt from a forgery—by careful examination supported by education and experience. The central importance of the discipline of anatomical pathology rests upon the provision of an accurate diagnosis. Diagnosis is the hub around which all subsequent therapeutic decisions turn. Medicine is often described as a blend of art and science, and as a medical subspecialty pathology might be perceived similarly. However, I would argue that pathology leans much more towards being a science than an art and its practice characterised by a meticulous and highly organised approach." See Jeremy R. Jass, *Understanding Pathology: From Disease Mechanisms to Clinical Practice* (Amsterdam, 1999), p. 13.

but also because it is a narrative report in a nonstandard format. Recommendations have been made as to the standard content of surgical pathology reports in certain conditions. However, in most cases the organization of a surgical report is as much a reflection of the institution at which the pathologist trained as anything else.

The implication then is that the subjectivity that is inherent to the surgical pathology diagnostic process may result in a lack of reproducibility among pathologists. Rigorous studies of the accuracy and reliability of histopathologic diagnosis, comparing surgical pathologists across a broad range of diseases, are rare.[109]

This frank assessment by Cote and Taylor of their own discipline is a reminder that, although pathology in general is a mature science, there are some specific areas within the general discipline that are less rigorous than others. Specifically, if replicability of experiments is a crucial aspect of a genuine science, then surgical pathology is not yet up to par. This fact does not condemn Boorse's general reply to Miller Brown, but it does reveal that there is room for scientific maturation within the field of pathology.

This section provided Margolis's and Miller Brown's objections to Boorse's concepts of health and disease. The basic criticism that they offer is that Boorse's concepts of health and disease are not really part of the practice of medicine. It was revealed that, through his discussion of the role of pathology in medicine, Boorse's overall reply to them is quite persuasive, even granting that his generalization about the scientific nature of pathology must be slightly modified.

*Bad Medicine Number 2*

The final critique of Boorse's concept of health comes from Germund Hesslow. In general, Hesslow thinks that Boorse's concepts of health and disease are correct, but they are useless and irrelevant with respect to medical decision-making.[110] Hesslow's three-part analysis unfolds as follows. First, he acknowledges that there are at least three good reasons for pursuing definitions of scientific terms. They are as follows:

1. Specific concepts (e.g., "force," "adaptation," "money") require precise definitions because they have important intellectual and practical benefits (e.g., the definition of "money supply" determines the empirical content of certain economic theories, and will affect predictions of future inflation as well as the choice of appropriate economic policy).
2. Clear definitions are crucial to understanding scientific theories (e.g., an understanding of space is crucial for understanding theories in physics.).
3. Clear definitions are useful for communicating within and across disciplines (e.g., it does not matter much from a theoretical point which processes are called *learning*, but it may be useful for scientific communication to have a common terminology.)[111]

---

[109] Richard J. Cote and Clive R. Taylor, "Immunohistochemistry and Related Marking Techniques," in Ivan Damjanov and James Linder (eds), *Anderson's Pathology*, p. 136.

[110] Germund Hesslow, "Do We Need a Concept of Disease?" *Theoretical Medicine*, 14/1 (1993): 6.

[111] Ibid., pp. 4–5 [my italics].

Second, after providing the above three reasons for needing definitions, he offers the following summary judgment:

> It is my contention that none of the above motives for conceptual analysis apply to the concepts of disease and illness. There is no biomedical theory in which disease appears as a theoretical entity and there are no laws or generalizations linking disease to other important variables. Therefore, there is no need for an analysis that makes a theory more determinate or understandable, and there is no need for operational definitions.[112]

Basically, Hesslow is arguing that there are neither theoretical nor practical reasons for offering a concept of health or a concept of disease. His rejection of theoretical reasons is based on his belief that there is no theory in medicine in which disease is understood as a theoretical entity. For example, the gene is a theoretical entity in biology. Atoms, quanta, and strings could be thought of as theoretical entities in physics. In medicine, however, Hesslow is claiming is that there is no corresponding entity, laws, or theoretical generalizations that connect disease states with other variables to understand bodily activities.

Moreover, he rejects practical reasons in favor of retaining the concepts of disease and health, because he sees no practical or important use for them. As Hesslow makes the point,

> The mere fact that a term is frequently used in a scientific discipline, however, does not mean that it is also theoretically or practically important, or that philosophers or scientists should spend time in clarifying its meaning. Ecologists frequently speak of forests and deserts, biologists of animals and plants, physiologists of cells and hormones and economists of money markets and industries. All of these terms are vague. Yet, neither scientists nor philosophers think it important to enquire about the meanings of industry, hormone, plant or forest (except, perhaps, when the need for operational definitions arise).[113]

Third, Hesslow is aware that there may be a number of other practical reasons that justify the importance of pursuing the concepts of health and disease. He notes the following four:

1. Medical treatment is motivated by disease.
2. Medical compensation through welfare schemes or insurance requires that it be known whether or not a disease is present in the person who is to be compensated.
3. A diseased person may be excused from certain moral obligations.
4. A diseased person (especially a mentally diseased person) may be excused from moral responsibility and legal liability.[114]

Hesslow rejects each of the above practical reasons that might be given in favor of retaining the concepts of health and disease. First, he replies that medical treatment is not motivated by disease. He mentions that many pathological conditions (e.g., benign

---

[112] Ibid., p. 5.
[113] Ibid., p. 5.
[114] Ibid., pp. 7–10.

tumors, birthmarks, and small fibromas) are not treated, while other pathological conditions (e.g., sterility) are intentionally induced. Given the different treatments for different pathological conditions, Hesslow thinks that patient discomfort or potential dangers to a patient motivate medical treatment. The concepts of health and disease, insists Hesslow, should be seen as unnecessary "straitjackets" with respect to the ultimate goals (According to Hesslow, these goals are the care and treatment for patient discomfort and suffering and treatments that can contend with potential dangers to patients) of clinical medicine.[115] Thus, Hesslow rejects the idea that medical treatment is motivated by refined concepts of health and disease.

Second, Hesslow argues that, although insurance companies need to guard themselves against exploitation, they only need to apply consistently a given definition of disease across cases. Moreover, he notes that the rationale of medical insurance schemes "is to spread risk more evenly for events which are costly, difficult or impossible to predict, outside the control of the individual and undesirable by most everyone."[116] He concludes that consistent application of a definition of a disease and how to contend with difficult cases with an eye to spreading risk "are certainly not dealt with by philosophical discussions about the true meaning of "disease.""[117]

Third, Hesslow claims that it is the long-term suffering, and not the concept of disease, that allows for people to be excused from their usual moral obligations. "If we take the right not to work ... it is not justified by disease *per se* but rather by the discomforts, pains or anxiety, or by the risk of future discomforts, that might result in not working."[118] Much like his comments about insurance schemes, Hesslow concludes that difficult cases are not solved by appealing to a particular concept of disease, but by the specifics of the job and the discomfort associated with continuing to work.

Fourth, Hesslow points out that it is the inability to calculate the future consequences of their actions that is the real justification behind giving moral and legal allowances to those people who are considered mentally ill.[119] According to Hesslow, punishment is designed to discourage potential criminals and to reinforce in felons the consequences of their actions. In the case of mentally ill individuals, it is frequently the case that neither can they be discouraged nor can they be punished for the consequences of their actions because they are unable to be affected by punishment. In the case of the mentally ill, according to Hesslow, punishment is meaningless suffering. The resolution in these cases is to relieve mentally ill people from social and legal responsibility and provide some other method of treatment or control. From these claims, Hesslow concludes that "[t]his way of justifying the relief from responsibility nowhere requires that we draw a line between the healthy and the mentally ill. The crucial line goes between those who are likely to be influenced by the responsibility and those who are not."[120]

---

[115] Ibid., pp. 7–8.
[116] Ibid., p. 8.
[117] Ibid., p. 9.
[118] Ibid., p. 9.
[119] Ibid., pp. 9–10.
[120] Ibid., p. 10.

*Boorse's reply to Hesslow*   Boorse provides a three-part rejoinder to Hesslow. First, he claims the following:

> I agree with almost all of Hesslow's observations, but not his conclusions from them ... I am simply not so pessimistic as he about the continued value of health concepts ... If disease is only as scientifically useful a concept as learning, memory, and intelligence are in psychology—his examples—that is still useful indeed ... Certainly, I am satisfied if "disease" is as much a theoretical term (and as value-free!) as "animal," "plant," "cell," and "hormone," and no worse a conceptual "straightjacket" than "organism."[121]

Second, with respect to therapy Boorse notes that

> Hesslow is right that disease status is unnecessary as a ground for medical treatment. In the social context, he also rightly denies that all and only diseases should be covered by insurance, exempt people from work or domestic duties, excuse crime, and so on. Even given a basic value framework, a theoretical disease judgment grounds no practical judgment, since the latter depend on details about a disease's severity and effect on a person's unique situation.[122]

Finally, regarding Hesslow's insistence that the concepts of health and disease should be abandoned, Boorse interjects the following reminder:

> [C]lear analysis is invaluable given the past and present role of the medical vocabulary. Since confusion and abuse of this vocabulary have sometimes been rife, especially in psychiatry, and no analytic consensus is yet in sight, there is more than enough reason to debate [my concept of health] and its competitors.[123]

So, in summary, Boorse thinks that the continued attempts to debate, defend, and accept certain concepts of health and disease (1) can be scientifically useful, (2) are not necessary (though can be useful) for the actual practices (i.e., treatment) of medicine, and (3) are helpful in both the prevention of confusion and abuse of technical terms within medicine.

Boorse's overall reply to Hesslow is reasonable, but the first part of his reply is not entirely satisfying because he omits a crucial part of Hesslow's criticism. Specifically, Hesslow claims that, although the meaning of terms like "intelligence," "memory," and "learning" play an important role of establishing terminological conventions within psychology, such a need for common terminology "is not usually regarded as philosophically very important, and it is not the same thing as a conceptual analysis."[124] In effect, because Boorse claims that he is satisfied if his concepts of health and disease are useful in the same way that "intelligence," "memory," and "learning" are useful in psychology, he is conceding that his account may be useful for establishing common terminology, but is not philosophically interesting.

---

[121] Boorse, "A Rebuttal on Health," pp. 53–4.

[122] Ibid., p. 55.

[123] Ibid. Note that Boorse also calls his concept of health "BST," which stands for "biostatistical." The bracketed addition is used in place of BST to avoid confusion.

[124] Hesslow, "Do We Need a Concept of Disease?," pp. 4–5.

Rather than conceding so much to Hesslow, Boorse should have relied on the third part of his reply as justification for offering his concepts of health and disease. That is, as Chapter 3 made clear, much of the health literature (especially the field of psychiatry) has had a tendency to collapse mental health and physical health into the same concept. It is the realization that mental health and physical health are distinct concepts that is of significance to both philosophers and medical professionals. Having made clear that the concepts of mental health and physical health are distinct, philosophers can then continue to tackle each concept independently or even offer an account of why the two concepts are not distinct. Moreover, medical practitioners can take advantage of such conceptual analysis as they go about making judgments concerning diagnosis, prognosis, and treatment. Thus, through the third part of his reply to Hesslow, Boorse does have the resources to claim that his concepts of health and disease are more than mere useful terminological conventions.

Finally, the second part of Boorse's reply to Hesslow is reasonable. Given that the treatment of disease reflects the interests, goals, and circumstances in which patients and practitioners find themselves, there is no necessary connection between theoretical disease judgments and corresponding treatments. Even if it is true that a person has lung cancer, it may be the case that, given the patient's age and related medical problems, treatment may not be advisable or the patient may reject treatment. Thus, Boorse agrees with Hesslow that, although the concepts of health and disease may be useful to the practice of medicine, they are not necessary for the treatment decisions associated with the practice of medicine.

In summary, this section has provided two criticisms that Boorse's concepts of health and disease are bad in the light of current medical practices. The first criticism, offered by Margolis and Miller Brown, is that Boorse's reliance on pathology to justify his concepts of health and disease is questionable because pathology is not really a science. Moreover, they claimed that Boorse's concepts of health and disease are suspect because they do not range over the practices of medicine. The ensuing discussion revealed that, for the most part, Boorse's rejoinder to these criticisms is successful. The second criticism, submitted by Hesslow, is that Boorse's concepts of health and disease are neither theoretically nor practically relevant to the practices of medicine. The assessment of this criticism revealed that, although Boorse may have conceded too much to Hesslow, his overall reply is on the mark.

## Conclusion

This chapter offered a critical analysis of the major criticisms of Boorse's naturalistic concept of health. Specifically, the following four categories of criticism were examined: (1) circular reasoning, (2) covert normativism, (3) bad biology, and (4) bad medicine. This analysis revealed that Boorse is on the mark in his reply to (1); successful in his rejoinder to (2), except for the fact that epistemic norms turn out to be part of his account; partly unpersuasive in his reply to (3) due to his inconsistent views about natural selection and the unsatisfactory role given to the environment in his concept of health; and largely convincing in his riposte to (4).

In general, this chapter has revealed that Boorse is fairly successful in deflecting most criticisms levied against his naturalistic concepts of health and disease. However, this chapter also showed that some of the criticisms identify serious weaknesses in Boorse's analysis. Specifically, Boorse's handling of both evolutionary and environmental factors with respect to his concept of health is unpersuasive. Moreover, Boorse is unconvincing in excluding epistemic values from the concept of health. Given these difficulties is not clear that Boorse's account, in its present form, "best explains medical disease judgments and our reactions to them."[125]

In the next concluding chapter, a modified version of Boorse's concept of health will be offered. It is to the details of this modified version that will occupy the remainder of this discussion.

---

[125] Boorse, "A Rebuttal on Health," p. 6.

Chapter 7
# An Evolutionary Concept of Health

**Introduction: Boorse and Beyond**

Boorse's concept of health includes a contextualist concept of function. With respect to the concept of health, he thinks that a dispositional part-functionalist concept of function is most appropriate (see Chapters 4 and 5). Boorse's naturalistic account purports to have three benefits: it is able to make sense of many disease processes without having to invoke any divine element; it is an objective account that includes, at most, epistemic norms; and it takes seriously that the concept of health must be qualified with respect to species, age, and gender.

Chapter 6, however, revealed a number of difficulties with Boorse's naturalistic concept of health. First, he is not consistent in how he understands the role of evolution with respect to his concept of function. Second, he is not able to distinguish genuine functions from mere accidents. Third, to the extent that Boorse acknowledges evolution in his reply to Engelhardt (see "covert normativism" section in Chapter 6), he does not explain convincingly why he thinks that the individual organism is the appropriate unit of selection. Fourth, Boorse does not address adequately the role of the environment in relation to the concept of health.

Despite the above difficulties, it is not necessary to reject Boorse's account entirely. Rather, there is reason to agree with William Bechtel's statement that, despite some reservations, he remains "sympathetic to [Boorse's] initial intuition that medical or physiological theory might provide an adequate grounding for an analysis of health."[1] So, in an attempt to resolve the difficulties facing Boorse's account, this chapter offers an evolutionary-homeostasis concept of health. Specifically, this chapter argues that an organism within a specific species, gender, and age group is in a state of health when its internal parts are functioning according to their evolved abilities. Crucial to understanding these evolved abilities is that they assist in both internal homeostasis and organism homeostasis.

This chapter unfolds as follows. First, a brief assessment of evolutionary senses of "function" will reveal that a mixed evolutionary-based propensity interpretation is the most plausible. Second, drawing on the discussion of homeostasis introduced in Chapter 2, a dual-homeostatic account, which includes intercellular homeostasis and (whole) organism homeostasis, will be explained. Third, the evolutionary-based propensity theory and the dual-homeostasis account will be brought together to offer an evolutionary-homeostasis concept of health. Fourth, five diseases are briefly examined to reveal the benefits of this concept of health. With reference to these

[1] William Bechtel, "A Naturalistic Concept of Health," in J. M. Humber and R. F. Almeder (eds), *Biomedical Ethics Review 1985* (Clifton, 1985), p. 144 [bracketed addition mine].

specific disease examples, this section argues that a number of apparent difficulties with the evolutionary-homeostasis account can be resolved. Finally, in order to acknowledge individual health from an evolutionary perspective, the last section will argue that it is reasonable to think that the "unit of selection" is the individual organism. The overall conclusion is that it is possible to offer a naturalistic concept of health that resolves the difficulties present in Boorse's analysis.

*A Return to Function*

The discussion of function in Chapter 4 revealed the following about the concepts of function defended by Wright and Boorse. Three key conclusions emerged from the discussion of Wright's account. First, his concept of function is able to exclude any sort of theological commitments. Second, his concept of function does not successfully range over organisms and artifacts. The basic problem is that he offers little justification for the claim that intentionally designed artifacts can be understood in the same way as organisms with natural functions. Third, Wright's concept of function is able to make sense of genuine functions from accidental effects, because of his emphasis on evolutionary causal history.

Three conclusions were also made manifest with respect to Boorse's concept of health. First, he was able to dismiss theological elements from his account. Second, he was able to offer an account that ranges over organisms and artifacts. Third, he was not able to offer an account that could distinguish genuine functions from mere accidental effects.

Thus, the limitations of Wright's and Boorse's accounts are as follows:

1. Wright's etiological concept of function cannot range over organisms and artifacts.
2. Boorse's concept of function cannot distinguish genuine functions from mere accidental effects.

Wright and Boorse are both determined to satisfy the adequacy condition of offering a concept of function that ranges over artifacts and organisms. Wright fails to meet this condition, and Boorse resolves it by defending a contextualist account of function. Yet, it is more reasonable to relax this requirement. There are two reasons—a theoretical one and a practical one—for doing so. First, the sources of functions and goals in organisms and artifacts are radically different. Intentional designers and users determine the functions of artifacts, but (disregarding divine designers) no such intentional designer is present in the case of biological entities. Rather, natural selection and other evolutionary forces are the relevant causes of organic functions.[2] Second, health judgments are not relevant to artifacts, but are relevant to whether or not an organism is functioning properly. Thus, it is reasonable to relax the

---

[2] It could be argued (as Wright does) that functions can range over organisms and artifacts because both rely on beneficial consequences. This claim, however, is not true in the case of artifacts. A person could create a device that has no benefit at all. For example, someone could invent a machine that counts grains of sand for no benefit at all. The function of the sand counter would still be to count sand, even if it does not have a benefit to the

requirement that a univocal concept of function necessarily must range over artifacts and organisms (note that the reason why relaxation of this adequacy condition does not salvage Wright's account will be made clear in the next section). Consequently, the naturalistic concept of function defended in this chapter will not range over both artifacts and organisms, although it will distinguish genuine functions from mere accidents with respect to biological features.[3] Moreover, given the advantages in both Boorse's and Wright's analyses, the concept of health defended in this chapter will include the etiological and dispositional elements in Wright's and Boorse's concepts of function as an alternative concept of function for the concept of health.

*Evolutionary Functional Naturalism*

Given that functions need only range over biological systems, which are the product of millions of years of evolution, evolutionary approaches to the concept of function are worth pursuing. To this end, a general description of *Evolutionary Functional Naturalism* (EFN hereafter) will prove useful. The following statement by Ernst Mayr is a good place to begin. Within the context of the importance of asking, "why does this feature of an organism exist?" Mayr tells us:

> Darwin's evolutionary theory necessitates this question [of asking "why?"]: No feature (or behavioral program) of an organism ordinarily evolves unless this is favored by natural selection. It must play a role in the survival and reproductive success of its bearer. Accepting this premise, it is necessary for the completion of causal analysis to ask for any feature, why it exists, that is what its function and role in the life of a particular organism is.[4]

To illustrate Mayr's claims in the above passage, consider the heart. According to Mayr, it is not only important to understand the details of *how* the heart is able to perform the pumping that it does, but a complete causal understanding of such a phenomenon requires that a persuasive defense of *why* it is the case that the heart makes manifest such behavior be provided. With respect to the heart, the answer a Darwinian like Mayr would give is that the blood-pumping activity of the heart is a behavior that is retained by natural selection not only because it circulates blood, but also because it ensures the survival and reproduction of the organism and the species to which it belongs (goal-directed element). Such an account, thinks Mayr, completes a causal explanation of why a feature is currently present in an organism and the reason why such a feature can correctly be thought of as a function for the organism. With this sketch in mind, the formal definition of EFN is as follows:

---

inventor or others. Thus, beneficial consequences are not necessary for functions to range over organisms and artifacts.

[3] Note that my argument for rejecting this adequacy condition is close to Boorse's account. For Boorse also thinks that naturally designed organisms and intentionally designed artifacts have to be analyzed differently—Boorse thinks that his contextualism can do this. Thus, Boorse and I are in basic agreement on this point. For discussion see Chapter 4.

[4] Ernst Mayr, "Teleological and Teleonomic, a New Analysis," *Boston Studies in the Philosophy of Science*, 14 (1974): 108.

*Evolutionary Functional Naturalism*: A naturalistic explanation that argues that a feature **X** has a function in an organism **O** if and only if activity **Y** of **X** produces effect **E** because **Y** and **E** were naturally selected (over some other causes and effects) and still continue to bring about the goals **G** of survival and reproductive success of **O**.

For example, the liver has a function of blood detoxification in mammals, because the activity of converting ammonia into the less toxic compound urea produces the effect of detoxified blood. Moreover, this activity and effect were naturally selected and still continue to be selected for the goals of survival and reproduction.

Note that there are more subtleties to Mayr's account than are captured in the above definition. Specifically, how to understand "selection" in the above definition is not made clear. Are features currently selected? Were they selected in the past? Will they be selected in the future? All of these questions will be addressed in the discussion that is to follow. Specifically, two philosophical approaches to understanding function within EFN will be distinguished: (1) the backward-looking *Etiological Functional Naturalism* and (2) the forward-looking *Propensity Functional Naturalism*. This section will argue that neither of these versions of EFN are adequate, but that a worthy alternative, *Mixed Evolutionary Functional Naturalism*, is available.

*Etiological functional naturalism*   On this interpretation, a feature performs a function in a system of an organism if and only if (1) the feature's presence in a system was useful with respect to the organism's reproductive success in previous generations and that (2) it is the result of evolutionary selection forces. Chapter 4 made clear that Larry Wright is a defender of this account. Recently, drawing on the insights of Wright, Ruth Millikan stands as one of the prominent defenders of the etiological version of EFN. She argues as follows:

> The functional trait must be one that is there in contrast to others that are not there, because of historic difference in the results of these alternative traits ... The difference between merely luckily or accidentally cycling through successive generations and having genuinely functional traits whose biological purpose is to contribute to such cycling lies in whether these traits were once selected from among other once extant traits due to their superior capacities to continue to cycle. Graphically, whether my shoulders have as a biological function to hold up my clothes depends not on what proportion of my ancestors used their shoulders that way to advantage but on whether there were once shoulderless people who died out because they had nothing to hang their clothes on.[5]

Valerie Hardcastle articulates this version of EFN by noting that it is a kind of "backward-looking" functional explanation "for why something is there in natural systems by picking out the property of that thing most valuable to previous generations plus some selecting mechanism."[6] The formal definition looks like this:

---

[5] Ruth Millikan, *White Queen Psychology and Other Essays for Alice* (Cambridge, 1993), p. 38. For a similar etiological account, see Karen Neander, "Functions as Selected Effects: The Conceptual Analyst's Defense," *Philosophy of Science*, 58/2 (1991a): 168–84 and "The Teleological Notion of 'Function'," *Australasian Journal of Philosophy*, 69/4 (1991b): 454–68.

[6] Valerie Hardcastle, "Understanding Functions: A Pragmatic Approach," in Valerie Hardcastle, ed., *Where Biology Meets Psychology* (Cambridge, 1999), p. 32. One of the most

Etiological Functional Naturalism: A kind of EFN explanation that argues that a feature **X** currently has a function in an organism **O** if and only if activity **Y** of **X** produces effect **E** because **Y** and **E** were naturally selected (over some other causes and effects) to bring about the goals **G** of survival and reproductive success of **O**.

With this general description in place, a specific health example is in order. In humans, iduronate sulfatase is the lysosomal enzyme that is designed to breakdown mucopolysaccharides (a gel-like substance found in the body of cells). For example, connective tissue outside of cells needs to be replaced on occasion. When this replacement occurs, iduronate sulfatase metabolizes the old connective tissue. On occasion, in males only, a genetic error occurs such that not enough iduronate sulfatase is present to breakdown the mucopolysaccharides that build-up from the remaining old connective tissue. The result of the build-up of mucopolysaccharides (in lysome cells) is the following multi-system collapse: hyperactivity, aggressive behavior, coarse facial features, enlargement of internal organs, dwarfism, stiffening of joints, progressive deafness, and severe mental retardation. This genetic disease is known as Hunter syndrome.[7]

From an EFN perspective, the function of these iduronate sulfatase enzymes is to metabolize mucopolysaccharides, because, ancestrally, there was selection pressure in favor of them doing just this to ensure survival and reproductive success. In severe cases, human males who either lack iduronate sulfatase enzymes or do not produce enough of them have multi-system dysfunction, rendering them physically unfit or unhealthy.

A quick glance at the etiological account might move one to consider this version of EFN credible. For, as part of its content, it appears to include both the necessary and sufficient conditions for what it means for **X** to have a function. As John Bigelow and Robert Pargetter affirm, "The big plus for the etiological theory is that it makes biological functions genuinely explanatory, and explanatory in a way most comfortable with the modern biological sciences."[8] Moreover, it provides a general framework for distinguishing genuine functions from mere accidents, because a feature of a biological system is a function if and only if it is the product of natural selection. All other features are accidents. Karen Neander provides the following technical description of the etiological account:

---

ardent defenders of etiological functional naturalism is Larry Wright. For example, he says that, "Given the background of natural selection ... natural functions ... can be understood in the very same terms as conscious functions ... For just as conscious functions provide a consequence-etiology by virtue of conscious selection, natural functions provide the very same sort of etiology as a result of natural selection." See Larry Wright, *Teleological Explanations: An Etiological Analysis of Goals and Functions* (Berkeley, 1976), p. 84.

[7] Note that there are two forms of Hunter syndrome. There is a severe form that occurs in juveniles (between ages 2–4) and a mild form that occurs in early adolescence (between ages 5–10). A more detailed account of Hunter syndrome can be found in Ramzi. S. Contran, Vinay Kumar, and Stanley L. Robbins, *Robbins Pathological Basis of Disease*, 4th edn (Philadelphia, 1989), pp. 149–51 and the following internet website: http://www.nlm.nih.gov/medlineplus/ency/article/001203.htm.

[8] John Bigelow and Robert Pargetter, "Functions," *Journal of Philosophy*, 84/4 (1987): 187.

It is the/a proper function of an item **X** of an organism **O** to do that which items of **X's** type did to contribute to the inclusive fitness of **O's** ancestors, and which caused the genotype, of which **X** is the phenotypic expression, to be selected by natural selection.[9]

Against the etiological account, scholars have offered four objections. First, some argue that the etiological account presupposes a rather unduly simplistic view of the evolution of traits. Specifically, the etiological account cannot guard against Panglossian-like "just-so-stories" about how a given feature *qua* trait **X** is retained as the fittest in a population as a result of the advantage conferred on **O** as a result of the fitness advantage had in an ancestral population. As Hardcastle makes the point,

> It is easy to spin "just-so stories" about why some [trait] **T** is maintained in [an organism **O**], but it is nearly impossible to fit these stories to our very complex biological world, even ignoring the difficulties of connecting phenotypes to genotypes ... Toss in pleiotropy, exaptations, random drift, and other forms of genetic hitchhiking, and we just can't assume in this world a natural selection of the fittest. That is but a toy model of evolution.[10]

Part of Hardcastle's criticism is uncharitable to the etiological account, which is not necessarily committed to the optimality interpretation of natural selection. The etiological account recognizes that not all traits are selected because they are optimal for a particular environment; rather, many traits are selected because they are superior or "just better" than other traits in contending with the existing environment. So, with respect to her claim that the etiological account assumes "a natural selection of the fittest," Hardcastle overstates her criticism.

Moreover, it is important to note that the adaptationist program need not be abandoned (although the optimality condition as a general requirement should be abandoned) in the light of epistemic limitations related to the complexity of historical entities like organisms. As Richard Lewontin recommends,

> Even if the assertion of universal adaptation is difficult to test because of simplifying assumptions and ingenious explanations can almost always result in an ad hoc adaptive explanation, at least in principle some of the assumptions can be tested in some cases. A weaker form of evolutionary explanation that explained some proportion of the cases by

---

[9] Neander, "Functions as Selected Effects: The Conceptual Analyst's Defense," p. 174.

[10] Hardcastle, "Understanding Functions: A Pragmatic Approach," p. 32 [bracketed additions mine; note that an upper case **O** has been substituted for a lower case **o** for the sake of consistency]. Briefly, "random drift" refers to the loss of variation that can occur by chance or by unpredictable changes of alleles. See Elliott Sober, *The Nature of Selection* (Cambridge, 1984), p. 24 fn. 11. "Pleiotropy" is a term used to describe the fact that a single gene can have multiple phenotypic effects or a cluster of genes may have several effects on a given phenotype. See Alexander Rosenberg, *The Structure of Biological Science* (Cambridge, 1985), p. 237. Finally, "exaptation" is the term used to suggest that it is possible for phenotypes to be co-opted from their present function in order to serve some other distinct function. See Stephen Jay Gould and Elizabeth Vrba, "Exaptation: A Missing Term in the Science of Form," *Paleobiology*, 8 (1982): 4–15. In his critique of the Wright-Millikan-Neander etiological concept of function, David Buller argues this point of Hardcastle in detail. See David J. Buller, "Etiological Theories of Function: A Geographical Survey," *Biology and Philosophy*, 13/4 (1998): 505–27.

adaptation and left the rest to allometry, pleitropy, random gene fixations, linkage and indirect selection would be utterly impervious to test. It would leave the biologist free to pursue the adaptationist program in the easy cases and leave the difficult ones on the scrap heap of chance. In a sense, then, biologists are forced to the extreme adaptationist program because alternatives, although they are undoubtedly operative in many cases, are untestable in particular cases.[11]

The point that can be drawn from Lewontin's account above is that it is safe to assume that most features of organisms are adaptive functions, even if particular features may not be adaptive. The reason is that there is no way to test whether or not a feature is the product of chance, but it is possible to test whether or not a feature is an adaptive function.[12] So, on the one hand, Hardcastle claims that epistemic constraints make it the case that the adaptationist program should be abandoned. On the other hand, Lewontin submits that epistemic constraints only give further support in favor of the adaptationist program.

The point that can be taken away from this discussion is that Hardcastle's concern about story telling in biology should be taken seriously, but is not a knockdown argument against the adaptationist program. Rather, it should be seen as a warning that the assumption that a given feature is an adaptive trait is tentative until empirical justification is forthcoming. Thus, Hardcastle's first criticism is not as successful as she insists and does not refute the etiological account of function, which relies on the adaptive history of traits.

Second, some have argued that the reasoning behind the etiological version of EFN is circular.[13] In general, a charge of circularity is the suggestion that one is attempting to defend or explain a particular conclusion by employing the very conclusion to be defended as a premise. Hardcastle notes the circularity criticism of the etiological account as follows:

[I]f we restrict our scope to functional explanations of T, and if we define functions in terms of the past selection of T, then we cannot use functions to explain the past selection of T for that would be using the past selection of T to explain the past selection of T. In other words, if we use a backward-looking approach to understanding functions, then we simply cannot give functional explanations of things we know are adaptations.[14]

Hardcastle's criticism is that the proponents of the etiological version of EFN include the historical function of **X** as part of their account for the historical selection for **X**. Restated, the reason why **X** is currently present is because **X** had a function at

---

[11] Richard Lewontin, "Adaptation," *Scientific American*, 239/3 (1978): 230.

[12] For an instructive discussion of the criteria (e.g., correlation between character and environment, results from altering a character, comparison of naturally occurring variants, etc.) needed to determine whether or not a feature is an adaptation, see Mary Jane West-Eberhard, "Adaptation: Current Usages," in David L. Hull and Michael Ruse (eds), *Philosophy of Biology* (Oxford, 1998), pp. 8–14.

[13] This criticism has been offered by Bigelow and Pargetter, "Functions," *Journal of Philosophy*, p. 190, and both Hardcastle, "Understanding Functions: A Pragmatic Approach," p. 33 and Bechtel, "A Naturalistic Concept of Health," p. 150.

[14] Hardcastle, "Understanding Functions: A Pragmatic Approach," p. 33.

some time in the past that was selected because of the function it had. For example, to argue that feathers currently function to help ensure thermal regulation in birds, because thermal regulation was selected for this function in the past, already builds into the analysis the idea that feathers had this function, for which it was then selected. The conclusion is that those who favor an etiological interpretation of function are smuggling into their defense the very thing they are trying to defend.

The etiological account can avoid this difficulty by making it clear that physiological feature **X** is a function of organism **O** if and only if **X** is selected not because it has a function, but because it is useful to the survival and reproduction of **O** and **X** is retained and passed on (genetically or behaviorally) to successive generations. On this version of the etiological account, the initial retention of **X** is not present because it already has a function, but because it is useful to the organism. It is only after **X** has been retained and transmitted to many successive generations that it acquires a function.[15] Beth Preston stresses this historical point when she notes that the etiological account "is a strong one, in the sense that a protracted period of time is required during which the performance of the trait is tested against alternatives and found successful, thus ensuring its own reproduction."[16] Thus, the combination of the usefulness of a feature and its successive propagation through reproductively established families tells against Hardcastle's charge of circularity.

Third, some argue that the etiological account is erroneously committed to the view that advantageous acclimations cannot be functions, because it allows only those activities that have a particular evolutionary history to be genuine functions.[17] In reply to those who subscribe to the etiological account, imagine a possible world in which the human lungs successfully acclimate to an atmosphere that has suddenly changed from being oxygen-rich to almost entirely carbon dioxide-rich. The function of lungs before the atmospheric shift was to inhale oxygen and exhale carbon dioxide, but in the new environment the lungs function to inhale and exhale carbon dioxide. According to the etiological account, this new activity of the lungs cannot be a genuine function of the lungs because it is not the product of natural selection. The point of this counterfactual is that the etiological account is forced to accept the counterintuitive view that many beneficial acclimations that help to keep an organism alive are not functions.[18]

---

[15] Although this is implicit in Neander's quotation provided above, Ruth Millikan explicitly emphasizes that "[t]he difference between merely luckily or accidentally cycling through successive generations and having genuinely functional traits whose biological purpose is to contribute to such cycling lies in whether these traits were once selected from among other once extant traits due to their superior capacities to continue to cycle." See Millikan, *White Queen Psychology and Other Essays for Alice*, p. 38.

[16] Beth Preston, "Why is a Wing Like a Spoon? A Pluralist Theory of Function," *The Journal of Philosophy*, 95/5 (1998): 227.

[17] Peter McLaughlin defends this criticism. See Peter McLaughlin, *What Functions Explain* (Cambridge, 2001), p. 90.

[18] This example is a variation on Joseph Margolis's version and this point about confusing function and evolution is offered by William Bechtel. See Joseph Margolis, "The Concept of Disease," *Journal of Medicine and Philosophy*, 1/3 (1976): 238–55 and Bechtel, "In Defense of a Naturalistic Concept of Health," pp. 131–70.

This third criticism seems to be the most damaging, but it is not clear that it is. What seems to be assumed within this criticism is that this counterintuitive implication of the etiological account renders it implausible. As McLaughlin claims, "The evolutionary etiological view asserts—counterintuitively—that newly advantageous traits have no functions."[19] Yet, intuitions do not resolve this issue. For example, imagine the first few instances in which birds used feathers for flight. The evolutionary etiologist would argue that these early instances of flight do not confer the function of flight on feathers, because such features have not been screened by natural selection—that is, they are not yet heritable. This sort of reasoning would apply to the claim that the thumb has the function of pressing the space bar on a keyboard. This activity is beneficial, but it is not the function of the thumb, because such an activity is not part of a natural selection history. It is only after such an accidental beneficial feature has been part of many cycles of generations and confers a fitness advantage is it the case that it becomes a genuine function. In this way, the etiologist can claim that this account best explains how to distinguish genuine functions from mere advantageous acclimations. It is able to do this based on its reliance on evolutionary theory, not intuitions about what appears to be a function and what does not appear to be a function. Thus, the etiological account can simply "bite the bullet" that mere advantageous acclimations, which do not have an evolutionary selective history, are not functions.

The fourth criticism is that the etiological account must attribute functions to those features that no longer have functions. For example, the appendix, which is part of the digestive organ known as the caecum, once had the function in early mammalian evolution to aid in digestion of certain plants with low nutritional value.[20] In hominid evolution, however, the appendix is still present but no longer has this digestive function; that is, it has not been maintained by natural selection. The problem for the etiological account is that it must accept that the function of the appendix still is to digest plants with low nutritional value, because that is what its evolutionary causal history designed it to do. Yet, it is clear that the human appendix is an evolutionary remnant that no longer has a function. The point is that, although the etiological account can distinguish genuine functions from accidents, it cannot distinguish between features that have genuine functions and those that once had, but no longer possess, genuine functions.[21]

This fourth criticism is one that the etiological account cannot evade. By relying solely on human evolution, the etiological account must ascribe functions to those features that no longer have functions. As Lowell Nissen correctly remarks, "Since history is forever, if functions are determined by their history, functions are forever.

---

[19] McLaughlin, *What Functions Explain*, p. 134.

[20] The function of the appendix is discussed by and Randolph M. Nesse and George C. Williams, *Why We Get Sick* (New York, 1994), pp. 129–30.

[21] Note that this criticism could also have been levied against Wright's etiological account. The reason it was suppressed is because Wright does not offer a rich enough of an evolutionary account to determine his considered view. Nonetheless, if Wright's account is to be understood in the same way as the evolutionary etiological account discussed in this section, then his analysis is open to this criticism.

New functions can be added, but old ones never die. That means that vestigial organs still have their original functions."[22] Thus, the etiological account is triumphant in distinguishing genuine functions from accidents because of its reliance on evolutionary causal history, but such an achievement proves to be a somewhat pyrrhic victory.

There is one final concern that needs to be noted. Some argue that the etiological account is committed to defining functions in terms of actual reproductive success. As it is described in this section, it is ambiguous whether or not such a commitment is entailed. Still, Bigelow and Pargetter note that some scholars argue that the etiological account assumes that fitness can be judged only retrospectively: that it is only after we have seen which creatures survived that we can judge which were the fittest; moreover, it assumes that the fact that certain creatures have survived, whereas others did not, is what constitutes their being fit.[23]

Clearly, this may be a serious problem with versions of the etiological account that are committed to the view that **Y** is a function of **X** if and only if **Y** contributes to *the actual* reproductive success of **O**. This leads to the absurd implication that only those things that actually perform their activity are functions. Imagine a case in which bananas are dangled above the heads of two monkeys. Assume that the hands of monkeys have evolved to grasp things; that is, grasping is an activity that contributes to reproductive success. Further imagine that as one monkey goes to grasp the dangling bananas, a lightning bolt strikes its hands, rendering them physically incapable of grasping. The other monkey, however, moves forward and grasps the bananas and proceeds to eat them. On the etiological account, the lightning-struck monkey's hand does not have the function to grasp, while the other monkey's hand does have the function to grasp, because the former monkey's (and not the latter's) hand can no longer actually contribute to the reproductive success of the monkey. In this case, it is obvious there is no difference between the two monkeys except for this accidental event, which is not in any way related to the adapted nature of the monkey's hand. The point is that it is absurd to confer a function on an organism or take away a function from an organism based on lucky or unlucky anomalous environmental perturbations, which are not part of the normal environment in which the organism has evolved.

It is this sort of example that lead Bigelow and Pargetter to claim that the "etiological theory is mistaken in defining functions purely retrospectively, in terms of actual survival."[24] So, if it is the case that the etiological account is committed to actual reproductive success, then this criticism is quite relevant. The point that can be taken away from this criticism is that it is better to say that **Y** is a function of **X** if and only if **Y** has *the capacity* its ancestors had to contribute to the reproductive success of **O**. By substituting "capacity" for "actuality," the problem of environmental

---

[22] Lowell Nissen, *Teleological Language in the Life Sciences* (Lanham, 1997), p. 185.
[23] Bigelow and Pargetter, "Functions," p. 190. A version of this criticism can be found in J. J. C. Smart, *Philosophy and Scientific Realism* (New York, 1963), p. 59.
[24] Bigelow and Pargetter, "Functions," p. 191. Note that Bigelow and Pargetter are aware that this criticism is not relevant to every version of the etiological account, but might be appropriate with respect to some versions.

anomalies disappears. This point is explicitly captured in the propensity interpretation of function.

*Propensity functional naturalism*   No doubt, there are many scholars who wish to distance themselves from relying on actual reproductive success. As a way of both maintaining EFN and contending with some of the criticisms put forth against the etiological interpretation of function, John Bigelow and Robert Pargetter advance what can be called *propensity functional naturalism*.[25] This account draws on the need to move away from the actual contributions to reproductive success toward the propensity or capacity to contribute to reproductive success. They articulate this "forward-looking" version of EFN by distinguishing it from the etiological explanation in the following manner:

> The etiological theory describes a character *now* serving a function, when it *did* confer propensities that improved the chances of survival. We suggest that it is appropriate, in such a case, to say that the character *has been serving that function all along*. Even before it had contributed (in an appropriate way) to survival, it had conferred a survival-enhancing propensity on the creature. And to confer such a propensity, we suggest, is what constitutes a function. *Something has a (biological) function just when it confers a survival-enhancing propensity on a creature that possesses it.*[26]

As Hardcastle explains, "Bigelow and Pargetter's solution [to the problems of the etiological account] is to use a forward-looking account of functions conjoined with the additional element that the functions were active in the past to explain evolution by natural selection. They claim that functions are dispositions or propensities to succeed under future selection pressures in a normal environment."[27] For example, the function of iduronate sulfatase enzymes is to metabolize mucopolysaccharides and not some other substance found in the body of cells, because creatures whose mucopolysaccharides are broken down by iduronate sulfatase enzymes have a greater disposition of surviving and reproducing than creatures whose mucopolysaccharides cannot be metabolized.

On this version of EFN, a function is tied to its predilection or disposition (as opposed to its actual) to have a certain degree of reproductive success with respect to acceptable environmental fluctuations. As Bigelow and Pargetter note, a propensity or disposition "is a subjunctive property: it specifies what will happen or what is likely to happen in the right circumstances, just as fragility is specified in terms of breaking or being likely to break in the right circumstances."[28] For example, the ear was selected in the past because it enhanced both predator/prey detection and the sense of body equilibrium, both of which confer a survival-enhancing propensity

---

[25] Ibid., pp. 191–4. An earlier version of the propensity view of function can be found in S. K. Mills and J. H. Beatty, "The Propensity Interpretation of Fitness," *Philosophy of Science*, 46/2 (1979): 263–86.

[26] Ibid., p. 192 [my italics].

[27] Hardcastle, "Understanding Functions: A Pragmatic Approach," p. 33 [bracketed addition mine].

[28] Bigelow and Pargetter, "Functions," p. 190.

on the organism. So long as similar (not exact) environmental pressures are present, one can be confident that, for example, the ear will continue to perform its functions for tokens of the species at any time in the life history of the tokens. The formal characterization of propensity functional naturalism looks like this:

> *Propensity Functional Naturalism*: A kind of EFN explanation that argues that a feature **X** has a function in an organism **O** by performing activity **Y** if and only if **Y** produces effect **E** because **Y** and **E** confer and will continue to confer a propensity **P** (within a certain range of environmental pressures) to bring about the goals **G** of survival and reproductive success of **O**.

For example, the reason iduronate sulfatase enzymes have a function in the human body is because their activity of metabolizing mucopolysaccharides confers a survival-enhancing propensity on the human body within a certain range of environmental pressures. Moreover, it will continue to confer a survival-enhancing propensity on the human body so long as the same range of environmental pressures is present.

It is this ability *qua* propensity of a feature to actualize a specific task(s) in the presence of a certain range of environmental perturbations that leads Bigelow and Pargetter to consider such a propensity as a survival-enhancing propensity and a biological function. Thus, Bigelow and Pargetter conclude that the function of a feature "generates propensities that are survival-enhancing in the creature's natural habitat."[29] For example, the gene that causes sickle-cell anemia is a highly adaptive feature of the immune system of people, who live in low altitudes, that defends them against malaria.[30] Notice that the natural habitat must include a low altitude, otherwise the harmful sickle-cell anemia effects "kick in." Natural habitat, then, is that in which adapted traits *were* selected (within a certain range of variation).

Within the context of the concept of health, William Bechtel endorses the analysis offered by Bigelow and Pargetter. He thinks that the propensity interpretation of function is the correct alternative to the etiological account, because it not only makes sense of what a function is, but it also specifies the correct sense of "function" with respect to a naturalistic concept of health. He explains as follows:

> There is [a] conceptually intermediate position that has been developed in philosophical reflections on evolutionary theory—a propensity interpretation of fitness. What the propensity interpretation of fitness does is define fitness in terms of propensity to reproduce, not reproductive success itself. This is all that is required for our purposes, *for we can now define something as functional if it increases the propensity of its bearer to reproduce* ...[31] The approach I am exploring directs one to engage in an engineering analysis to identify how the physiological organization of the system equips it to deal with the selection forces working upon it. A healthy state of the system is one in which it makes best use of its physiological endowments in responding to selection pressures.[32]

---

[29] Ibid., p. 192.
[30] The details of sickle-cell anemia will be discussed in a later section of this chapter.
[31] Bechtel, "In Defense of a Naturalistic Concept of Health," p. 151 [my italics].
[32] Ibid., p. 154. Note that Bigelow and Pargetter understand health in terms of the propensity interpretation. See Bigelow and Pargetter, "Functions," pp. 192–3 [bracketed addition mine].

However, the propensity interpretation faces a number of objections. The first concern is noted by Peter Godfrey-Smith, who claims that the propensity interpretation of function "draws on the historical facts it sought to avoid."[33] The point is that the propensity interpretation is designed to resolve the problem faced by the etiological account of relying on biological history to make sense of what is and is not a function. Indeed, after arguing that it would be a mistake to insist that the existence of functions must be based on the contingent truth of evolution, Bigelow and Pargetter claim,

> We have the intuition that the concept of biological function, and views about what functions biological characters have, are not thus contingent upon the acceptance of the theory of evolution by natural selection and on discovering what led to the evolutionary development of a trait.[34]

The problem is that Bigelow and Pargetter appear to rely on just this history when they claim that

> [i]f a character is no longer survival enhancing, because of a sudden and recent change in environment, we may continue to refer its natural habitat to the past. Consequently, our propensity theory will continue to tie functions to what would be survival-enhancing in the past habitat. In such cases, there will be no conflict between the judgments of our theory and those of the etiological theory.[35]

It is this sort of reply that can make sense of Godfrey-Smith's claim that, for Bigelow and Pargetter, it appears that natural habitat "is understood historically."[36] Primarily, Bigelow and Pargetter want to make sure they can keep functions and mere accidents (i.e., acclimations) distinct. Yet, they are clearly committed to the view that a feature already has a function *qua* propensity independent of *historical* notions of survival.

Rather than thinking that Bigelow and Pargetter are committed to the historical element they hoped to avoid, it is better to claim that their account is ambiguous with respect to how they understand "past habitat." That is, they want to distance themselves from including evolutionary selection mechanisms as part of their propensity interpretation of function. However, they also *appear* to concede that evolutionary selection mechanisms are part of their propensity account when they claim that some of their judgments about function do not conflict with the judgments made by proponents of the etiological theory. It is this claim that drives Godfrey-Smith to insist that Bigelow and Pargetter are committed to an evolutionary sense of "past habitat." Yet, this is not the case. Bigelow and Pargetter are only committed to the claim that their function ascriptions are compatible with (i.e., do not conflict) those function ascriptions that are rendered from an etiological perspective. To avoid this confusion, they need only make clear that "past habitat" refers to the recent past habitat in which the survival-enhancing propensity is relevant. In fact,

---

[33] Peter Godfrey-Smith, "A Modern History Theory of Functions," *Noûs*, 28/3 (1994): 352.
[34] Bigelow and Pargetter, "Functions," pp. 188–9.
[35] Ibid., 196.
[36] Godfrey-Smith, "A Modern History Theory of Functions," p. 352.

their propensity account makes clear that a propensity is understood within the context of a certain range of environmental fluctuations. Radical environmental changes simply mean that a particular trait does not have a survival-enhancing propensity in the existing radical environment. This reply is quite in keeping with their overall account. Thus, although Bigelow and Pargetter are ambiguous in how they understand the term "past," it is clear that they can overcome this objection by Godfrey-Smith and embrace (as they would like to do) an evolutionary history-free propensity interpretation of function. The implication is that, contrary to Godfrey-Smith, Bigelow and Pargetter are not committed to the evolutionary history they are trying to avoid.

The second criticism is raised by Hardcastle, who argues that propensity functional naturalism is open to the very circularity problem that it is designed to avoid. Much like the etiological approach, the propensity version of EFN assumes that evolved functions will continue to be selected for now and in the future. Since, for Bigelow and Pargetter, "function" means "propensity to enhance survival," they are claiming that, for example, the function of the ear will proceed to be selected because it will go on to be selected. As Hardcastle warns, "if we define functions in terms of future selection of [trait] **T**, then we cannot use functions to account for the future selection of **T** for that would be using the future selection of **T** to explain the future selection of **T**."[37]

Hardcastle's point is that the propensity interpretation defends a conclusion by incorporating the conclusion within the defense. The difficulty with this criticism is that it assumes that, according to the propensity account, functions are defined in terms of future selection. This, however, is not the case. The propensity theory is committed to the view that feature **X** is a function only if **X** has a survival-enhancing propensity. As Bigelow and Pargetter make clear, "On our theory, the character already has a function, and by bad luck it might not survive, but with luck it may survive, and it may survive because it has a function."[38] Their point is that function *qua* propensity is independent of any sort of selection mechanisms. So, for Hardcastle to insist that the propensity interpretation is committed to defining functions in terms of the future selection of some character is to ignore the priority that Bigelow and Pargetter give to function over selection. Thus, the propensity interpretation does not fall prey to the charge of circularity levied by Hardcastle.

The third problem with the propensity interpretation of function is that it takes function as ontologically prior to selection—a move that begs the question of how they are able to determine what is and is not a function. As Bigelow and Pargetter note, "On our theory, *the character already has the function*, and by bad luck it might not survive, but with luck it may survive, and it may survive *because* it has a function."[39] Similarly, in response to the etiological account, Bechtel claims, "The

---

[37] Hardcastle, "Understanding Functions: A Pragmatic Approach," p. 34. For further criticisms of the propensity theory approach, see Sandra Mitchell, "Dispositions or Etiologies? A Comment on Bigelow and Pargetter," *Journal of Philosophy*, 90/5 (1993): 249–59.

[38] Bigelow and Pargetter, "Functions," p. 195.

[39] Ibid., p. 192 [my italics].

correct order is to claim that *those things that are functional will evolve*, rather than to claim that those things that evolve are functional."⁴⁰

The above claims by Bigelow, Pargetter, and Bechtel are problematic. The obvious problem with giving priority to function over selection is that it begs the question of *why* it is the case that **X** has the function in the first place. **X** has the function to do **Y**, because **X** yields a survival-enhancing propensity on **O**. But why does **X** have the function *qua* survival enhancing propensity that it has? Surely, they cannot rely on propensity here, because propensity and function are one and the same once selection is no longer part of the concept of function. That is, if Bigelow, Pargetter, and Bechtel presume (as they do) that character **X** "already has the function" prior to selection, then this means that **X** already has a propensity prior to selection. If not selection, then what confers "having a propensity" that makes it the case that **X** is a function? They could respond by claiming that a propensity is a property or capacity of a trait to do **X**. Yet, this leads to a regress problem. For now it can be asked, how is it the case that a property or capacity "already" exists in a creature without introducing some sort of causal history to account for the capacity? As it stands, Bigelow, Pargetter, and Bechtel have no answer, because a capacity or property is an unexplained metaphysical element of their analyses. Natural selection, on the other hand, is a physical force or process (like gravity). Are propensities thought to be the same? This seems unlikely, because Bigelow and Pargetter have already ruled out the possibility that propensity relies on contingent natural phenomena. The upshot of this overall objection is that Bigelow, Pargetter, and Bechtel have not offered a persuasive account of what a function is. Thus, it is not at all clear that giving priority to propensity over selection is preferable.

Bigelow, Pargetter, and Bechtel might object to the above criticism by claiming that "What is a function?" is different from the question "What causes functions to be present?" For example, if Bigelow and Pargetter find a watch, they can claim to know it's a watch first and then ask who made it. Obviously, they know that they have to give a causal history to account for its function, but that is different from defining what a function is. That is, they could argue that they do not have to answer the second question in order to answer the first. However, this reply is vulnerable to the next criticism.

This final objection to the ahistorical propensity account is that it cannot distinguish genuine functions from mere side effects. For example, imagine that the metabolic activities of iduronate sulfatase enzymes not only breakdown mucopolysaccharides, but they also have the accidental benefit of improving the sense of smell. On the propensity interpretation, both the metabolic activities and the improved sense of smell would have to be considered genuine functions because the former (directly) confers a survival-enhancing propensity and the latter (accidentally) confers a survival-enhancing propensity. Peter McLaughlin voices a somewhat similar concern about the propensity account as follows:

"The function of [**X**] is **Y**" is true, not only when **X** does **Y** due to its propensity, but also when it has a strong propensity to do **Y**, but happens to do it by accident and not due to its

---

⁴⁰ Bechtel, "A Naturalistic Concept of Health," p. 150 [my italics].

propensity ... Furthermore, if low probabilities were to count as low propensities, then it would seem that even accidents occur on account of a propensity.[41]

The implication of the above account leads McLaughlin to conclude correctly that those who embrace the history-free propensity interpretation of fitness are "forced to attribute a function to more or less everything."[42] Indeed, this criticism reveals why they must address the question "What causes functions to be present?" Thus, the history-free propensity interpretation of function should be rejected on the grounds that it cannot distinguish genuine functions from mere side effects.

*Mixed evolutionary functional naturalism* Thus far, the general conclusion is that neither the etiological account nor the propensity account is a way to understand what a function is. The etiological account suffers from focusing on actual reproductive success and not being able to allow an entity to lose its function, whereas the propensity interpretation cannot distinguish genuine functions from fortuitous accidents and it cannot justify giving priority to function over selection.

The more defensible alternative combines these two accounts. The propensity interpretation has the advantage that it is not committed to the actual reproductive success of a trait, but only to the disposition of such a trait to enhance reproductive success. The advantage of the etiological account is that it is able to distinguish genuine functions from mere side effects because it takes causal history into account. In the spirit of unification, the appropriate account of function will give priority to natural selection, but claim that selection ranges over propensities to survive and reproduce. In full, a feature of an organism is a function if and only if it confers a propensity to enhance the goal of survival and reproductive success on an organism and that such a propensity is established through natural selection. The formal characterization of this mixed account is as follows:

*Mixed Evolutionary Functional Naturalism*: A kind of EFN explanation that maintains that a feature **X** has a function in an organism **O** by performing an activity **Y** if and only if **Y** produces effect **E** and both **Y** and **E** confer a survival enhancing propensity **P** on **O** (within a certain range of environmental pressures) and will continue to confer **P** on **O** (so long as a certain range of environmental pressures is present). And, moreover, **P** is currently present, because, ancestrally, there was natural selection in favor of retaining **P** to bring about the goals **G** of survival and reproduction.

A return to the enzyme example will help to explain the above account. Recall that iduronate sulfatase is the lysosomal enzyme that is designed to breakdown mucopolysaccharides. With respect to the mixed account above, iduronate sulfatase is a function of the human organism (and other species), because its ability to metabolize mucopolysaccharides confers a survival-enhancing propensity on the human organism. Moreover, the reason why it currently confers such a propensity

---

[41] McLaughlin, *What Functions Explain*, p. 126.
[42] Ibid., p. 128.

is because, ancestrally, there was natural selection in favor of retaining such a propensity for the sake of survival and reproduction.[43]

This section has addressed the missing element to Boorse's concept of function. It agrees with Boorse that a dispositional account is reasonable, but insists that it must be understood within the context of natural selection. Indeed, after revealing the inadequacies of both the etiological and the propensity interpretations of function, this section concluded that a mixed etiological/propensity account is a cogent concept of biological function. With the relevant concept of function determined, it is now possible to turn to the second section on homeostasis.

*Homeostasis*

Chapter 2 revealed that Boorse acknowledges that his naturalistic concept of health assumes homeostasis as a necessary condition. Recall that Boorse concedes as follows:

> Though I did not stress the dynamism [i.e., the process of homeostasis] of normal physiology in presenting [my naturalistic concept of health], I always assumed it ... Obviously, no fact is more pervasive than what is often called "dynamic equilibrium" of normal physiology: the normal functional variation within organisms acting and reacting to their environment. The normal level of almost all part-functions varies with what an organism is doing, what other part-functions are being performed, and the environment ... A common pattern is that environmental stress evokes short-term compensatory functions that maintain homeostasis up to a point, but beyond that point the coping mechanisms break down and a discontinuity, a discrete state of illness, results.[44]

It is now appropriate to sketch the framework of a homeostatic system. The general idea is that an individual organism's internal environment is in homeostasis if it responds appropriately to various stimuli from the internal and external environment. Specifically, recall from Chapter 2 that, on the physiological level, the following internal physical states must be kept stable for the intercellular fluid to be in homeostasis:

---

[43] Godfrey-Smith has suggested that "ancestrally" must refer not to the geologic past, but to the recent past. His justification is that a feature may have evolved in the recent past by natural selection to have a different function than it had in the geologic past. For example, it is likely that feathers evolved in the geologic past to ensure thermal regulation in birds. In the recent past, however, feathers have evolved to aid in flight. Godfrey-Smith's point is that by looking only at the geologic past would result in an erroneous account of the function of a particular feature. This suggestion is reasonable. In the light of this suggestion, "ancestrally" refers to both or either historical past—the deep geologic past or the more recent evolutionary past—to accommodate a feature having a new function or multiple functions. Note, however, that contrary to Godfrey-Smith, this account does not dismiss the geologic past in favor of the recent evolutionary past, because this would leave out the possibility that the geologic function and the more recent evolutionary function could co-exist. See Godfrey-Smith, "A Modern History Theory of Functions," pp. 355–9.

[44] Christopher Boorse, "A Rebuttal on Health," in James M. Humber and Robert F. Almeder (eds), *What is Disease?*" (Totowa, 1997), pp. 78–9 [bracketed additions mine].

1. The chemical composition of the intercellular fluid (e.g., constant level of glucose in the bloodstream)
2. The osmotic pressure of the intercellular fluid (determined by the relative amounts of water and solutes)
3. The level of carbon dioxide in the intercellular fluid
4. The temperature of the intercellular fluid
5. The elimination of waste from the intercellular fluid [45]

If the above five states of the intercellular fluid are held fairly constant, then the internal environment is considered to be in homeostasis. Recall that homeostasis is maintained by both positive and negative feedback. Many organs and organ systems of the body are designed by natural selection to secure intercellular homeostasis. For example, it is crucial that intercellular temperature be within a certain range so that metabolic processes can occur. To this end, overall body temperature must remain at a certain level to ensure that intercellular homeostasis is maintained. This example is a glimpse into the interconnected and hierarchical nature of the human body. As a way of elaborating on the discussion in Chapter 2, Figure 7.1 from Charles Seidel offers a pictorial look at the five elements of a standard homeostatic system:[46]

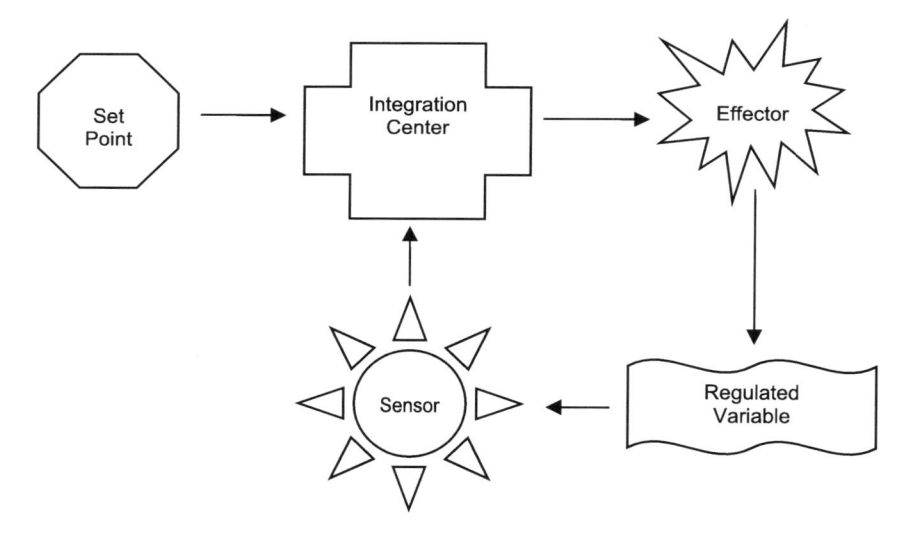

Figure 7.1   Standard Homeostatic System

Through the example of body temperature, the above five components can be summarized as follows:[47]

---

[45] These five elements of intercellular fluid are taken from M. B. V. Roberts, *Biology: A Functional Approach*, 4th edn (Surrey, 1986), p. 201.

[46] This diagram of a homeostatic system is taken from Charles Seidel, *Basic Concepts in Physiology* (New York, 2002), p. 3.

[47] This summary is taken from ibid., pp. 205–10.

1. *Regulated Variable* is a variable that is kept constant. For example, the following are regulated variables: body temperature, blood pressure, and the blood content of glucose, oxygen, and potassium ions. (Note that heart rate, cardiac resistance, urine output, and breathing rate are not regulated outputs. Rather, they are usually understood as *effectors*, which are designed to maintain set point levels.)
2. *Set Point* is a quantitative value for the regulated variable. For example, 98°F is the approximate temperature of the interior of the human body.
3. *Sensor(s)* assesses the current status of the regulated variable. The anterior hypothalamus and the skin are the temperature-sensor organs of the human body.
4. *Integration Center* compares current conditions with the set point. The anterior hypothalamus is organ that acts as the integration center for the human body. It receives the information about surface body temperature from skin nerve endings. It compares this information with the set point.
5. *Effector* brings current status of regulated variable into line with the set point. With respect to body temperature, this feedback process is also initiated by the hypothalamus and is an effector along with the anterior and posterior hypothalamus. If the body temperature is above the set point (i.e., overheated) then sweat production is initiated and the shivering center is inhibited in order to return the body's temperature to its set point. If the body temperature is below the set point (i.e., underheated), then cellular metabolism is increased through the anterior hypothalamus and shivering is increased through the posterior hypothalamus in order to return the body's temperature to its set point. If there is a foreign invader (e.g., bacteria), body temperature can rise in an attempt to destroy it. In the case of a fever, the set point itself increases as well.

The above elements of homeostasis are relevant to the various organs and organ systems of the body. The result is a feedback loop between the intercellular fluid and many of the other structures of the body.

What about the physiological functions of the body as a whole? Boorse hints at this concern in the above quotation when he defines dynamic equilibrium as "the normal functional variation within organisms acting and reacting to their environment." Then he goes on to claim that "the normal level of all part-functions varies with *what the organism is doing*."[48] Boorse's use of "within organism" suggests that he is concerned with how the internal part-functions of organisms react to their environment, but his use of *"what the organism is doing"* suggests that internal part-functions maintain their dynamic equilibrium *qua* homeostasis with respect to the physiological activities of the organism. For example, eating, waste removal, sleeping, running, walking, etc. are functions of the body (not merely any particular part) as a whole that help to sustain intercellular fluid. Where this analysis departs from Boorse is that intercellular homeostasis, which is associated with the integrated internal activities of the body, is distinct from the external behaviors of the

---

[48] My italics.

body. These external behaviors are distinct evolved patterns that are not only being influenced by intercellular fluid, but are also influencing intercellular homeostasis. Therefore, the idea is that there is a dual homeostatic interaction between behavioral activities of organisms as a whole and their intercellular activities.

For example, sleeping, eating, and waste removal are necessary for regaining lost energy. Energy restoration is crucial not only for carrying out intercellular processes, but also for the organism as it contends with daily environmental disturbances. Importantly, these physiological activities are *coordinated activities* of the organism as a whole as it interacts with its environment—they cannot be understood in terms of parts alone. What part of the body pumps blood? What part of the body has the function of walking? What part of the body has the function of sleeping? The answer to the first question is the heart. The remaining questions do not have such a straightforward answer. The reason is that walking, sleeping, eating, reproducing, swimming, etc. are evolved coordinated activities of an organism as a whole in relation to its environment. It is the body as a whole that walks. In general, the legs, the arms, and torso coordinate to create a pattern of activity called walking. Similarly, it is the body as whole that reproduces. It is the body as a whole that sleeps. It is these sorts of physical activities of the whole body that cannot be captured by Boorse's part-functionalism or intercellular homeostasis, but might be relevant to his *"what the organism is doing."* It is to these sorts of activities that "organism homeostasis" refers.

In defense of this holistic notion of body movement, Kurt Goldstein, says that when humans make a certain movement

> we do not innervate individual muscles or muscle groups, but a change in the present state of *innervation* of all the body muscles takes place. Thus, a *pattern* of innervation results, in which one definite single contraction, namely, the one which is intended, stands in the foreground. For the appropriate contraction of one muscle group, i.e. for that contraction by which a definite effect results, a certain state of innervation of the remaining body muscles is requisite. To be sure, we do not notice this state of innervation, because it seems to be insignificant for the intention of that movement. But it is not at all insignificant, it rather *enables the organism* to execute the movement correctly.[49]

As Goldstein makes clear, specific body movements require that all (he probably means most) body muscles (in addition to the specific muscles of a particular movement) be coordinated or stimulated to ensure that the specific body movement is accomplished. The pattern of movement that emerges is in conjunction with the pressures from the external environment. Drawing from Goldstein's account, it is this pattern of movement in response to environmental stress that is the product of natural selection. For example, the overall patterns of swimming motion of fishes or flying patterns in birds are evolved patterns that are crucial to survival and reproductive success. It is these sorts of behavioral patterns that allow organisms to interact in an

---

[49] Kurt Goldstein, *The Organism, A Holistic Approach to Biology Derived from Pathological Data in Man* (Boston, 1963), pp. 229–30. For the sake of this discussion, Goldstein's inclusion of intentions can be ignored. The concern is only with making sense of the coordination of bodily activities [my italics].

energetically balanced way with their environments. It is the energy balance created by these coordinated behaviors that is here being called organism homeostasis. On this view, organisms share a close relationship with their environment such that energy balance is part of understanding organisms as ecologically oriented creatures. David Depew makes this point quite persuasively as follows:

> That bounded, informed, autocatalytic dissipative systems are by definition parts of ecological communities, and that the information which they store and use is subject to dynamics that are inseparably both competitive and cooperative, are facts that Darwinians have ignored at their peril ... For natural selection can play the deep, essential, and above all creative roles suggested by their theories only when organisms are treated ecologically.[50]

Thus, along with intercellular homeostasis, organism homeostasis must be included in the discussion of homeostasis. That is, since it is the overall organism that directly contends with the environment, intercellular homeostasis can be viewed as a necessary condition for overall physiological homeostasis, which is crucial to both intercellular homeostasis and survival and reproduction. For instance, walking, running, sleeping, jumping, grasping, and other evolved behavioral activities can be viewed as effectors that are crucial to maintaining an organism's life (i.e., energy balance maintenance) under a certain range of environmental influences. Bechtel hints at this sense of "organism homeostasis":

> The idea that living organisms incorporate a complex organization that makes them homeostatic systems provides an important element needed in a satisfactory physiological concept of health. In terms of it, one can define a healthy system as one that is at or near its designed equilibrium state. Significant deviations, especially those in which some external agency is required to restore the system to the equilibrium state, are disease states.[51]

According to Bechtel, the complexity of the human body is sufficient to understand it as a homeostatic system. Notice that this claim is distinct from the idea that the human body is composed of homeostatic systems. The first claim refers to what is here being called organism homeostasis, while the second claim refers to internal homeostasis. To this end, the physical activities of the brain (or specific parts) can be seen as the integration centers that assist in fight-flight responses, resting responses, bathing responses, etc. These overall physical functions of the body are not easily captured in Boorse's strict part-functionalist account, although he does hint at such functions. Rather, this requirement of dual-homeostasis reveals that there are functions that can be attributed to the organism as a whole (without including mental phenomena and non-epistemic norms). The upshot is that, once the discussion on health includes homeostasis, organic functional holism is compatible with Boorse's part-functionalism.

---

[50] David Depew, "Darwinism and Developmentalism: Prospects for Convergence," in Gertrudis van de Dijver, Stanley N. Salthe, and Manuela Delpos (eds), *Evolutionary Systems: Biological and Epistemological Perspectives on Selection and Self-Organization* (Dordrecht, 1998), p. 31.

[51] Bechtel, "A Naturalistic Concept of Health," p. 149.

This section has offered a brief glimpse into the concept of homeostasis. It included a discussion of both intercellular homeostasis, organism homeostasis, and a general explanation of the different elements that comprise a homeostatic system. The general conclusion that should be gleaned from this section is that homeostasis should include not only the internal intercellular balances of the body, but also the many behavioral activities of the body designed to contend directly with the environment.

*Combining Function and Homeostasis: An Evolutionary Concept of Health*

An obvious objection to understanding health in terms of homeostasis alone is that there is little reason to think that the body works towards maintaining physiological homeostasis. Bechtel notes, "The problem with the physiological perspective when taken on its own is that it failed to show why any premium should be placed on maintaining a system at its homeostatic equilibrium."[52] After noting this problem, Bechtel goes on to offer "the anchor" to ground physiological homeostasis:

> Within an evolutionary scenario, we can recognize the homeostatic design with its set equilibrium point as both a product of natural selection and, more importantly, as likely to enhance future survival. Maintaining the system in such a condition becomes important in aiding the survival and reproductive success of an organism ... [53]

As Bechtel notes, the idea of thinking of the body (for the most part) as a homeostatic system is justified by way of natural selection. Specifically, keeping intercellular fluid and the physical activities of the body as a whole in homeostasis has been selected because it helps to ensure higher-end goals of survival and reproduction. So, it is quite reasonable to think that physiological homeostasis is a necessary condition for health.

In terms of the mixed evolutionary concept of function developed in the earlier section of this chapter, regulated variables, set points, sensors, integration centers and effectors are functions, because their specific propensities to ensure homeostasis and survival and reproduction are the product of natural selection. For instance, inflammation is an excellent example of the fruitfulness of the mixed account of function combined with homeostasis. Stephen Chensue and Peter Ward offer the following summary:

> Inflammation is best defined in teleologic terms. Specifically, it is a series of molecular and cellular responses *acquired during evolution designed to eliminate foreign agents and promote repair of damaged tissues*. Unfortunately, these responses are not infallible. Pathogens have concurrently evolved mechanisms to avoid elimination; new pathogens occasionally emerge from the environment, and under some circumstances aberrant immunoinflammatory responses damage the host. The complexity of the immunoinflammatory system is a reflection of millions of years of environmental changes.[54]

---

[52] Ibid., p. 151.
[53] Ibid.
[54] Stephen W. Chensue and Peter A. Ward, "Inflammation," in Ivan Damjanov and James Linder (eds), *Anderson's Pathology*, 10th edn (St. Louis, 1996), p. 387 [my italics].

Chensue and Ward make clear that there is a goal-directed element involved in inflammation. For example, a fluid inflammatory response, known as edema (accumulation of water in tissues), is an attempt by the host body to "dilute the insulting agent, thus reducing the concentration of harmful molecules."[55] Moreover, by eliminating the harmful molecules, intercellular homeostasis is maintained. In this process, a set of cell-types (e.g., cytokines, leukocytes, macrophages, eosinophils, etc.) interacts to defend the body from the invader. In order to coordinate different cell-types, molecular mediators, known as cytokines, direct the various stages (initiate, recruit, remove, and repair) of the inflammatory response. That is, the goal of cytokines is to bring to fruition each of these stages of inflammation in order to weaken or eliminate the invading agent and to repair damaged tissue.

From the perspective of homeostasis, the regulated variables associated with the inflammatory response are those associated with intercellular fluid (osmotic pressure, chemical composition, temperature, waste, etc.). The set points will be those that are relevant to each regulated variable of the intercellular fluid. The main sensors in the inflammatory response are the bone marrow and lymph nodes. When it is necessary, the bone marrow produces the different sorts of leukocytes and the lymph nodes produce the various lymphocytes. Both the bone marrow and the lymph nodes act as sensors and integration centers, monitoring current conditions with respect to the various set points of the intercellular fluid. Finally, cytokines and the other cell-types that defend and repair the body are the effectors, which are working to return the intercellular fluid to its overall set point.

After intercellular homeostasis occurs, it is possible for the functions of the organism as a whole to be brought into a homeostatic state as well. For example, after edema of the legs subsides, regular walking, sleeping, and eating patterns return. Indeed, once these patterns have returned, intercellular homeostasis is also maintained. From this perspective, intercellular homeostasis and organism homeostasis act as feedback loops for maintaining one another. Each of these activities has its set points, regulated variables, sensors, and integration centers. Finally, these overall physiological activities are crucial with respect to survival and reproduction. The picture of what is here being called *dual-homeostasis* is as follows:

**Intercellular Homeostasis ⇔ Organism Homeostasis ⇒ Survival and Reproduction**

The double arrow between intercellular homeostasis and organism homeostasis represents the feedback interrelationship between the two. The single arrow between organism homeostasis and survival and reproduction represents the idea that the various elements that comprise both intercellular homeostasis and organism homeostasis (set points, effectors, etc.) are adaptive functions that confer a survival and reproductive-enhancing propensity on the individual organism. With the above analysis in place, it is now possible to give an account of what health is. Basically, health, which includes the mixed evolutionary concept of function and the physiological concept of homeostasis discussed above, is the propensity of an

---

[55] Ibid.

organism and its parts to maintain intercellular and organism homeostasis for the sake of ensuring survival and reproduction.

Note, however, the following four qualifications (also made by Boorse) need to be introduced into the analysis. First, the condition of intercellular homeostasis will vary from species to species. Different species will have evolved distinct propensities for different set points, regulated variables, sensors, and integration centers to ensure the maintenance of intercellular homeostasis for the sake of survival and reproduction. Second, since evolution has produced features in women that are not present in men (e.g., lactation and ovulation), this evolutionary-homeostatic concept of health must be further qualified to accommodate gender differences. Third, not only are species and gender differences part of this account, but general age differences must also be included. For the proper function of many physiological systems are only fully functional between a certain age range. For example, life cycle development (which is an evolved feature) reveals that certain systems are functional in newborn infants (e.g., respiratory system), but leaves others systems rather undeveloped (e.g., visual systems and reproductive systems). These developmental differences are included in this account of health. Fourth, environmental factors are ineliminable from this evolutionary account. Since proper functioning is tied to the evolved propensity to perform certain activities, such activities are the product of a certain range of environmental variation. This variation will include the geologic environments and the recent evolutionary environments of which the human species is a product. Consequently, the health status of human functions must be understood within the context of the relevant range of environmental variations.

With the above four qualifications included in the analysis, the evolutionary concept of health defended in this chapter can be summarized as follows:

> *Evolutionary-Homeostatic Concept of Health*: An organism—within a certain species, gender, age group, and environment—is in a state of health if and only if its relevant parts and overall behavioral activities have and retain evolved functional propensities to secure dual-homeostasis, which in turn confers a survival enhancing functional propensity on the organism as a whole.

The implication of the evolutionary-homeostatic concept of health noted above (EHCH hereafter) is that health is a state that admits of degree. Different internal and external factors that disrupt various parts of the homeostatic system may only reduce various propensities slightly, rendering an organism only slightly unhealthy. Alternatively, internal and external factors may disrupt parts of the homeostatic system and reduce various propensities tremendously, rendering an organism extremely unhealthy. A turn to a number of actual "diseases" will reveal the fruitfulness and possible limitations of the EHCH developed in this section.

*Case Studies*

*Case 1: tuberculosis* Tuberculosis (a respiratory infection once called "consumption") is an infectious disease. It is caused by two different organisms: *Mycobacterium tuberculosis* and *Mycobacterium bovis*. The first of these passes from person to

An Evolutionary Concept of Health            197

person by way of the respiratory system. The second infects domestic animals, but can infect humans who consume the infected animals or their by-products (e.g., milk from cows). J. N. Hays offers the following explanation of tuberculosis:

> The causative "germ," whether M. tuberculosis or M. bovis, lodges in the human body. Immunological reactions shortly begin, and a walled-off "tubercle" results that contains the bacillus and prevents its further spread through the body. The person so infected may be said to "have" tuberculosis, if by that word is meant a positive reaction to a tuberculin test; but in many cases no clinical symptoms ever develop, so that if the tuberculin test were not administered no assumption of tuberculosis would ever be made. In some individuals, however—and here the etiological puzzles arise—the body's immune systems fail to contain the spread of the bacillus, and different clinical manifestations of tuberculosis results, sometimes rapidly, more often much more gradually.[56]

After examining the history of tuberculosis, Hays offers the following summary judgment about the decline of this disease in the nineteenth century:

> Much of the explanation of that decline, which began in the nineteenth century, therefore necessarily relies on environmental and social changes. The regulation of workplaces [increased and improved] ... More important, housing improved after the horror-filled first generation of industrial cities ... [R]educed birthrates certainly made several important contributions: healthier women, healthier babies, greater possibility of improving a family's standard of housing and diet alike, perhaps less stress. It is therefore likely that the decline in incidence of tuberculosis in the second half of the nineteenth century was chiefly caused by increasing individual powers of resistance, for which several environmental and social factors must receive credit ... Those individual powers of resistance may have been further strengthened by heredity, as exposure stimulated antibody activity in successive generations.[57]

There are five points that need to be made clear from the above descriptions:

1. Tuberculosis in humans is caused by two kinds of organisms that invade the body either through the air (from person to person) or by way of certain foods.
2. Many people's immune systems are able to sterilize the bacilli or "control" them for an extended period of time by encapsulating them in a sort of protective "capsule" called granuloma or tubercle, but some people's immune systems cannot bring this defense to fruition.[58]

---

[56] J. N. Hays, *The Burdens of Disease: Epidemics and Human Response in Western History* (New Brunswick, 1998), p. 161.

[57] Ibid., p. 176 [bracketed addition mine].

[58] Thomas Daniel explains this fantastic defense mechanism as follows: "The body of a person infected with tubercle bacilli responds to this invader mobilizing an immune system that is elegant in its specificity and complex in its action. Many cells are involved, under the control of CD4⁺ T-lymphocytes that secrete cytokines that direct other cells to form granulomas and carry out other immunologic processes. This complex immune system produces resistance to infection and defends the body against the invasion of the tubercle

3. Some people whose immune systems can contain the bacilli eventually succumb to them after many years of dormancy.
4. Susceptibility to the bacilli varies among people.
5. Environmental conditions influence the spread of tuberculosis.

It is not difficult to make sense of what Hays calls "the etiological puzzle" of tuberculosis once a Darwinian perspective is taken. Randolph Nesse and George Williams explain as follows:

> Dangerous bacteria, most notably those that cause tuberculosis and gonorrhea, are now more difficult to control with antibiotics than they were ten or twenty years ago. Bacteria have been evolving defenses against antibiotics just as surely as they have been evolving defenses against our natural weaponry and that of fungi throughout their evolutionary history.[59]

Basically, because bacteria can replicate by the millions so quickly, they are able to make manifest advantageous variations and mutations. Host defenses cannot counteract these variations quickly enough to eradicate the new strains. Moreover, some people's immune systems will react to invasion better than others. Thus, the immune system effectors, which have evolved to handle certain kinds of bacteria, cannot thwart the onslaught of certain new variations. The effect is a breakdown in both intercellular and organism homeostasis, resulting in an unhealthy or diseased condition. This explains points 4 and 5 above. Certain environmental conditions noted by Hays (e.g., low levels of dust and sunshine) along with certain variations of the tuberculosis bacteria coupled with the immune systems of certain people can help to reduce susceptibility to certain strains of the virus. However, certain environmental conditions (e.g., dusty and dark close quarters) in conjunction with certain variations of the virus in association with certain immune systems will render a body very susceptible to tuberculosis.

What can be said about points 2 and 3? That is, 90% of people's immune systems are able to bring about this defensive response, but about 10% are not able to do so. Why can some people, but not others, bring forth the relevant effectors (e.g., CD4+ T-lymphocytes) to produce the granulomas that defensively encase the bacilli? There are numerous answers to this question. In some people, the immune response simply fails with respect to the production of the relevant lymphocytes due to age or congenital mishap. In other people, the presence of other viruses or bacteria (e.g., HIV), which directly attack the CD4+ T-lymphocytes, prevent the immune system from functioning in a coordinated fashion. Still, others have compromised immune systems associated with drug and alcohol abuse. Children appear to be more susceptible to the bacilli. Any of these factors combined with poor environmental conditions (e.g., dusty or poorly ventilated work areas) make people more susceptible to the tuberculosis bacilli.[60]

---

bacillus." See Thomas M. Daniel, *Captain of Death: The Story of Tuberculosis* (Rochester, 1997), p. 150.

[59] Nesse and Williams, *Why We Get Sick*, p. 53.
[60] This summary is drawn from Anonymous, "Tuberculosis," http//:www.Tuberculosis.net.

The tubercle bacilli, when they are in an active stage (they can lay dormant in the tubercle for years without detection), can destroy the lungs, liver, kidneys, brain, bone, and other organs. To some extent, the body defense system can build a wall around the bacilli (the way a scab forms around a cut), but when the bacilli become active, they can destroy this wall and disrupt physiological homeostasis.[61] With respect to the EHCH developed in this chapter, the particular effectors that attempt to destroy the bacilli do not have the evolved propensity to do so (as a result of both congenital and environmental factors noted above), eventually resulting in massive disruption of intercellular homeostasis. Such disruption then leads to the destruction of various organs and these effects produce organism homeostasis imbalance. The result is that the evolved propensity for physiological homeostasis—both intercellular and organism—can be considerably destroyed, resulting in a very unhealthy organism.

Tuberculosis is an example of an infectious disease that can be understood through EHCH. Basically, humans have evolved immune responses to contend with viral infections within certain environmental ranges. A person can be considered unhealthy when overall homeostasis is compromised by immune system dysfunction in conjunction with environmental factors. Since there is a constant evolutionary battle between humans and other viruses, the propensity to defend against such invaders will be limited to certain types of invaders. The rates of evolutionary change at the viral level make it nearly impossible for human adaptive structures to retaliate appropriately to all variations and mutants. So, poor health is not the result of immune system dysfunction, but the disruption of intercellular homeostasis.

Finally, note that, from the EHCH perspective, a person infected with the tuberculosis virus is not automatically considered unhealthy. The following conditions help make sense of this case. If the appropriate immune system response functions properly (i.e., destroys the bacilli) within its designed constraints, then homeostasis will not be disturbed and the person will be considered healthy. If a person is not able to produce properly the relevant immune response when infected by the virus, then the person would be deemed unhealthy to the degree that homeostasis is compromised. If a person is able to control the virus through immune response, but the bacilli are not destroyed, then it is likely that either the immune response is faulty or the virus is a mutant strain that cannot be destroyed. In such cases, the virus lays dormant for many years. It is only when the bacilli awaken, escape from the tubercles and disrupt homeostasis is the person considered unhealthy. The point is that the presence of a virus by itself is neither necessary nor sufficient to render a person physically unhealthy or diseased. According to the EHCH, it is the evolved propensities of homeostatic systems that must be disrupted for physiological conditions to be unhealthy or diseased.

---

[61] The effects of the tubercle bacilli is wonderfully described in Chapter 9 of Rene and Jean Dubos's *The White Plague: Tuberculosis, Man and Society* (Boston, 1952) and the overall history and story of this disease is clearly narrated by Daniel, *Captain of Death: The Story of Tuberculosis*.

*Case 2: allergies*  Allergies are another set of conditions to consider with respect to the EHCH. There are many types of allergies. They can be partially categorized as follows: (1) injected allergies (drugs, venom), (2) ingested allergies (foods), (3) inhaled allergies (pollen and animal dander), and (4) skin allergies (plants).[62] Allergies, which occur in varying degrees, are responses by the immune systems. In some cases, a minor allergic reaction can result in itchy eyes, mild sneezing, or slight inflammation of the tongue, having little or no serious effect on the dispositional properties of physiological homeostasis.[63] The result is that an organism with a mild allergy is a relatively healthy organism. For example, some people are mildly or severely allergic to cat hair. In an environment where cats are present, people will be considered unhealthy or healthy to some degree, depending upon how their systems react to cats. Indeed, some people have no allergic reaction to cats. Of course, severe allergic reactions (e.g., bee stings in some people) can result in acute respiratory and pulmonary distress. In these sorts of cases, the organism is extremely unhealthy, because the dispositional properties of physiological homeostasis have been greatly reduced in the particular environment. Different sorts of allergies reveal that health is a state that not only admits of degree, but may also admit of duration and vary with local environmental conditions.

A further qualification about allergies is needed. Many allergic reactions are immune system responses governed by the immunoglobin-E (IgE) system. Some have argued that allergy is a vestigial system that is beneficial in other species, but simply damages tissue in humans and should be viewed as an immune-response error. Thus, much like the appendix, the IgE system can cause physiological problems, but has no present function. In response, Margie Profet has argued that the IgE system is a specialized evolved back-up system to remove toxins from the body. As she notes, "The evolutionary persistence of the allergic capability, despite its physiological costs, implies the existence of an adaptive benefit for this capability that outweighs the costs; this undermines the view that allergy is an immunological error."[64] The idea is that the body does have various toxin-fixing antibodies and enzymes that can decompose various sorts of chemical toxins. Yet, there are some toxins (e.g., venom, industrial pollutants, phenolic acids, and alkaloids) that are able to bypass these defenses. Profet argues that the IgE system is a second round of defense designed to eliminate these sorts of toxins that have evaded initial detection. In her own words, "[A]llergy is designed to be a last line of defense against toxins; that is, the allergic response is triggered when individual's primary antitoxin defense mechanisms have proven on a previous occasion to be insufficient in preventing a specific toxin from persisting in the bloodstream and damaging cells."[65] Randolph

---

[62]  Margie Profet, "The Function of Allergy: Immunological Defense Against Toxins," *Quarterly Review of Biology*, 66/1 (March 1991): 36–40. See also Kathleen C. Barnes, George J. Armelagos, and Steven C. Morreale, "Darwinian Medicine and the Emergence of Allergy," in Wenda R. Trevathan, E. O. Smith, and James J. McKenna (eds), *Evolutionary Medicine* (New York, 1999), pp. 209–43.

[63]  Allergies were briefly discussed in the "strong normativism" section of Chapter 3 and the "function versus accident" section of Chapter 4.

[64]  Ibid., pp. 24–5.

[65]  Ibid., p. 27.

Nesse and George Williams offer the following summary of Profet's theory about certain allergic reactions:

> [An allergy] gets toxins out of you in a hurry. Shedding tears gets them [i.e., toxins] out of the eyes. Mucous secretions and sneezing and coughing get them out of the respiratory tract. Vomiting gets them out of the stomach. Allergic reactions act quickly to expel offending materials. This fits the rapidity with which toxins can cause harm. A few mouthfuls of those beautiful foxgloves in your garden can kill you a lot faster than a phone call can summon aid. Appropriately for Profet's theory, the only part of our immunological system that seems to be in a great hurry is that which mediates allergy. Other aspects of allergy that she mentions in support of her theory include the propensity to be triggered by venoms and by toxins that bind permanently to body tissue, the release of anticoagulants during allergic inflammation to counteract coagulant venoms, and the apparently erratic distribution of allergies to specific substances.[66]

With respect to EHCH, allergies may seem problematic. For the IgE system has an evolved propensity to fight off certain toxins, but it does so by disrupting homeostasis. That is, the IgE system is a biological function that can render an organism unhealthy.

The reply to the above difficulty is a reminder that evolutionary systems are not perfect systems. In an attempt to resolve one problem, biological systems can have disrupting side effects. This is simply the result of the body as a bundle of evolutionary compromises. With respect to homeostasis, the IgE system is an effector that has the evolved propensity of maintaining intercellular homeostasis. In order to do this it must (to some degree) disrupt organism homeostasis at times. (A fever is an effector in much the same way.) According to EHCH, allergic responses (and fevers) can render an organism mildly or severely unhealthy (depending upon their degree of disturbance to intercellular and organism homeostasis) in the short run, so that both intercellular and organism homeostasis can be secured in the long run. This example stands as reminder that biological features that appear to reduce the health status of people may have evolutionary functions that are not obvious. These sorts of examples require that the health judgment that is made be qualified for short term and long term benefits. The EHCH perspective is respectful and alert to such scenarios. So, rather than telling against EHCH, allergies (i.e., biological functions that can cause harm) validate it.

*Case 3: Down's syndrome* Down's syndrome (Trisomy 21) is one of the most common autosomal abnormalities. It is the result of having more than the usual number of chromosomes (aneuploidy).[67] This occurs during meiosis, when homologous chromosomes do not separate into distinct cells (this phenomenon is known as non-disjunction). People with Down's syndrome have some combination of the following physiological characteristics in differing degrees: slit-eyed appearance, skeletal abnormalities, disruption of metabolism, reduced resistance to

---

[66] Nesse and Williams, *Why We Get Sick*, p. 163 [bracketed additions mine].

[67] Down's syndrome and other genetic disorders are discussed by David T. Purtilo, *A Survey of Human Diseases* (Menlo Park, 1978), pp. 174–90.

infection, defects of the heart, slowness of movement, and many other physiological birth deformities. According to David Purtilo, "It is thought that these deformities are the result of an increased dose of an enzyme from the extra chromosome 21."[68]

A person with Down's syndrome is unhealthy because both intercellular and organism homeostasis are disrupted. Intercellular homeostasis is disturbed because (in part) the additional chromosome, which assists in excessive enzyme production, is toxic to developing cells. Organism homeostasis is disrupted because the propensity to contend with normal environmental variations can be greatly limited, depending upon the severity of a particular case. So, the degree to which a person with Down's syndrome is unhealthy depends upon the severity of the genetic defect on both intercellular and organism homeostasis.

With respect to this disease, age is relevant to the extent that it is a defect present at birth and throughout life. There does not appear to be much gender bias (unlike, for example, Klinefelter's syndrome, which occurs in males only), and, although the exact causal factors of this non-disjunction are unknown, maternal age is strongly correlated with the genetic error. Finally, the influence of the external environment on the phenotypic expression of Down's syndrome is very difficult to establish.[69] It appears that Down's syndrome can occur in just about any environmental context, but the severity of it may vary, because the person is more "susceptible to other genetic and environmental insults, leading to the features, diseases, and conditions associated with Down's syndrome."[70] Thus, since environmental factors cannot be ruled out in the case of Down's syndrome-related diseases, the degree to which a person is unhealthy will be somewhat environmentally sensitive.

In summary, the evolutionary concept of health is able to make sense of both the genetic and phenotypic aspects of Down's syndrome and can likely make sense of other inherited disorders. As was suggested through the example of Hunter disease explained earlier and Down's syndrome discussed here, a cogent concept of health will need to be sensitive to age, gender, and environmental factors before health judgments can be formed.

*Case 4: sickle cell anemia*  Sickle cell anemia is a blood disorder caused by a gene that is also beneficial. This disorder occurs mostly in people from Africa (and some parts of India), where malaria is a major cause of death. To understand sickle cell anemia, a few definitions related to genetics need to be made clear. First, alleles are alternative forms of a particular gene that affect a specific trait in different ways. For example, consider eye color. Assume that brown eyes are "dominant" over blue eyes. "B" refers to a dominant allele. "b" refers to a recessive allele. The gene for brown-

---

[68] Ibid., p. 182.

[69] It turns out that the severity of Down's syndrome is related to the interaction of a host of genes. As Len Leshin notes, "[I]t would be a mistake to assume that the clinical features of Down's syndrome are only due to a handful of genes being overexpressed. You can think of the overexpressed gene products interacting with a number of normal gene products, each product individualized by the person's unique genetic makeup, and thus being 'thrown out of genetic balance'" See Len Leshin, "Trisomy 21: The Story of Down Syndrome," http://www.ds-health.com/trisomy.htm.

[70] Ibid.

colored eyes includes the following set of alleles: **BB** and **Bb**. The alleles for blue eyes are **bb**. **BB** is a condition known as *homozygous dominant*. This means that so long as **BB** alleles are present, brown colored eyes will always be present over any other colored eyes. **Bb** is the condition known as *heterozygous*. In this case, a person has both a dominant and a recessive gene. In heterozygous cases, the dominant allele swamps the effects of the recessive allele. So, **Bb** will produce brown eyes, even though a recessive gene is present. Finally, **bb** refers to the condition known as *homozygous recessive*. In this case, a person has two recessive alleles. With respect to eye color, **bb** will produce blue eyes.

In principle, sickle cell anemia occurs in a similar way, but the effect under consideration is red-blood cell modification with respect to malaria parasites. Assume that **RR** is the homozygous dominant condition, **Rr** is the heterozygous condition, and **rr**, is the homozygous recessive condition. Genetically, the three conditions produce the following effects:

1. *Homozygous Dominant*: These people carry two of the same forms of the gene (alleles), and are not able to modify the shape of their red blood cells. Although there are no detrimental side effects, these people are unable to defend against malaria parasites.
2. *Homozygous Recessive*: These people carry two recessive alleles that are able to modify the shape of their red blood cells. However, as result of this modification, they also suffer crippling side effects. This group of people is said to have *sickle cell disease*.
3. *Heterozygous*: These people carry one dominant and one recessive allele. The recessive gene **r** is able to modify the shape of the red blood cells. Moreover, the combination of **Rr** defends against malaria without any serious crippling effects in certain environments.

Nesse and Williams report on people with the homozygous recessive condition as follows: "Their red blood cells twist into a crescent or sickle shape that cannot circulate normally, thus causing bleeding, shortness of breath, and pain in bones, muscles, and the abdomen."[71] Again, these people are said to have the *sickle cell disease*. Those who are homozygous dominant for this gene have normal red blood corpuscles, but are unable to defend themselves against malaria. However, those who are heterozygous for the gene have the *sickle cell trait*. These people have a hemoglobin structure that is able to remove the infected malaria parasites before they cause serious damage to the body.[72] Much like Down's syndrome, sickle cell

---

[71] Nesse and Williams, *Why We Get Sick*, p. 99. Note that the genetic account of sickle cell anemia presented here has been simplified. For a detailed discussion, see Anonymous, "How Does Sickle Cell Cause Disease?" http://sickle.bwh.harvard.edu/scd_background.html.

[72] Stanley N. Salthe explains this ingenious mechanism of the heterozygote condition as follows: "The kind of adaptation that was constructed does not interfere with the insertion of parasites into the blood stream of mosquitoes. Nor does it interfere with the ability of parasites to feed on hemoglobin. And it did not bolster the ability of the human organism to withstand any of the many symptoms of malaria. What it did was to modify hemoglobin in such a way that, when oxygen concentration within the red cell becomes lowered by the metabolic

anemia (the homozygous recessive condition) is a genetic disease and can only be acquired through the genes of parents.

With respect to those who have the homozygous recessive genes, they are deemed unhealthy from the perspective of EHCH. Both intercellular fluid and organism homeostasis are greatly disrupted, rendering these people very unhealthy. In contrast, people who are homozygous dominant become unhealthy only if they contract malaria. In the case of those who are homozygous dominant it is clear that the role of the environment is crucial to their health. So long as these people do not live in malaria infested areas they will have no health concerns with respect to their genetic condition. In contrast, the homozygous recessive condition will render a person very unhealthy in just about any environmental condition, because the deformation of the hemoglobin is an inevitable consequence of being homozygous recessive.

Now, the heterozygous condition must be assessed. At first glance, it appears that this condition is healthy, since malaria can be destroyed. Within an evolutionary perspective, Nesse and Williams offer the following summary judgment:

> The sickle-cell gene thus illustrates *heterozygote advantage*. Because of their resistance to malaria, heterozygotes are favored over both kinds of homozygotes: Homozygotes [who are recessive] for the sickle-cell allele have low fitness resulting from sickle-cell disease, while homozygotes [who are dominant] for the normal allele have low fitness resulting from their vulnerability to malaria.[73]

One additional point needs to be made explicit concerning the above description. Specifically, these fitness claims by Nesse and Williams must be qualified with respect to the environment, because *adaptation* means *adaptation to local environments*. So, the fitness advantage that heterozygotes have over both sets of homozygotes is relative to the low-altitude environment in which malaria is present. If, however, people with each of these conditions were placed in an environment where no malaria existed and the altitude was very high, then the fitness advantages would change. Although the heterozygotes and the homozygote dominant people would still have a fitness advantage over the homozygote recessive people, the heterozygote people would no longer have a fitness advantage over the homozygote dominant people. The reason is that the heterozygote condition in high altitudes does not confer its propensity advantage in such places. That is, the high altitude causes the red blood cells to be modified. The result of this modification is hypoxia, which can produce fainting spells and other physically harmful conditions.[74] In such a scenario, the

---

activity of increasing numbers of the aerobic parasite, it would precipitate, its crystals then deforming the red cell in such a way that it would lyse, releasing the parasites into the blood stream at a developmental stage when they are not ready to survive there." See Stanley N. Salthe, "The Role of Natural Selection Theory in Understanding Evolutionary Systems," in Gertrudis van de Dijver, Stanley N. Salthe, and Manuela Delpos (eds), *Evolutionary Systems: Biological and Epistemological Perspectives on Selection and Self-Organization*, p. 15.

[73] Nesse and Williams, *Why We Get Sick*, p. 99 [bracketed additions mine].

[74] In general, heterozygote women are more prone to urinary tract infections than homozygote dominant women. Note that the extent to which the heterozygote condition is

homozygous dominant people would have a fitness advantage over the heterozygote people. Restated, in the low-altitude/malaria environment, the heterozygote people are healthier than both sets of homozygote people, because the evolved survival/ reproduction propensity is present. Moreover, if it is true that there are side effects from the heterozygote condition even in this environment, then these people may still be somewhat unhealthy, but healthier than both homozygous people. The point is that adaptive traits need to be understood in relation to local environments in making health judgments. The EHCH is sensitive to such nuances created by natural selection.

*Case 5: osteoporosis (degenerative disease)*  Osteoporosis is a degenerative bone disease usually found in elderly people. It is characterized by low bone mass and structural deterioration of bone tissue, leading to bone fragility and an increased susceptibility to fractures, especially of the hip, spine, and wrist. It is most common (80%) among women over the age of 50 (in their post-menopausal years), but it is also present (20%) in men over the age of 50.

For the sake of this discussion, osteoporosis poses two problems for EHCH. First, osteoporosis is a sort of "silent disease," because bone loss occurs without symptoms. Restated, osteoporosis does render a person unhealthy, but does so without compromising the propensities associated with intercellular homeostasis. The problematic implication of the concept of health developed in this chapter is that people with osteoporosis are healthy, because this sort of deterioration does not effect intercellular homeostasis.

The reply to the above account is that EHCH not only ranges over the intercellular fluid, but it also ranges over the overall behavioral activities of organisms. For example, locomotion is an integral part of the human organism's ability to maintain overall physiological homeostasis as it interacts with the environment. On this account, locomotion is an effector that helps to return the body to overall physiological homeostasis. Since osteoporosis can greatly limit mobility (in women this can occur due to a lack of estrogen, which acts as an effector to maintain bone density. In men it is a lack of testosterone that leads to decreased bone density), it directly reduces the propensity of locomotion to contribute to overall physiological homeostasis. Moreover, since there is a feedback relationship between organism homeostasis and intercellular homeostasis, a reduction in mobility could reduce access to food resources. For example, people who hunt for their meals would not be able to do so. The result is that nutritional deficiencies could occur, disrupting intercellular homeostasis.

The point is that if either the propensity to secure intercellular homeostasis or organism homeostasis is reduced, then an organism will be unhealthy to some degree. Admittedly, in many cases the person may be trivially unhealthy. This is why many disabilities (deafness, blindness, loss of limbs, etc.) render a person unhealthy

---

physically harmful with respect to exercise and other scenarios is unclear or controversial from the data collected and studied. For the experiments and other physical ailments associated with the heterozygote condition, see John Kark, "Sickle Cell Trait," http://sickle.bwh.harvard.edu/sickle_trait.html.

to some degree, even if intercellular homeostasis is not compromised. Thus, a person with osteoporosis would be unhealthy to some degree, depending upon the severity of the osteoporosis.

Assume that the first problem above has been resolved. The second more serious problem is that EHCH is deeply tied to the process of evolution. Specifically, conditions that afflict people after their reproductive years or people who have inoperative reproductive systems would not have any impact on the evolved survival/reproduction-enhancing propensity of their functions. For example, maintaining a certain set point bone density is relevant with respect to reproductive success, but is irrelevant in cases where reproductive success is not a factor. Alternatively, since osteoporosis is a natural condition of post-menopausal women and some men, there is nothing unhealthy about such a feature. Much as it is healthy (or not unhealthy) for a newborn human baby not to be able to walk and a ninety year-old human to be able to see well, it is healthy (or not unhealthy) *qua* normal for elderly people to have osteoporosis. Thus, the possible implications of EHCH are:

1. The concept of health is not relevant to people who are not capable of reproducing.

or

2. The concept of health must treat putatively unhealthy states of certain species and age groups as "normal" features of those species and age groups, suggesting that such features are healthy.

No doubt, this is a serious objection. Neither of the above alternatives is satisfying. Embracing an evolutionary foundation for the concept of health does have the benefit of distinguishing genuine functions from mere side effects, taking environmental factors seriously, and even acknowledging certain aspects of life-span development. It appears, however, that it has the bizarre implication of insisting that the concept of health does not range over a certain class of people who are not capable of reproducing or renders some of their conditions healthy when they are unhealthy. Note that even if it is assumed that most people over a certain age will develop osteoporosis, this statistical fact in no way resolves the problem. They are putatively regarded as unhealthy, but EHCH cannot acknowledge this to be the case.

This objection could be resolved by indicating that the account offered here is species-specific and includes both geologic and recent evolutionary factors. One of the recent evolutionary factors in humans is the emergence of culture from early nomadic clan activities. The result of culture is that the various functions individual humans now possess include activities beyond basic subsistence and reproduction. This is the move suggested by Bechtel. He argues that "evolution," which includes the mechanisms of variation, selection, and retention, refers not only to strict biological evolution, but also to any phenomenon that has these three mechanisms in place. Conceding that "universal selection" is both speculative and controversial, Bechtel offers the following proposal:

Many more of the characteristics of humans could be construed as adaptive when one extends one's focus beyond the inheritance of genes to the inheritance of cultural entities. Within this broader evolutionary framework, health involves those characteristics that make one adaptive in one's endeavors to propagate oneself or one's culture, and so on, when judged against a variety of selection forces, and disease is whatever deters from such adaptedness.[75]

The implication of the above general application of the evolutionary perspective, according to Bechtel, is that "anything can be understood as evolving as long as it has mechanisms for variation, selection, and retention. Thus, any human product—ideas, cultural patterns, values—that can be selectively propagated can be construed as evolving."[76]

Although it is difficult not to be sympathetic with Bechtel's attempt, it runs into a few obstacles. First, by having such a broad (or watered-down) account of evolution, the concept of function becomes trivial. Any personal activity that is retained (in the light of other activities) becomes a function of those people who retain it so long as it has the propensity to enhance their lives and projects within their cultural environment. For example, if some people choose shuffleboard over basketball on a regular basis, then one of their functions is to play shuffleboard, if shuffleboard playing has a survival-enhancing propensity within the context of their cultural environment. Alternatively, if they choose basketball over shuffleboard the following week, then their function is to play basketball. The problem is that what counts as retention is left to the capricious *choices and values* of people such that functions become unreasonably ephemeral and arbitrary. Moreover, this proposal must acknowledge that it is not possible for that which is selected to be neutral with respect to survival-enhancing propensity. For example, if one were to pick a certain brand of pen over others because of its appearance and price, such a pen (on this general selectionist account) would have a survival-enhancing propensity, when it is clear that it is most likely neutral with respect to having a survival-enhancing propensity. No doubt, it is this concern that leads Bechtel to make the following concession:

> [E]mploying such a generalized concept of evolution in the endeavor to define health may open Pandora's box. One can view almost any human product as capable of selective replication (including, for example, pornography). If health is whatever promotes generalized evolutionary success, it must be directed toward promoting all of these modes of replication.[77]

Second, propagating oneself and propagating one's culture are two distinct functions that can come into conflict. For example, cigarettes are cultural artifacts. Engaging in activities that ensure the production of sales of cigarettes, however minutely, contributes to the propagation of culture. However, it turns out that cigarettes are a leading cause of death to a large number of people every year. As a

---

[75] Bechtel, "A Naturalistic Concept of Health," p. 153.
[76] Ibid.
[77] Ibid., p. 154.

result, one may wish to prevent the production and sale of cigarettes. In this attempt to prevent the proliferation of cigarettes, one would be reducing (however minutely) the propagation of culture in favor of individual health. On Bechtel's account, such an anti-cigarette campaign would render a person's culture unhealthy, but individual health would be enhanced. Thus, the cigarette would be a disease to the individual, but a health-producing feature of a culture. The point is that cultural evolution and biological evolution can come into tension, because the former will include all sorts of values and ideologies not present in the latter. Again, Bechtel accedes by noting that "[if a health judgment] ultimately has to be ideological in character, then one has foresaken a naturalistic framework."[78] Bechtel's point is that if health were to be determined by cultural ideological views, then all sorts of cultural norms would have to be included in the concept of health. Yet, such an implication is anathema to a naturalistic concept of health. Thus, it is clear that Bechtel is correct not to be persuaded that such a generalized account of selection is appropriate to a naturalistic concept of health. Indeed, it follows that drawing on cultural evolution to save naturalism and offer a concept of health that can range over the entire life span of people is ineffective.

As an alternative to Bechtel's account, it is possible to return to the propensity aspect of functions to help the EHCH to range over the entire life span of an organism. Specifically, even if it is the case that an organism is not able to actualize one of its goals, it does not follow that the parts that contribute to such goals have lost their propensity with respect to those goals. For example, even if the ignition switch of a car cannot actually turn on a car because the engine does not work, it does not follow that the ignition switch has lost its propensity to start the car. Indeed, it is possible to transfer the ignition switch to a car of the same model with an engine that actually works, and it will be able to start this car. Similarly, a heart retains its survival/reproduction-enhancing propensity even if actual reproductive success is impossible. The point (as mentioned in Chapter 4) is that the propensity that $X$ confers on $Y$ can only be eliminated through the elimination or major modification of $X$ (e.g., the appendix), not $Y$. This is evident by transferring the heart from a brain-dead person to a patient that needs a heart and can reproduce. In the same way, then, the bones or skeletal structures of people with osteoporosis are unhealthy to whatever degree they reduce the survival/reproduction-enhancing propensity bones confer. This same sort of reasoning holds for evolved parts of organisms and the physical activities of the organism as a whole. Therefore, it is possible to consider osteoporosis-like degenerative diseases through the EHCH.

Some people may not be persuaded by the above salvage efforts. One could argue that once the ultimate goals of functions are eliminated, the functions themselves cease to exist. So, if the ultimate goals of biological functions are to confer a survival and reproductive-enhancing propensity on the organism as whole, such functions cease to exist if all of the goals of the function cannot be actualized in a normal range of environmental variations. In such scenarios, since no biological function exists, the state of health also no longer exists. So, it could be argued that it is a mistake to

---

[78] Ibid.

think that survival-enhancing propensities are relevant. What follows from this reply is that EHCH may still fail to range over the entire life span of an organism.

In reply, the above objection relies on a very narrow interpretation of reproductive success. Reproduction includes not only sexual reproduction, but also rearing of children. That is, natural selection favors life expectancy beyond reproductive years and includes child-rearing years. Indeed, the need for child rearing explains why parents live after a child is born. Since reproductive years in women continue until around the age of forty five, an additional fifteen years can be added to accommodate child rearing. So, reproductive success in women continues until around the age of sixty. In men, the age may be closer to seventy. The point is that it is possible for the EHCH to treat dysfunctions as diseases within this age range.

Beyond this age range, EHCH would treat degenerative conditions, like osteoporosis, as the product of medical advances. That is, the fact that many people live beyond their child-bearing and child-rearing age is because of the assistance from medical technology. The result is that social forces, not biological ones, control advanced aging. The implication is that the EHCH accepts the view that osteoporosis (and other degenerative conditions), when it occurs in women after the age of sixty and men after the age of seventy, is not a disease. The reason is that late aging and its effects are no longer strictly part of biological functional analysis.[79] However, the EHCH is able to handle many cases like osteoporosis because it acknowledges that health judgments must be qualified to handle natural life-span transitions.

This section has offered a number of diseases and conditions that give further support to the benefit of the EHCH. The combination of evolution and homeostasis as a way of understanding the body helps to make sense of a wide range of physical conditions, including infectious diseases, degenerative conditions, allergic immunity, and genetic abnormalities due to error during meiosis or genetic differences due to evolution. Note, however, certain cases related to aging (e.g., osteoporosis and decreased virility) require special treatment. Specifically, the EHCH would not view these cases as disease cases when they involve patients of advanced age, and treatment regiments (e.g., hormone therapy in osteoporosis or viagra in decreased virility) would be considered "performance-enhancing" interventions. The ability of the EHCH to handle the range of cases (with sensitivity to age, gender, and the environment) presented here suggests that it is a naturalistic concept of health worth taking seriously.

---

[79] Arthur L. Caplan makes a similar comment when he argues as follows: "Aging exists ... as a consequence of lack of evolutionary foresight; it is simply a bi-product of selective forces working to increase the chances of reproductive success in the life of the individual organism. Senescence has no function; it is simply the inadvertent subversion of organic function, later in life, in favor of maximizing reproductive advantage, early in life." See Arthur L. Caplan, "The 'Unnaturalness' of Aging—A Sickness Unto Death?" in Arthur L. Caplan, H. Tristram Engelhardt Jr., and James J. McCartney (eds), *Concepts of Health and Disease: Interdisciplinary Perspectives* (London, 1981), p. 731.

## A Final Concern: The Units of Selection Problem

The previous chapter argued that Boorse's reply to the units of selection problem posed by Engelhardt is unpersuasive. To summarize, Boorse argues that the unit of selection that is relevant to the concept of health is the individual organism, because this is the part of the "teleological pie" in which pathologists or medical physiologists are interested. This move is unpersuasive, however, without further explanation of why pathologists or medical physiologists believe that natural selection ranges over individual organisms. For even granting Boorse's contextualism about function, this does not resolve the units of selection problem. This is not to suggest that Boorse is mistaken. But a brief defense is required, if one is going to entertain seriously the prospect of an evolutionary concept of individual health.[80]

*Groups versus genes*  Engelhardt argues that if health is to be understood in terms of the individual organism, then relying on evolution is a mistake because evolution would favor the health of groups. That is, he thinks that natural selection favors groups, not individuals:

> Unlike evolution, which is a group- or species-centered concept, definitions of human health and disease tend to be individually oriented. Such definitions may not, therefore, include certain individual problems as states of health, even if those problems contribute to the survival advantage of the species.[81]

Engelhardt's concern is that an evolutionary perspective, which focuses on features of groups and/or survival and reproduction of groups, excludes those topics, like health, that are relevant to individuals.[82] For example, there seems to be some

---

[80] Given the scope of this project a full account of the units of selection problem is impossible. All that is required is some justification in favor of thinking that individuals cannot be ignored in the process of natural selection in favor of genes or groups. If it can be shown that individuals are the unit of selection with respect to genes, then it does reveal that groups are not the *only* unit of selection. This is enough to tell against Engelhardt's criticism. Still, this section will argue that the theory of group selection is not a very plausible account.

[81] H. Tristram Engelhardt, "Health and Disease: Philosophical Perspectives," in W. T. Reich (ed.), *Encyclopedia of Bioethics* (New York, 1978), pp. 601–2. This quotation is taken from Bechtel, "A Naturalistic Concept of Health," p. 151. Note that one of the best attempts to defend group selection is put forth by Elliott Sober and David Sloan Wilson, *Unto Others: Evolution and Psychology of Unselfish Behavior* (Cambridge, 1999).

[82] Although her concern is more focused on species design, Anne Gammelgaard argues as follows: "The problem of determining the unit of selection has immediate bearings on the prospects of grounding the concept of species design in evolutionary biology. Until that problem is resolved, we cannot determine the functional organization of the human organism from the perspective of evolutionary biology. We do not know whether to determine the functional organization of the body in relation to the genes, the cell or the organism. In other words, we cannot identify such a species design on the basis of evolutionary biology. It follows that if we cannot understand species design from an evolutionary perspective, then it would be impossible to render meaningful health judgments about species design from this

evidence that gestational diabetes benefits the baby, but harms the mother.[83] From an individual perspective, the mother is unhealthy. However, from an evolutionary perspective, since gestational diabetes helps keep the group alive, it would have to be accepted as a healthy condition. Thus, the implication of Engelhardt's claims above is that evolution would be of little assistance in understanding individual health.

On the other extreme, Richard Dawkins has argued that only genes—and neither individuals nor groups—are the units of selection.[84] As Dawkins proclaims, "We are survival machines—robot vehicles blindly programmed to preserve the selfish molecules known as genes ..."[85] David Hull summarizes Dawkins's position as follows:

> Dawkins raised a series of objections to selection occurring even at the level of the "individual"—that is, particular organisms. Dawkins argued that selection occurs almost exclusively at the level of individual genes or, more generally, replicators. In its most extreme form, gene selectionism is the view that ultimately the only things that compete with each other are alleles at the same locus. Genes at different loci cannot compete with each other in the relevant sense. In this sense, gene selectionism is an extremely monistic view of evolution.[86]

So, if Dawkins were correct, health judgments would have to be restricted to the survival and reproductive success of genes, not individuals. Alternatively, if Engelhardt is correct, health judgments are restricted to the survival and reproductive success of groups, not individuals. Under either scenario, individuals are left "out in the cold" with respect to judgments about health.

*The Case against Genes and a Defense of the Individual*

It is this penchant to exclude the individual organism from natural selection by the group selectionists and the genic selectionists that requires some defense of individual selectionism in human beings. This section will offer a defense of individual selectionism by way of Stephen Jay Gould's *visibility argument* and his *causal complexity argument*.

---

perspective." See Anne Gammelgaard, "Evolutionary Biology and the Concept of Disease," *Medicine, Health Care and Philosophy*, 3/2 (2000): 113.

[83] See D. Haig, "Genetic Conflicts in Human Pregnancy," *Quarterly Review of Biology*, 68 (1993): 495–532.

[84] Dawkins has made this claim in numerous places, but it is most famously articulated in his *The Selfish Gene* (New York, 1976). This view is implied by Randolph Nesse, "On the Difficulty of Defining Disease: A Darwinian Perspective," *Medicine, Health Care and Philosophy*, 4/1 (2001): 37–46.

[85] Ibid. This quotation is taken from Stephen Gould, "Caring Groups and Selfish Genes," in Stephen Jay Gould, *The Panda's Thumb* (New York, 1980), p. 89.

[86] David Hull, "Introduction to Part II," in David L. Hull and Michael Ruse (eds), *The Philosophy of Biology* (Oxford, 1998), p. 149.

*The argument from visibility* To start, in an attempt to defend Boorse's individuality thesis and argue against Engelhardt's group selectionist account, Bechtel argues as follows:

> Engelhardt's objection ... feeds on a misconception of contemporary evolutionary theory. He treats evolution as concerned with the promotion of species, whereas the dominant tradition in evolutionary thinking has been to view selection as promoting individuals. For the most part, group selection has been the object of derision, and some evolutionists have gone so far in the opposite direction as to insist that the proper focus of an evolutionary analysis is the single gene. Only recently have a few biologists argued for viewing selection as working at the group or species level, as well as the individual level, but they certainly have represented a minority perspective. Moreover, all philosophers and biologists arguing for higher levels of selection also grant that selection occurs at lower levels, such as the level of the individual.[87]

Much of what Bechtel says above is true, but he has not really offered a reply to Engelhardt's criticism. All he has accomplished is to note that group selection is a minority view and that individual selectionism is possible from a multi-level perspective. What is needed, however, is a justification for thinking that individual selection should be taken seriously for human beings,[88] so that group selection is implausible. What is needed for the task at hand is an account of why the individual should be viewed as the unit of selection. If this can be done, it will reveal that Engelhardt's insistence that the unit of selection is only the group or species is false.

Stephen Jay Gould hints at just such a justification when he offers a version of what can be called the visibility argument. In reply to Richard Dawkins's insistence that the unit of selection can only be the gene, Gould replies as follows:

> I find a fatal flaw in Dawkins's attack from below. No matter how much power Dawkins wishes to assign to genes, there is one thing that he cannot give them—direct visibility to natural selection. Selection simply cannot see genes and pick among them directly. It must use bodies as an intermediary. A gene is a bit of DNA hidden within a cell. Selection views bodies. It favors some bodies because they are stronger, better insulated, earlier in their sexual maturation, fiercer in combat, or more beautiful to behold.[89]

Gould's point is that it is the phenotype (interactor) that makes a direct contribution to whether or not certain alleles are transmitted to the next generation. Even if it is the case that genes "use" bodies to do their dirty work, it is still the body and its features that are being screened by the natural world. Genes cannot be the unit of selection, because nature cannot "see" such inconspicuous entities. As Gould notes,

---

[87] Bechtel, "A Naturalistic Concept of Health," p. 152.

[88] Note that a decisive argument against group selection is not needed here. For there may very well be cases of group selection for certain species, but such cases do not rule out the possibility of individual selection in certain species.

[89] Gould, "Caring Groups and Selfish Genes," in S. J. Gould, *The Panda's Thumb*, p. 90.

"If, in favoring a stronger body, selection acted directly upon a gene for strength, then Dawkins might be vindicated."[90]

In summary, Gould is arguing that, because of both the visibility problem and the complex causal factors involved in constructing phenotypes, the individual body is the unit of selection. Even if one conceded that genes create all phenotypes (this is not the case), it is still the overall organism *bauplan* that maintains the existence of genes. That is, it is the transformation (translation) of genes into morphological, physiological, and behavioral units with which natural selection comes in contact.

*The argument from causal complexity* Thinking of the units of selection problem within the framework of Ockham's razor may be of help to see why Gould wins this argument. Ockham's razor is the principle of parsimony, the idea that entities should not be postulated without necessity and that the best explanation is one that posits the fewest number of entities. Since both Dawkins and Gould disagree as to what is the single unit of selection (Dawkins argues for the gene, while Gould argues for the individual organism), parsimony is not relevant to this part of the discussion. Where parsimony is relevant is in terms of the causal relationship(s) between genes and phenotypes. Dawkins is suggesting that the only entity that need be postulated is the gene with respect to natural selection, because of its unique causal role in creating phenotypes for its own selfish "motives."

Yet, as Gould correctly notes, these various units "are channeled through a kaleidoscopic series of environmental influences: embryonic and postnatal, internal and external. Parts are not translated genes, selection doesn't even work directly on parts. It accepts or rejects entire organisms because suites of parts interacting in complex ways, confer advantages."[91] The point to be gleaned from this comparison is that Gould postulates, contrary to Dawkins, a complex host of causal factors for understanding bodies—this is as parsimonious as one can be with respect to biological entities. With respect to Ockham's razor, Dawkins has cut off more than he is allowed. Gould, on the other hand, has correctly postulated multiple causal factors, employing Ockham's razor judiciously. From this fact about multiple causal factors in constructing organisms, Gould concludes that causal uniqueness is not present in genes, making it the case that genes cannot be the unit of selection. Rather, he thinks that it is the result of such multiple causal factors in constructing organisms (and their parts) that leads to the conclusion that individual organisms (not even their parts) are the units of selection. Thus, the combination of the visibility argument and

---

[90] Ibid., pp. 90–91. Robert Brandon makes this same point when he claims that "reproductive success is determined by phenotype irrespective of genotype. Intuitively, selection 'sees' a 4-foot-tall plant as a 4-foot-tall plant, not as a 4-foot-tall plant with genotype g. This idea can be made precise by using the probabilistically defined notion of *screening off*. The basic idea behind the notion of screening off is this: if $A$ renders $B$ statistically irrelevant with respect to some outcome $E$, but not vice versa, then $A$ is a better causal explainer of $E$ than is $B$." See Robert N. Brandon, "Levels of Selection," in David L. Hull and Michael Ruse (eds), *Philosophy of Biology* (Oxford, 1998), p. 180.

[91] Ibid., p. 91. Of course, Dawkins is well aware of this causal complexity, but does not give it its proper place within the units of selection debate. Dawkins's "genes-eye view" rhetoric may be obscuring his considered view.

the causal complexity argument reveals that it is quite reasonable to consider the individual as the appropriate unit of selection.[92]

To summarize, Gould not only rejects the idea that genes are the units of selection, but also that parts of organisms are the units of selection. His defense of this view is that genes cannot be the unit of selection because they are invisible to selection. Moreover, he notes that parts of organisms cannot be the units of selection, because their existence is the product of a host of environmental forces that act on a set of parts "interacting in complex ways." Thus, it is reasonable to consider the individual organism as the unit of selection. The further upshot of this conclusion is that, contrary to Engelhardt's criticism, it is not unreasonable to talk about individual health within the context of evolution.[93] Indeed, the EHCH offered in this chapter has attempted to do just that.

*The Case against Groups*

Note that Engelhardt could reply that the above analysis has only shown that genes cannot be the units of selection. It has not shown that groups cannot be the units of selection. Thus, as it stands, the unit of selection could be either the individual organism or the group. This is a reasonable reply, but it can be answered. Indeed, there are two arguments that help validate the implausibility of group selection.

To start, it is important to get clear on what group selection is. The general idea is that there is a group adaptation, which is a property of the group that benefits the survival and reproduction of the group as a whole. As Robert Brandon explains, "group selection is natural selection acting at the level of biological groups. And natural selection is the differential reproduction of biological entities that is due to the differential adaptedness of those entities to a common environment."[94] For example, V.C. Wynne-Edwards argued that some species curtail their reproduction

---

[92] Speaking in rather general terms, it should be noted that Kim Sterelny and Philip Kitcher have tried to defeat Gould's visibility argument by insisting that phenotypic traits do not screen off genotypic traits. They argue that the allelic environment must be tampered with in order to show that phenotypic traits do screen off genotypic traits. Yet, they claim that the tampering of the allelic environment reveals that fitness varies more with changes in the genotype than the phenotype. They concede, however, that "mixing orthodox concepts of the environment with ideas about genic selection is a recipe for trouble ..." The result of this concession is that it is not at all clear that they have defeated Gould's visibility argument. Moreover, even if their response is persuasive, it leaves the complexity argument untouched. See Kim Sterelny and Philip Kitcher, "The Return of the Gene," in David L. Hull and Michael Ruse (eds), *The Philosophy of Biology* (Oxford, 1998), pp. 153–75.

[93] The intention is not to deny that group selection as a possible occurrence. Whether or not it is relevant to hominid evolution is also not necessarily being denied. Rather, the goal of this section is simply to provide a reasonable justification for thinking that the individual organism is the unit of selection, because group selection is not a powerful enough force. It is worth noting, however, that most cases of group selection have been interpreted as forms of kin selection or reciprocal altruism, rendering the idea that the unit of selection can be (or is) the group as very controversial.

[94] R. N. Brandon, "The Levels of Selection," p. 183.

in relation to local food supply.[95] If all individuals in a group reproduced at their maximum capacity, then their offspring would consume all the food supply in the local area. As result of over-consumption, the group could suffer extinction. The group could avoid such a fate by collectively restraining their reproduction. However, traditionally understood, natural selection on individuals does not favor reproductive constraint. An individual that increases its reproduction will automatically have an advantage relative to individuals who have fewer offspring. Within a group, if some individuals produce more offspring than others do, the former will proliferate. Three questions emerge from this scenario:

1. Can individual selection within the group be overcome by selection between groups?
2. Is there a strong likelihood that selection between groups can out-compete selection within groups?
3. Even if group selection is possible, how strong of a process is it?

The answer to the first question is that it is theoretically possible for selection between groups to out-compete selection within groups so long as (i) migration rates are low and (ii) group extinction rates are high. For example, a group that controls its reproduction can continue to maintain this behavior so long as (i) migration into the population by those individuals who reproduce at maximum rates is limited (because such reproducers will quickly take over the population in favor of individual selection) and (ii) the group dies off quickly so that another group can continue the same birth control behaviors. If the group survives too long, then invasion from high-level breeders is inevitable, eventually eliminating the group-level behavior.

The answer to question 2 is that it is not likely that selection between groups can out-compete selection within groups. Moreover, the answer to question 3 is that, even if group selection is possible, it is a rather weak force. There are two arguments—*The Argument from Speed* and *The Argument from Heritability*—that justify these answers to questions 2 and 3. A look at each argument will reveal the implausibility of group selection.

*The argument from speed* The first criticism is that group selection is a weak force compared to individual selection, because of the slow life cycle of groups with respect to individuals. Individuals reproduce at a much faster rate than groups do. As a result of relatively fast reproduction, individuals can migrate in and out of different groups. The result is that, at any given time, individual adaptations will dominate over any group level trait. In the reproduction example, it is very unlikely that the group level feature of controlling reproduction could ever survive because groups live too long compared to individuals. Either from new offspring or invasion from an outsider, individuals who reproduce at maximum rates would eventually take over the group before it could die out and form a new group. Thus, in answer to question 2, it is unlikely that between group selection could out-compete individual selection

---

[95] V. C. Wynne-Edwards, *Animal Dispersion in Relation to Social Behavior* (Edinburgh, 1962).

within groups. Consequently, Engelhardt's claim that groups are the unit of selection is unpromising.

In terms of selfish individuals infiltrating a group of altruists, Mark Ridley offers the following summary judgment in reply to question 3:

> Most biologists suppose that group selection is a weak force in opposition to individual selection because of the slow life-cycles of groups as compared with individuals. Individuals die and reproduce once per generation. As a result, groups go extinct at a much slower rate. The amount of time it will take for selfish individuals to infect and proliferate in a group represents only a small part of the group's life span. At any one time, therefore, individual adaptations will predominate.[96]

Ridley is arguing that even if group selection is a process in the natural world, its success would be very short lived, because individuals reproduce much faster than groups reproduce. Thus, although group selection could be maintained for a few generations of groups, such maintenance is short-lived. It is this short-lived aspect of group selection that, according to Ridley, renders it a weak force compared to individual selection. So, if Ridley's reply is on the mark, then it is unreasonable to think (as Engelhardt does) that the dominant unit of selection is the group.

*The argument from heritability* The second argument against group selection is based on rejecting the idea that there are heritable features distinct to groups that are not simply features of individuals that comprise the groups. As Brandon makes the point, "In order for differential selection to be group selection (i.e. selection at the group level), there must be some group property (the group phenotype) that screens off all other properties from group reproductive success."[97] The problem is that it is very difficult to make sense of a group having a phenotype in any real sense that can be inherited by another group. Moreover, it has to be the case (as Brandon notes) that the group level property can screen-off all non-group level properties from group reproductive success. Yet this is impossible to do, since the group level phenotype really is the composite phenotype of all the individual phenotypes that comprise the group. It is just this point that leads Brandon to state the following concern:

> It is not completely clear what sort of things should count as group properties ... properties that might be selectively relevant are less obviously group properties. For instance, we may want to count the ability to avoid predation as a group property. Whether or not that is a group property depends on whether or not the group's ability to avoid predation is something "over and above" the ability of each individual to avoid predation—that is, whether there is some group effect on the individuals' abilities to avoid predation.[98]

Brandon is arguing that it is an empirical question as to whether there are group-level properties beyond individual properties, but he is clear that some effect by the

---

[96] Mark Ridley, *Evolution*, 2nd edn (Cambridge, 1996), p. 326. This same criticism can be found in John Maynard Smith, "Group Selection," *Quarterly Review of Biology*, 51 (1976): 277–83.
[97] Brandon, "The Levels of Selection," p. 184.
[98] Ibid., footnote 8.

group on the individual would have to be at work. Brandon's point is correct, but not only must there be some effect by the group on the individual, but the effect must also be heritable at the group level. As Ridley notes, "units in nature that show adaptations are the units that show heritability. For example, mutations that influence the phenotype of a unit must be passed on to the offspring of that unit in the next generation. In such a case, natural selection can act to increase the mutation's frequency."[99] In the case of groups, there is no mechanism that is able to pass along a group-level advantageous feature, because groups reproduce by way of individual reproduction within groups. It is this lack of a mechanism that leads Ridley to claim that "[a] genetic variant that increases a group's chance of success tends not to be inherited." Thus, it is this heritability element (along with whether or not groups actually possess properties) that makes group selection implausible. If this argument from heritability is cogent, then it tells against Engelhardt's claim that groups are the unit of selection.

This section has offered a brief glimpse into the units of selection debate. This explication revealed that it is implausible to think that either genes or groups are the unit of selection. Genes cannot be the unit of selection, because they do not directly interact with the selecting environment. Moreover, groups cannot be the unit of selection because of the heritability concern. However, in the rare cases that group selection could possibly occur, it is, at best, a weak process relative to individual selection. The result is that the individual is the reasonable unit of selection. The implication is that it is possible to offer an evolutionary concept of health with respect to individuals.

## Conclusion

*Part 1: Chapter 7 Summary*

This chapter began by noting some of the difficulties with Boorse's analysis and suggesting that a modified naturalistic concept of health could do better in contending with these difficulties. To this end, an evolutionary propensity interpretation of function was defended in favor of other evolutionary accounts. Moreover, given the importance of homeostasis to basic cellular processes, a dual-homeostasis account was developed to make sense of cellular-level homeostasis and overall organismic homeostasis. Then, the next section argued that both levels of homeostasis are composed of elements that are functions in the evolutionary propensity sense. This section went on to conclude that an organism is in a state of health if and only if it is able to maintain the survival/reproduction-enhancing propensities that both intercellular homeostasis and organism homeostasis confer on the organism as a whole. The next section examined a number of "diseases" as a way of revealing the fruitfulness and implications of an evolutionary-homeostasis concept of health. Finally, the last section defended the idea that it is possible to offer an evolutionary concept of health that makes sense of the health of individual organisms.

---

[99] Ridley, *Evolution*, p. 329.

*Part 2: Final Conclusion*

This work has offered a glimpse into the concept of health literature through the work of Christopher Boorse. In preparation for Boorse's own naturalistic concept of health, Chapter 2 provided his critique of various naturalist accounts of health, Chapter 3 explicated his rejection of particular normative concepts of health, and Chapter 4 made clear Boorse's contextualist concept of function. With these chapters in place, Chapter 5 explicated Boorse's naturalistic concept of health. This analysis revealed that Boorse thinks that health is the absence of pathological conditions of parts of organisms, a condition that is understood as an ideal dispositional-functional state of parts of organisms of a particular species, gender, and age group. Chapter 6 examined the many criticisms of Boorse's concept of health. This chapter made manifest that, although Boorse is mostly successful in his reply to his critics, there are a number of difficulties associated with evolution, epistemic norms, and the environment. Finally, Chapter 7 offered a modification of Boorse's concept of health, the EHCH, which is able to address the difficulties with his account. The EHCH argues that an organism—within a certain species, gender, age group, and environment—is in a state of health if and only if its relevant parts and overall behavioral activities have evolved propensities to secure dual-homeostasis, which in turn confers a survival enhancing propensity on the organism as a whole.

The upshot of this analysis is that the difficulties with Boorse's analysis have been resolved. First, a definitive evolutionary concept of function was defended and embraced as part of a naturalistic concept of health. This concept of function overcomes Boorse's lack of justification for objective functions and helps to makes sense of the goal-directed complex structure of biological systems. Second, this evolutionary concept of function is able to distinguish genuine functions from mere side effects, because of its reliance on natural selection. Third, the various disease examples reveal how the EHCH developed here acknowledges the role of the environment when making health judgments. Specifically, the health status of people is partly determined by the combination of their susceptibilities and the environment with which they interact. This discussion revealed that health and disease admit of degree, depending upon environmental conditions. Finally, an argument was offered that the individual organism is the unit of selection. This allows for the possibility of an evolutionary concept of health to acknowledge individual organisms. If this work has, in fact, filled these lacunas in Boorse's account, then the EHCH is a reasonable perspective from which to understand human physical health.

# Bibliography

Agassi, Joseph, "Mechanistic and Holistic Models in Psychiatry," *Nature and System*, 3 (1981): 143–52.
Agich, George, J., "Disease and Value: A Rejection of the Value-Neutrality Thesis," *Theoretical Medicine*, 4/1 (1983): 27–41.
—— and Charles E. Begley (eds), *The Price of Health* (Dordrecht: D. Reidel Publishing Company, 1986).
Ahmed, Paul I. and George V. Coelho (eds), *Toward a New Definition of Health* (New York: Plenum Press, 1979).
Alexander, Samuel, *Space, Time and Deity*, vol. 2 (London: Macmillan, 1927).
Anonymous, "Hunter syndrome," http://www/nlm.nih.gov/medlineplus/ency/article/ 01203.htm.
——, "Tuberculosis," http//:www.Tuberculosis.net.
Aristotle, *Parts of Animals*, trans. A. L. Peck (Cambridge: Harvard University Press, 1937).
Aronowitz, Robert A., *Making Sense of Illness: Science, Society, and Disease* (New York: Cambridge University Press, 1998).
Ayala, Francisco J., "Teleological Explanations in Evolutionary Biology," *Philosophy of Science*, 37/1(1970): 1–15.
——, "Teleological Explanations," in Michael Ruse, ed., *The Philosophy of Biology* (London: Hutchinson & Co. Ltd., 1973), pp. 187–95.
Barnes, Kathleen C., George J. Armelagos, and Steven C. Morreale, "Darwinian Medicine and the Emergence of Allergy," in Wenda R. Trevathan, E. O. Smith, and James J. McKenna (eds), *Evolutionary Medicine* (New York: Oxford University Press, 1999), pp. 209–43.
Beauchamp, Tom L. and LeRoy Walters (eds), *Contemporary Issues in Bioethics*, 5th edn (Belmont: Wadsworth Publishing Company, 1999).
Bechtel, William, "In Defense of a Naturalistic Concept of Health," in Humber, J. M. and Almeder, R. F. (eds), *Biomedical Ethics Review 1985* (Clifton: Humana Press, 1985), pp. 131–70.
Beckner, Morton, *The Biological Way of Thought* (New York: Columbia University Press, 1959).
——. "Function and Teleology," *Journal of the History of Biology*, 2/1 (1969): 151–64.
Behe, Michael J., "Self–Organization and Irreducibly Complex Systems: A Reply to Shanks and Joplin," *Philosophy of Science*, 67/1 (2000): 155–62.
Bengt, Brülde, "On How to Define the Concept of Health: A Loose Comparative Approach," *Medicine, Health Care and Philosophy*, 3 (2000): 305–8.
Bernard, Claude, *Introduction to the Study of Experimental Medicine*, trans. H. C. Green (New York: Dover, 1957).

Bigelow, John and Robert Pargetter, "Functions," *Journal of Philosophy*, 84/4 (1987): 181–96.
Blackmore, Susan, *The Meme Machine* (Oxford: Oxford University Press, 1999).
Block, Ned J., "Are Mechanistic and Teleological Explanations of Behavior Incompatible?" *The Philosophical Review*, 21/83 (1971): 109–17.
Boorse, Christopher, "On the Distinction Between Disease and Illness," *Philosophy and Public Affairs*, 5/1 (1975): 49–68.
——, "Wright on Functions," *The Philosophical Review*, 85/1 (1976): 70–86.
——, "What a Theory of Mental Health Should Be," *Journal of the Theory of Social Behavior*, 6/1 (1976): 61–84.
——, "Health as a Theoretical Concept," *Philosophy of Science*, 44/4 (1977): 542–73.
——, "Concepts of Health," in Donald Van DeVeer and Tom Regan (eds), *Health Care Ethics: An Introduction* (Philadelphia: Temple University Press, 1987), pp. 359–93.
——, "A Rebuttal on Health," in James M. Humber and Robert F. Almeder (eds), *What is Disease?* (Totowa: Humana Press, 1997), pp. 1–134.
Brackenridge, R. D. C. and W. John Elder (eds), *Medical Selection of Life Risks* (New York: Stockton Press, 1998).
Braithwaite, Richard, *Scientific Explanation* (Cambridge: Cambridge University Press, 1964).
Brandon, Robert N., "Levels of Selection," in David L. Hull and Michael Ruse (eds), *The Philosophy of Biology* (Oxford: Oxford University Press, 1998), pp. 180–97.
Broad, C. D., "Mechanism and Emergentism," in Jaegwon Kim and Ernest Sosa (eds), *Metaphysics: An Anthology* (Oxford: Blackwell, 1999), pp. 487–98.
Brothwell, Don R., *Diseases in Antiquity: A Survey of the Diseases, Injuries, and Surgery of Early Populations* (Springfield: C. C. Thomas, 1967).
Brown, W. Miller, "On Defining 'Disease'," *Journal of Medicine and Philosophy*, 10 (1985): 311–28.
Buller, David J., "Etiological Theories of Function: A Geographical Survey," *Biology and Philosophy*, 13/4 (1998): 505–27.
Bunzl, Martin, "Discussion: Comment on 'Health as a Theoretical Concept'," *Philosophy of Science*, 47/1 (1980): 116–18.
Burian, Richard M., "Adaptation: Historical Perspectives," in Evelyn Fox Keller and Elisabeth A Lloyd (eds), *Keywords in Evolutionary Biology* (Cambridge: Harvard University Press, 1992), pp. 7–12.
Byerly, Henry, "Teleology and Evolutionary Theory: Mechanisms and Meaning," *Nature and System*, 1 (1979): 157–76.
Canfield, John, "Teleological Explanations in Biology," *British Journal for the Philosophy of Science*, 14/56 (1964): 285–95.
Cannon, Walter B., *The Wisdom of the Body* (New York: Norton, 1939).
Caplan, Arthur L., "The "Unnaturalness" of Aging—A Sickness Unto Death?" in Arthur L. Caplan, H. Tristram Engelhardt Jr., and James J. McCartney (eds), *Concepts of Health and Disease: Interdisciplinary Perspectives* (London: Addison-Wesley Publishing Company, 1981), pp. 725–37.

——, "Concept of Health and Disease," in R. M. Veatch (ed.), *Medical Ethics* (Boston: Jones and Bartlett, 1989), pp. 49–62.
——, "Does the Philosophy of Medicine Exist?" *Theoretical Medicine*, 13/1 (1992), pp. 67–77.
Caws, Peter, *The Philosophy of Science* (Princeton: D. Van Nostrand Company, Inc., 1965).
Chensue, Stephen, W. and Peter A. Ward, "Inflammation," in Ivan Damjanov and James Linder (eds), *Anderson's Pathology*, 10th edn, vol. 1 (St. Louis: Mosby 1996), pp. 387–415.
Chopra, Deepak, *Creating Health: Beyond Prevention, Toward Perfection* (Boston: Houghton Mifflin Company, 1987).
Clouser, K. D., C. M. Culver, and E. Gert, "Malady: A New Treatment of Disease," *The Hasting Center Report*, 11 (1981): 29–37.
Cockerham, William C., *Medical Sociology* (Upper Saddle River: Prentice Hall, 1998).
Cohen, Morris R., and Ernest Nagel, *An Introduction to Logic and Scientific Method* (New York: Harcourt, Brace, and World, Inc., 1934).
Copeland, B. Jack, "Narrow Versus Wide Mechanism: Including a Re-Examination of Turing's Views on the Mind-Machine Issue," *Journal of Philosophy*, 96/1 (2000): 5–32.
Copp, David, "Why Naturalism?" *Ethical Theory and Moral Practice*, 6/2 (2003): 179–200.
Cote, Richard J. and Clive R. Taylor, "Immunohistochemistry and Related Marking Techniques," in Ivan Damjanov and James Linder (eds), *Anderson's Pathology*, 10th edn, vol. 1 (St. Louis: Mosby), pp. 136–75.
Cotran, Ramzi S., Vinay Kumar, and Stanley L. Robbins, *Robbins Pathologic Basis for Disease*, 4th edn (Philadelphia: W. B. Saunders, Co.,1989).
Cottingham, John, Robert Stoothoff and Dugald Murdoch, trans. and eds, *The Philosophical Writings of Descartes* (2 vols, Cambridge: Cambridge University Press, 1985).
Csányi, Vilmos, "Evolution: Model or Metaphor?" in Van De Vijver, Gertrudis, Stanley N. Salthe and Manuela Delpos (eds), *Evolutionary Systems: Biological and Epistemological Perspectives on Selection and Self-Organization* (Dordrecht: Kluwer Academic Publishers, 1998), pp. 1–12.
Cummins, Robert "Functional Analysis," in Elliott Sober (ed.), *Conceptual Issues in Evolutionary Biology*, 2nd edn (Cambridge: MIT Press, 1994), pp. 49–69. This essay was originally published in *Journal of Philosophy*, 72 (1975): 741–64.
D'Amico, Robert, "Is Disease a Natural Kind?" *Journal of Medicine and Philosophy*, 20 (1995), pp. 551–69.
Dalrymple, Willard, *Foundations of Health* (Boston: Allyn and Bacon, Inc., 1959).
Daniel, Thomas M., *Captain of Death: The Story of Tuberculosis* (Rochester: University of Rochester Press, 1997).
Daniels, Norman, *Just Health Care* (Cambridge: Cambridge University Press, 1985).
Davey, Basiro (ed.), *Birth to Old Age: Health in Transition* (Buckingham: Open University Press, 1995).

——, Alastair Gray, and Clive Seale (eds), 2nd edn, *Health and Disease: A Reader* (Buckingham: Open University Press, 1995).

—— and Tim Halliday (eds), *Human Biology and Health: An Evolutionary Approach* (Buckingham: Open University Press, 1994).

Dawkins, Richard, *The Selfish Gene* (New York: Oxford University Press, 1976).

de Sousa, Ronald B., "The Politics of Mental Illness," *Inquiry*, 15 (1972): 187–201.

DeMarco, Joseph P., *Moral Philosophy: A Contemporary Overview* (Boston and London: Jones and Bartlett Publishers, 1996).

Dennett, Daniel C., *Darwin's Dangerous Idea: Evolution and the Meanings of Life* (New York: Simon & Schuster, 1995).

Depew, David J., "Darwinism and Developmentalism," in Gertrudis van de Dijver, Stanley N. Salthe, and Manuela Delpos (eds), *Evolutionary Systems: Biological and Epistemological Perspectives on Selection and Self-Organization* (Dordrecht: Kluwer Academic Publishers, 1998), pp. 21–32.

—— and Bruce H. Weber, *Darwinism Evolving: System Dynamics and the Genealogy of Natural Selection* (Cambridge: The MIT Press, 1995).

Descartes, René, *The Philosophical Writings of Descartes*, eds and trans. John Cottingham, Robert Stooothoff, and Dugald Murdoch (2 vols, Cambridge: Cambridge University Press, 1985).

Des Chene, Dennis, *Spirits and Clocks: Machine and Organisms in Descartes* (Ithaca: Cornell University Press, 2002).

DeVries, Raymond and Janardan Subedi (eds), *Bioethics and Society* (Upper Saddle River: Prentice Hall, 1998).

Dubos, René, *Mirage of Health* (New York: Harper Colophon Books, 1979).

—— and Jean Dubos, *The White Plague: Tuberculosis, Man and Society* (Boston: Little, Brown and Company, 1952).

Elveback, Lila R., et al., "Health, Normality, and the Ghost of Gauss," *JAMA*, 211/1 (1970): 69–75.

Engel, George L., "Homeostasis, Behavioral Adjustment and the Concept of Health and Disease," in Roy R. Grinker (ed.), *Mid-Century Psychiatry* (Springfield: Charles C. Thomas Publisher, 1953), pp. 33–59.

Engelhardt, H. Tristram, Jr., "The Concepts of Health and Disease," in H. Tristram Engelhardt, Jr., and S.F. Spicker (eds), *Evaluation and Explanation in the Biomedical Sciences: proceedings of the First Trans-Disciplinary Symposium on Philosophy and Medicine Held at Galveston*, (Dordrecht: D. Reidel Publishing Co., 1975), pp. 125–41.

——, "Ideology and Etiology," *Journal of Medicine and Philosophy*, 1/3 (1976): 256–68.

——, "Human Well-Being and Medicine: Some Basic Value Judgments in the Biomedical Sciences," in H. Tristram Engelhardt Jr. and Daniel Callahan (eds), *Science, Ethics, and Medicine* (New York: Hastings Center, Institute of Society, Ethics, and Life, 1976), pp. 120–39.

——, "Health and Disease: Philosophical Perspectives," in W. T. Reich (ed.), *Encyclopedia of Bioethics* (New York: Macmillan, 1978), pp. 599–606.

——, "Clinical Problems and the Concept of Disease," in Lennart Nordefelt and B. Ingemar B. Lindahl (eds), *Health, Disease, and Causal Explanations in Medicine* (Dordrecht: D. Reidel Publishing Company, 1984), pp. 27–41.
——, *The Foundations of Bioethics* (New York: Oxford University Press, 1986).
——, "Germ-Line Genetic Engineering and Moral Diversity: Moral Controversies in a Post-Christian World," *Social Philosophy & Policy*, 13/ 2 (1996): 47–62.
Erde, Edmund L., "Philosophical Considerations Regarding Defining "Health," "Disease," etc., and Their Bearing on Medical Practice," *Ethics and Science in Medicine*, 6 (1979): 31–48.
Fassbender, William, *You and Your Health*, 3rd edn (New York: John Wiley & Sons, 1984).
Fedoryyka, Kateryna, "Health as a Normative Concept: Towards a New Conceptual Framework," *Journal of Medicine and Philosophy*, 22/2 (1997): 143–60.
Fodor, Jerry, "Peacocking," *London Review of Books*, 18 April 1996.
Friedli, Georges-Louis, *Interaction of Deamidated Soluble Wheat Protein (SWP) with Other Food Proteins and Metals* (Ph.D. Thesis), http://www.friedli.com/research/PhD/PhD.html#contents?
Fuchs, Victor R., "Concepts of Health—An Economist's Perspective," *The Journal of Medicine and Philosophy*, 1/3 (1976): 229–37.
Fulford, K. W. M., *Moral Theory and Medical Practice* (New York: Cambridge University Press, 1989).
Gammelgaard, Anne, "Evolutionary Biology and the Concept of Disease," *Medicine, Health Care and Philosophy*, 3/2 (2000): 109–16.
Garrett, Thomas, M., Harold W. Baillie, and Rosellen M. Garrett, *Health Care Ethics: Principles and Problems*, 3rd edn (Upper Saddle River: Prentice Hall, 1998).
Giaimo, Susan, *Markets and Medicine: The Politics of Healthcare Reform in Britain, Germany, and the United States* (Ann Arbor: The University of Michigan Press, 2002).
Glennan, Stuart S., "Mechanism and the Nature of Causation," *Erkenntnis*, 44/1 (1996): 49–71.
Godfrey-Smith, Peter, "A Modern History Theory of Functions," *Noûs*, 28/3 (1994): 344–62.
Goldstein, Kurt, *The Organism, A Holistic Approach to Biology Derived from Pathological Data in Man* (Boston: Beacon Press, 1963).
Goosens, William K., "Values, Health, and Medicine," *Philosophy of Science*, 47/1 (1980): 100–115.
Gould, Stephen Jay, "Caring Groups and Selfish Genes," in Stephen Jay Gould, *The Panda's Thumb* (New York: Norton, 1980), pp. 85–92.
——, *The Mismeasure of Man* (New York: Norton, 1981).
—— and Elizabeth Vrba, "Exaptation: A Missing Term in the Science of Form," *Paleobiology*, 8/1 (1982): 4–15.
Gray, Alastair (ed.), *World Health and Disease* (Buckingham: Open University Press, 1993).
Green, Brian, *The Elegant Universe* (New York: W. W. Norton & Company, 1999).
Greenberg, Jerrod S. and George B. Dintiman, *Exploring Health: Expanding the Boundaries of Wellness* (Englewood Cliffs: Prentice Hall, 1992).

Grmek, Mirko D. (ed.), *Western Medical Thought from Antiquity to the Middle Ages* (Cambridge: Harvard University Press, 1997).

Haig, David, "Genetic Conflicts in Human Pregnancy," *Quarterly Review of Biology*, 68/4 (1993): 495–532.

Halama, Kenneth J. and David N. Reznick, "Adaptation, Optimality, and the Meaning of Phenotypic Variation in Natural Populations," in Steven Hecht Orzack and Elliott Sober (eds), *Adaptationism and Optimality* (Cambridge: Cambridge University).

Hardcastle, Valerie, "Understanding Functions: A Pragmatic Approach," in Valerie Hardcastle (ed.), *Where Biology Meets Psychology* (Cambridge: The MIT Press, 1999), pp. 27–43.

Hare, R. M., "Health," *Journal of Medical Ethics*, 12/4 (1986): 174–81.

Hartmann, Heinz, *Psychoanalysis and Moral Values* (New York: International Universities Press, 1960).

Hays, J. N., *The Burdens of Disease: Epidemics and Human Response in Western History* (New Brunswick: Rutgers University Press, 1998).

Hekht, Muze'on Re'uven ve`ldit, *Illness and Healing in Ancient Times* (Haifa: University of Haifa, 1996).

Hempel, Carl, "Fundamentals of Concept Formation in Empirical Science," in Otto Neurath, Rudolf Carnap, and Charles Morris (eds), *International Encyclopedia of Unified Science: Foundations of the Unity of Science* (2 vols, Chicago: Chicago University Press, 1952), vol. 2, no. 7, pp. 1–93.

——, "The Logic of Functional Analysis," in Carl Hempel, *Aspects of Scientific Explanation* (New York: Free Press, 1965), pp. 297–330.

Hesslow, Germund, "Do We Need a Concept of Disease?" *Theoretical Medicine*, 14/1 (1993): 1–14.

Hull, David, "The Effect of Essentialism on Taxonomy: Two Thousand Years of Stasis," *British Journal of the Philosophy of Science*, 15/60 (1965): 314–26.

——, "Individuality and Selection," *Annual Review of Ecology and Systematics*, 11 (1980): 311–32

——, "Introduction to Part II," in David L. Hull and Michael Ruse (eds), *The Philosophy of Biology* (Oxford: Oxford University Press, 1998), pp. 149–52.

Humber, James M. and Robert F. Almeder (eds), *What is Disease?* (Totowa: Humana Press, 1997).

Humphreys, Paul, "Aspects of Emergence," *Philosophical Topics*, 24/1 (1996): 53–70.

——, "How Properties Emerge," *Philosophy of Science*, 64/1 (1997): 1–17.

Jass, Jeremy R., *Understanding Pathology: From Disease Mechanisms to Clinical Practice* (Amsterdam: Harwood Academic Publishers, 1999).

Johnson, Kenneth D., David L. Rayle, and Hale L. Wedberg, *Biology: An Introduction* (Menlo Park: The Benjamin/Cummings Publishing Company, Inc., 1984).

Jolly, Alison, *Lucy's Legacy: Sex and Intelligence in Human Evolution* (Cambridge: Harvard University Press, 1999).

Kark, John, "Sickle Cell Trait," http://sickle.bwh.harvard.edu/sickle_trait.html.

Kass, L. R., "Regarding the End of Medicine and the Pursuit of Health," *Public Interest*, 40 (1975): 11–42.

Keller, Evelyn Fox and Elisabeth A. Lloyd (eds), *Keywords in Evolutionary Biology* (Cambridge: Harvard University Press, 1992)

Kelley, David E., *et al.*, "Thyrotoxic Periodic Paralysis," *Archives of Internal Medicine*, 149/11 (1989): 2597–600.

Kendell, R. E., *The Concept of Disease and Its Implications for Psychiatry* (Edinburgh: University of Edinburgh, 1975).

Khushf, George, "Why Bioethics Needs the Philosophy of Medicine: Some Implications of Reflection on Concepts of Health and Disease," *Theoretical Medicine*, 18/1–2 (1997): 145–63.

——, "Expanding the Horizon of Reflection on Health and Disease," *The Journal of Medicine and Philosophy*, 20/5 (1995): 461–73.

King, C. Daly, "The Meaning of Normal," *Yale Journal of Biology and Medicine*, 17 (1945): 493–501.

Kitcher, Philip, "Species," *Philosophy of Science*, vol. 51/3 (1984): 308–33.

Kopp, Peter, "Thyroid Diseases," in Marlene B. Goldman and Maureen C. Hatch (eds), *Women and Health* (San Diego: Academic Press, 2000), pp. 655–73.

Kovács, József, "The Concept of Health and Disease," *Medicine, Health Care, and Philosophy*, 1/1 (1998): 31–9.

Kuhn, Thomas H., *The Copernican Revolution* (Cambridge: Harvard University Press, 1957).

——, "Metaphor in Science," in Andrew Ortony (ed.), *Metaphor and Thought*, 2nd edn (Cambridge: Cambridge University Press, 1993), pp. 533–42.

Kuzma, Jan W., *Basic Statistics for the Health Sciences*, 2nd edn (Mountain View: Mayfield Publishing Company, 1992).

Lacey, Hugh, *Is Science Value-Free?* (London: Routledge, 1999).

Lawrence, Peter, *The Making of a Fly: the Genetics of Animal Design* (Oxford: Blackwell Science, 1992).

Ledermann, E. K., "Mechanism and Holism in Physical Medicine," in David Lamb, Teifion Davies, and Marie Roberts (eds), *Explorations in Medicine Volume 1*, (Aldershot: Avebury), pp. 39–58.

Lennox, James G., "Health as an Objective Value," *Journal of Medicine and Philosophy*, 20/5 (1995): 409–511.

Leshin, Len, "Trisomy 21: The Story of Down's Syndrome," health.com/trisomy.htm.

Lewontin, Richard C., *Biology as Ideology: The Doctrine of DNA* (New York: Harper Perennial, 1992).

——, "Adaptation," *Scientific American*, 239/3 (1978): 212–30.

Longino, Helen E., *Science as Social Knowledge* (New Jersey: Princeton University Press, 1990).

Machamer, Peter, Lindley Darden, and Carl F. Craver, "Thinking About Mechanisms," *Philosophy of Science*, 67/1 (2000): 1–25.

Malcolm, Norman, "The Conceivability of Mechanism," in A. P. Martinich and Ernest Sosa (eds), *Analytic Philosophy: An Anthology* (Oxford: Blackwell Publishers, 2001), pp. 287–300.

Margolis, Joseph, "The Concept of Disease," *Journal of Medicine and Philosophy*, 1/3 (1976): 238–55.

——, *Psychotherapy and Morality* (New York: Random House, 1966).
——, "Illness and Medical Values," *The Philosophy Forum*, 8 (1959): 55–76
Markin, Rodney S. and James Linder, "Informatics," in Ivan Damjanov and James Linder (eds), *Anderson's Pathology*, 10th edn, vol. 1 (St. Louis: Mosby), pp. 110–19.
Marmor, Judith, "Homosexuality and Cultural Value Systems," *American Journal of Psychiatry*, 130/11 (1973): 1208–9.
Mayr, Ernst, "Teleological and Teleonomic, a New Analysis," *Boston Studies in the Philosophy of Science*, 14 (1974): 91–117.
——, "Typological Versus Population Thinking," in Ernst Mayr, *Evolution and the Diversity of Life* (Cambridge: Harvard University Press, 1976), 26–9.
McLaughlin, Peter, *What Functions Explain* (Cambridge: Cambridge University Press, 2001).
McManus, Bruce M. and Shelina Babul, "The Autopsy," in Ivan Damjanov and James Linder (eds), *Anderson's Pathology*, 10th edn, vol. 1 (St. Louis: Mosby), pp. 15–32.
Megill, Allan (ed.), *Rethinking Objectivity* (Durham: Duke University Press, 1994).
——, "Four Senses of Objectivity," in Allan Megill (ed.), *Rethinking Objectivity* (Durham: Duke University Press, 1994), pp. 1–20.
Miller, Stuart (ed.), *Essays and Sketches of Mark Twain* (New York: Barnes & Noble Books, 1995).
Millgram, Elijah, *Practical Induction* (Cambridge: Harvard University Press, 1997).
Millikan, Ruth, *White Queen Psychology and Other Essays for Alice* (Cambridge: MIT Press, 1993).
Mills, S. K. and J. H. Beatty, "The Propensity Interpretation of Fitness," *Philosophy of Science*, 46/2 (1979): 263–86.
Milyo, Jeffrey D. and Jennifer M. Mellor, "Is Inequality Bad for Our Health?" *Critical Review*, 13/3–4 (2000): 359–72.
Mitchell, Sandra, "Dispositions or Etiologies? A Comment on Bigelow and Pargetter," *Journal of Philosophy*, 90/5 (1993): 249–59.
Moore, John A., *Science as a Way of Knowing: The Foundations of Modern Biology* (Cambridge, Harvard University Press, 1993).
Mordacci, Robert, "Health as an Analogical Concept," *Journal of Medicine and Philosophy*, 20/5 (1995): 475–97.
Morris, William (ed.), *The American Heritage Dictionary of the American English Language: New College Edition* (Boston: Houghton Mifflin Company, 1978).
Munson, Robert (ed.), *Intervention and Reflection: Basic Issues in Medical Ethics*, 5th edn (Belmont: Wadsworth Publishing Company, 1996).
Nagel, Ernest, *The Structure of Science* (New York and Burlingame: Harcourt Brace & World, 1961).
Neander, Karen, "Functions as Selected Effects: The Conceptual Analyst's Defense," *Philosophy of Science*, 58/2 (1991a): 168–84.
——, "The Teleological Notion of 'Function'," *Australasian Journal of Philosophy*, 69/4 (1991b): 454–68.

Nesse, Randolph, M., "On the Difficulty of Defining Disease: A Darwinian Perspective," *Medicine, Health Care and Philosophy*, 4/1 (2001): 37–46.

——, and George C. Williams, *Why We Get Sick* (New York: Times Books, 1994).

Nezelof, Christian and Thomas A. Seemayer, "A History of Pathology: An Overview," in Ivan Damjanov and James Linder (eds), *Anderson's Pathology*, 10th edn (St. Louis: Mosby, 1996), pp. 1–11.

Nissen, Lowell, *Teleological Language in the Life Sciences* (Lanham: Rowman & Littlefield Publishers, Inc., 1997).

Nordenfelt, Lennart and B. Ingemar B. Lindahl (eds), *Health, Disease, and Causal Explanations in Medicine* (Dordrecht: D. Reidel Publishing Company, 1984).

Oreskes, Naomi, and Homer Le Grand (eds), *Plate Tectonics: An Insider's History of the Modern Theory of the Earth* (Boulder: Westview Press, 2001).

Ozar, David T., "What Should Count as Basic Health Care?" *Theoretical Medicine*, 4/2 (1983): 129–41.

Paley, William, *Natural Theology, or Evidences of the Existence and Attributes of the Deity Collected from the Appearances of Nature* (London: Fauldner, 1802). Reprinted by Westmead: Gregg International, 1970.

Panksepp, Jaak, *Affective Neuroscience: The Foundations of Human and Animal Emotions* (New York: Oxford University Press, 1998).

Parson, Talcott, "Definitions of Health and Illness in the Light of American Values and Social Structure," in Arthur L. Caplan, H. Tristram Engelhardt Jr., and James J. McCartney (eds), *Concepts of Health and Disease: Interdisciplinary Perspectives* (London: Addison-Wesley Publishing Company, 1981), pp. 57–81.

Paul, William E. (ed.), *Fundamental Immunology*, 4th edn (Philadelphia: Lippincott-Raven, 1999).

Payne, Wayne A. and Dale B. Hahn, *Understanding Your Health*, 3rd edn (St. Louis: Mosby-Year Book, Inc., 1992).

Pellegrino, Edmund D., "What the Philosophy *Of* Medicine *Is*," *Theoretical Medicine and Bioethics*, 19/4 (1998): 315–36.

Plunkett, Richard J. and Aladine C. Hayden (eds), *Standard Nomenclature of Diseases and Operations*, 4th edn (New York: Blakiston, 1951).

Poincaré, Henri, *The Value of Science* (New York: Dover, 1920/1958).

Prabhu, S. R., D. F. Wilson, D. K. Daftary, and N. W. Johnson, *Oral Diseases in the Tropics* (New York: Oxford University Press, 1992).

Preston, Beth, "Why is a Wing Like a Spoon? A Pluralist Theory of Function," *The Journal of Philosophy*, 95/5 (1998): 215–54.

Profet, Margie, "The Function of Allergy: Immunological Defense Against Toxins," *Quarterly Review of Biology*, 66/1 (1991): 23–54.

Purtilo, David T., *A Survey of Human Diseases* (Menlo Park: Addison-Wesley Publishing Company, 1978).

Reeve, C. D. C., *Practices of Reason: Aristotle's Nicomachean Ethics* (Oxford: Clarendon Press, 1995).

Reznek, Lawrie, *The Nature of Disease* (London: Routledge and Kegan Paul, 1987).

Ricker, W.E., "Changes in the Average Size and Average Age of Pacific Salmon," *Canadian Journal of Fisheries and Aquatic Science*, 38 (1981): 1636–56.

Ridley, Mark, *Evolution*, 2nd edn (Cambridge: Blackwell Science, 1996).
Rieff, Philip, *Freud: The Mind of the Moralist* (New York: Viking, 1959).
Roberts, M. B. V., *Biology: A Functional Approach*, 4th edn (Surrey, UK: ELBS with Nelson, 1986).
Root-Bernstein, Robert, "On Defining a Scientific Theory: Creationism Considered," in Ashley Montagu (ed.), *Science and Creationism* (Oxford: Oxford University Press, 1984), pp. 64–94.
Rosenberg, Alexander, *The Structure of Biological Science* (Cambridge: Cambridge University Press, 1985).
Rosenberg, Jay. F., *Thinking Clearly About Death*, 2nd edn (Indianapolis: Hackett Publishing Co., 1998).
Rubin, Emanuel and John L. Farber, *Pathology* (Philadelphia: J. B. Lippincott Co., 1988).
Rueger, Alexander, "Physical Emergence, Diachronic and Synchronic," *Synthese*, 124/3 (2000): 297–322.
Ruse, Michael, *Mystery of Mysteries: Is Evolution a Social Construction?* (Cambridge: Harvard University Press, 1999).
——, "Defining Disease: The Question of Sexual Orientation," in James M. Humber and Robert F. Almeder (eds), *What is Disease?* (Totowa: Humana Press, 1997), pp. 137–71.
Ryle, J. A., "The Meaning of Normal," *The Lancet*, 249/6436 (1947): 1–5.
Salthe, Stanley N., "The Role of Natural Selection Theory in Understanding Evolutionary Systems," in Gertrudis van de Dijver, Stanley N. Salthe, and Manuela Delpos (eds), *Evolutionary Systems: Biological and Epistemological Perspectives on Selection and Self-Organization* (Dordrecht: Kluwer Academic Publishers, 1998), pp. 13–20.
Scadding, J. B., "Health and Disease: What Can Medicine Do for Philosophy?" *Journal of Medical Ethics*, 14/3 (1988): 118–24.
Schaffner, Kenneth F. and Robert S. Cohen (eds), *PSA 1972* (Dordrecht-Holland: D. Reidel Publishing Company, 1974).
Scheffler, Israel, "Thoughts on Teleology," *British Journal for the Philosophy of Science*, 9/36 (1959): 265–85.
Schmidtz, David, *Rational Choice and Moral Agency* (New Jersey: Princeton University Press, 1995).
Scriven, Michael, "The Exact Role of Value Judgments in Science," in Kenneth F. Schaffner and Robert S. Cohen (eds), *PSA 1972* (Dordrecht-Holland: D. Reidel Publishing Company, 1974), pp. 219–47.
Sedgwick, Peter, *Psycho Politics* (New York: Harper & Row, 1982).
Seedhouse, David., "The Need for a Philosophy of Health," in David Lamb, Teifion Davies, and Marie Roberts (eds), *Explorations in Medicine Volume 1* (Aldershot: Avebury 1987), pp. 123–51.
Seidel, Charles, *Basic Concepts in Physiology* (New York: McGraw Hill, 2002).
Shanks, Niall and Karl H. Joplin, "Redundant Complexity: A Critical Analysis of Intelligent Design in Biochemistry?" *Philosophy of Science*, 66/2 (1999): 268–82.
Silverstein, Arthur M., *A History of Immunology* (San Diego: Academic Press, 1989).

Simon, Herbert A., "The Architecture of Complexity," *Proceedings of the American Philosophical Society*, 106/6 (1962): 467–82.
Smart, J. J. C., *Philosophy and Scientific Realism* (New York: Random House, 1963).
Smith, John Maynard, "Group Selection," *Quarterly Review of Biology*, 51 (1976): 277–83.
——, "How to Model Evolution," in John Dupré (ed.), *The Latest on the Best: Essays on Optimality and Evolution* (Cambridge: MIT Press, 1987), pp. 119–31.
Sober, Elliott (ed.), *Conceptual Issues in Evolutionary Biology*, 2nd edn (Cambridge: The MIT Press, 1994).
——, *The Nature of Selection* (Cambridge: The MIT Press, 1984).
—— and David Sloan Wilson, *Unto Others: Evolution and Psychology of Unselfish Behavior* (Cambridge, Mass.: Harvard University Press, 1999).
Soll, Ivan, *An Introduction to Hegel's Metaphysics* (Chicago: The University of Chicago Press, 1969).
Sommerhoff, Gerd, *Analytical Biology* (Oxford: Oxford University Press, 1950).
Sonntag, Susan, *Illness as Metaphor* (New York: Vintage Books, 1979).
Stempsey, William E., *Disease and Diagnosis* (Dordrecht: Kluwer Academic Publishers, 1999).
——, "A Pathological View of Disease," *Theoretical Medicine*, 21/ 4 (2000): 321–30.
Sterelny, Kim and Philip Kitcher, "The Return of the Gene," in David L. Hull and Michael Ruse (eds), *The Philosophy of Biology* (Oxford: Oxford University Press, 1998), pp. 153–75.
—— and Paul E. Griffiths, *Sex and Death: An Introduction to the Philosophy of Biology* (Chicago: The University of Chicago Press, 1999).
Stuart, James and Donald Scherer, *Logical Thinking: An Introduction to Logic*, 2nd edn (New York: McGraw Hill, 1997).
Thoday, J. M., and J. B. Gibson, "Isolation by Disruptive Selection," *Nature*, 193 (1962): 1164–6.
Thomasma, David C., "The Role of the Clinical Medical Ethicist: The Problem of Applied Ethics and Medicine," in Michael Bradie, Thomas W. Attig, and Nicholas Rescher (eds), *The Applied Turn in Contemporary Philosophy*, Vol. V (Bowling Green: The Applied Philosophy Program Bowling Green State University, 1983), pp. 136–57.
Toulmin, Stephen, "From Clocks to Chaos: Humanizing the Mechanistic World-View," in Hermann Haken, Anders Karlqvist, and Uno Svedin (eds), *The Machine as Metaphor and Tool* (Berlin: Springer-Verlag, 1993), pp.139–53.
Twain, Mark, "Concerning Tobacco," in Stuart Miller (ed.), *Essays and Sketches of Mark Twain* (New York: Barnes & Nobles Books, 1995), pp. 151–3.
Ulizzi, L. and L. Terrenato, "Natural Selection Associated with Birth Rate," *Annnals of Human Genetics*, 56 (1992): 113–18.
Underwood, J. C. E. (ed.), *General and Systematic Pathology*, 2nd edn (New York: Churchill Livingstone, 1996).
van der Steen, Wim J., and P. J. Thung, *Faces of Medicine: A Philosophical Study* (Dordrecht: Kluwer Academic Publishers, 1988).
Van Valen, L., "Morphological Variation and the Width of Ecological Niche," *American Naturalist*, 99/3 (1965): 377–90.

Veatch, Robert M., "Generalization of Expertise: Scientific Expertise and Value Judgments," *Hastings Center Studies*, 1 (1973): 29–40.

Virchow, Rudolf, "One Hundred Years of General Pathology," in Rudolf Virchow, *Disease, Life, and Man: Selected Essays of Rudolf Virchow*, trans., Lelland J. Rather (Stanford: Stanford University Press, 1958), pp. 170–215.

Wakefield, Jerome C., "The Concept of Mental Disorder: On the Boundary Between Biological Facts and Social Values," *American Psychologist*, 47/3 (1992): 373–88.

Weiner, Jonathan, *The Beak of the Finch* (New York: Knopf, 1994).

Welcowitz, Joan, Robert B. Ewen, and Jacob Cohen, *Introductory Statistics for the Behavioral Sciences*, 4th edn (San Diego: Harcourt Brace Jovanovich, 1991).

West-Eberhard, Mary Jane, "Adaptation: Current Usages," in David L. Hull and Michael Ruse (eds), *Philosophy of Biology* (Oxford: Oxford University Press, 1998), pp. 8–14.

Wilson, Edward O., *Consilience: The Unity of Knowledge* (New York: Knopf, 1998).

Wimsatt, William C., "The Ontology of Complex Systems: Levels of Organization, Perspectives, and Causal Thickets," in M. Mathen and R. X. Ware (eds), *Biology and Society: Reflections on Methodology* (Calgary: University of Calgary Press, 1994), pp. 207–74.

World Health Organization, "Constitution of the World Health Organization," *Chronicle of the World Health Organization*, 1/1–2 (1947): 29–43.

Wright, Larry, "Functions," in Elliott Sober (ed.), *Conceptual Issues in Evolutionary Biology* (Cambridge: MIT Press, 1994), pp. 27–47. [This article was published originally in *Philosophical Review*, 82/1 (1973), pp. 139–68.]

——, *Teleological Explanations* (Berkeley and Los Angeles: University of California Press, 1976).

Wuketits, Franz M., "Organisms, Vital Forces, and Machines: Classical Controversies and the Contemporary Discussion of 'Reductionism VS. Holism'," in Paul Hoyningen-huene and F. M. Wuketits (eds), *Reductionism and Systems Theory in the Life Sciences* (Dordrecht: Kluwer Academic Press, 1989), pp. 3–28.

Wynne-Edwards, V. C., *Animal Dispersion in Relation to Social Behavior* (Edinburgh: Oliver and Boyd, 1962).

# Index

('concept of health' is abbreviated to 'coh', except for its own main entry where it is written out)

accident, function, distinction 58–9
adaptation
    and coh 19–37
    Kovács on 21
    Lewontin on 178–9
Agich, George
    Boorse
        covert normativism charge 145–50
        reply 150–56
    on normative coh 3
albumin example, normal distribution 16–18
allergies
    EHCH case 200–201
    and IgE system 200
    Nesse and Williams on 201
    types 200
allergy example
    function, accident distinction 59
    part-functionalism 104
    statistical coh 15
    strong normativism 41–2
    weak normativism 46
appeal to authority fallacy 139–40, 141
Aristotle, on human function 101–2
Aronowitz, Robert, on disease 112

Babul, Shelina 166
bacteria
    evolution, and tuberculosis 198
    Nesse and Williams on 198
baldness example, disease 133, 134, 135
Bechtel, William 20, 173, 186–7, 212
    on body homeostasis 194
    Boorse
        circularity charge 127–9
        reply 129–31
    on cultural evolutionism 207–8
    on organism homeostasis 193
    on propensity functional naturalism 184

Bernard, Claude, on homeostatic coh 28–9, 35fn63
Bigelow, John, and Robert Pargetter 177, 182
    on propensity functional naturalism 183, 184, 185–6, 187
biology, evolutionary, Ruse on 153
biology example, analytic philosophy 7
body
    Descartes on 97fn4
    homeostasis, Bechtel on 194
    as homeostatic system 194
    intercellular fluid 189–90
    movements, Goldstein on 192
Boorse, Christopher
    coh 8–11, 95–124, 174
        acclimation-adaptation 24, 25–7
        criticism of 125–72
            bad biology/reply 156–63
            bad medicine/reply 163–71
            circularity/reply 125–31
            covert normativism/reply 131–56
            Stempsey's 139–40, 141
    on disease 122–3, 130
        illness, distinction 44–5
    on dynamic equilibrium 191
    on evolutionary-adaptation coh 20–23
    on function 57–8, 84–92, 112–13, 162, 163, 164
        etiological 64–84
    on health and disease 95–6
    on homeostatic coh 34–7, 189
    on naturalism 13–14
    on naturalistic coh 8–11, 13–14, 95–124
        criticism of 125–72
    on normativism 39–40
        functional 54–6
        moral 51–3
        strong 42–5
        thick/thin distinction 49fn30

weak 46–9
  on objectivism 112–15
  as objectivist 107–15
  on part-functionalism 136
  as part-functionalist 104–7, 193
  on pathology 164–5
  on species design 23, 157
  on statistical coh 15, 18–19
  on units of selection 136, 210–11
Braithwaite, Richard, on goal-directed systems 84–5
Brandon, Robert 214
  on group selection 216–17
Byerly, Henry 101

cancer, description, Sontag on 154
Cannon, Walter B. 28
  on homeostatic coh 29
causal complexity, argument from, Gould on 213–14
Caws, Peter 6, 148
Chensue, Stephen, and Peter Ward, on inflammation 194–5
cigarettes example, and cultural evolutionism 207–8
Cohen, Morris R. 148
compatibilist approach, to coh 5, 6, 7
concept of health (coh)
  acclimation-adaptation 24–5
    Boorse on 24, 25–7
    negative version 24–5
    positive version 24
  and adaptation 19–37
  approaches to 4–7
  Boorse 8–11, 95–124, 174
  clinicians' understanding of 15
  compatibilist approach 5, 6, 7
  consilience, lack of 2
  disease 122–3
  evolutionary-adaptation 19–20
    Boorse's reply 20–3
  evolutionary-homeostasis see EHCH
  function see function
  history 4–5
  homeostatic 28–34
    Bernard on 28–9, 35fn63
    Boorse on 34–7
    Engel on 28, 29–34, 35–6
    external environment 31
    intercellular fluid 31, 32
    internal environment 31
    mechanisms 32–3
    negative feedback 33, 34
    positive feedback 33, 34
    psychological aspects 32, 34
    social factors 34
  importance of 1
  mechanistic analogy 97–8
  and mental causation 36fn65
  naturalist see naturalism
  naturalists 3
    vs normativists 2–4
  Nodernfelt on 1–2
  normal function 115–19
  normative see normativism
  normativists 3
  philosophy, contribution of 5–7
  as physical health 8
  reference class 115–19
    thyroid example 117, 118
  statistical 14–19, 160–1
    allergy example 15
    Boorse on 15, 18–19
consilience, lack of 2
constructivists, vs destructivists 146
Cote, Richard, and Clive Taylor, on surgical pathology 166–7
Cotran, Ramzi S. 140, 141
Cummins, Robert, on function 120

Daly King, C. 128
Damjanov, Ivan 165
Dawkins, Richard, on genes as units of selection 211, 212, 213
Depew, David, on organism homeostasis 193
Des Chene, Dennis, on mechanism 99–100, 106
Descartes, René
  on the body 97fn4
  *Treatise of Man* 97fn4
disease
  Aronowitz on 112
  baldness example 133, 134, 135
  Boorse on 122–3, 130
  coh 122–3
  concept, Engelhardt on 4, 110, 143, 161
  and health
    Boorse on 95–6
    Hesslow on 168–9
  Hesslow on 168
illness

## Index

absence in natural world 43
  distinction, Boorse on 44–5
    Sedgwick on 43–4
      Boorse's critique 44–5
  Margolis on 163–4
  Miller Brown on 164
  naturalist, vs normative theories ix
  ontologist, vs physiologist theories ix
  and pathology 166
  *see also* health
Down's syndrome
  EHCH case 201–2
  Purtilo on 202
dynamic equilibrium, Boorse on 191

EFN (etiological functional naturalism) 176–83
  criticisms of 178–83
    circularity 179
  definition 177
  Hardcastle on 176, 179–80
  Hunter syndrome example 177
  lungs function example 180
  McLaughlin on 181
  Millikan on 176
  Neander on 177–8
  Preston on 180
EHCH (evolutionary-homeostasis coh) 173, 194–209, 217, 218
  age differences 196
  allergies example 200–201
  case studies 196–209
  definition 196
  Down's syndrome example 201–2
  environmental factors 196
  gender differences 196
  osteoporosis example 205–9
  sickle cell anemia example 202–5
  species variations 196
  tuberculosis example 196–9
Engel, George 28
  on homeostatic coh 28, 29–34, 35–6
  on psychology of anger 31
Engelhardt, H. Tristram
  Boorse
    bad biology charge 157–8, 161
      reply 158–9, 161–2
    covert normativism charge 135–6
      reply 136–44
  on disease 4, 110, 143, 161
  on weak normativism 45–6

entropy, Schrödinger on 109
Evolutionary Functional Naturalism 175–88
  definition 176
  *see also* EFN; mixed evolutionary functional naturalism; propensity functional naturalism
evolutionism
  cultural
    Bechtel on 207–8
    cigarettes example 207–8
  Hardcastle on 178
  heart example 175
  Mayr on 175
  Ruse on 151
  Wakefield on 161

Farber, John L. 141
Fodor, Jerry 154
Freud, Sigmund 32
Fulford, K.W.M., Boorse, covert normativism charge 131–2
  reply 132
function
  accident
    allergy example 59
    distinction 58–9
    heart example 58–9
  adequacy conditions 58–60, 62–3, 89–92
  Boorse on 57–8, 84–92, 112–13, 162, 163, 174
  conscious, vs natural 59–60
  contextualist conception 87, 93, 119, 120, 129
  Cummins on 120
  debate, coh 57–93
  definition 84
  dispositional concept 120
  divine element, exclusion 58, 60, 174
  etiological concept
    Boorse's critique 64–84
    'common connection' criticism/reply 80–4
    equivocation criticism/reply 65–9
    examples 61–3
    necessary and sufficient conditions criticism/reply 70–80
    tautology criticism/reply 64
  Kass on 128
  lungs example 120
  mast cells example 84–5

Nissen on 181–2
Wright on 58–63, 93, 162, 174
see also EFN
functionalism see part-functionalism

Gammelgaard, Anne, on units of selection 210fn82
genes 21–2
  as units of selection 137, 211
  vs the individual 211–13
Glennan, Stuart 100
  on part-functionalism 103fn20
goal-directed systems, Braithwaite on 84
Godfrey-Smith, Peter 185
Goldstein, Kurt, on body movements 192
Gould, Stephen Jay
  causal complexity argument 213–14
  visibility argument 211, 212–13
Graves' disease 118
Greene, Brian 100
Griffiths, Paul 21
group selection 210–11
  argument
    from heritability 216–17
    from speed 215–16
  Brandon on 216–17
  case against 214–17
  Ridley on 216, 217
  vs genes 210–11

Hardcastle, Valerie 186
  on EFN 176, 179–80
  on evolutionism 178
Hare, R.M., Boorse, covert normativism charge 133
  reply 134–5
Hays, J.N., on tuberculosis 197
health
  definition 195–6
  dimensions 8
  and disease
    Boorse on 95–6
    Hesslow on 168–9
  elements of 96
  judgements, therapeutic judgements, distinction 52
  as objective condition 97
  Parson's definition 3–4, 24
  philosophy of, disciplines xi
  statistical coh 14–19

WHO definition 2
see also concept of health; disease
heart example, evolutionism 175
Hempel, Carl 58
Hesslow, Germund 163
  Boorse
    bad medicine charge 167–9
    reply 170–71
  on disease 168
  and health 168–9
  on need for scientific definitions 167–8
holism, organic functional 101–3
  definition 102
homeostasis 189–94
  body, Bechtel on 194
  Boorse on 34–7, 189
  and coh 28–37
  of organisms
    Bechtel on 193
    Depew on 193
  see also homeostatic system; intercellular homeostasis
homeostatic system 190–94
  body as 194
  components 190–91
  effector 190, 191
  integration center 190, 191
  internal physical states 190
  regulated variable 190, 191
  sensor 190, 191
  set point 190, 191
homosexuality, Marmor on 42, 43
  Boorse's critique 42–3
human function, Aristotle on 101–2
Hunter syndrome example, EFN 177

IgE system
  as effector 201
  Profet on 200
individual, vs genes 211–13
inflammation, Ward and Chensue on 194–5
instinctual needs 30
intercellular fluid, body homeostasis 189–90
intercellular homeostasis 191–2, 193
  and organism survival 195
  and osteoporosis 205–6
  species variations 196

Kant, Immanuel, *Critique of Pure Reason* 111

Kass, Leon R., on function 128
Kovács, József, on adaptation 21
Kumar, Vinay 140, 141
Kuzma, Jan, on normal distribution 16

Lacey, Hugh, on science 147
Ledermann, E.K., on mechanism 97–8, 99
Lennox, James G., on functional normativism 53–4
Lewontin, Richard, on adaptation 178–9
Linder, James 165, 166
Longino, Helen, on science 146
lungs example
    EFN 180
    function 120

Machamer, Peter 101
McLaughlin, Peter
    on EFN 181
    on propensity functional naturalism 187–8
McManus, Bruce 166
Margolis, James 163
    Boorse
        bad medicine charge 163–4
            reply 164–7
    on disease 163–4
    on medicine 163–4
    moral normativism 50–51
Markin, Rodney 165, 166
Marmor, Judith, on homosexuality 42, 43
mast cells example, function 84–5
Mayr, Ernst 160
    on evolutionism 175
mean, statistical 16fn11
    tooth decay 19
mechanism
    criticism of 100–101
    definition 100
    Des Chene on 99–100, 106
    Ledermann on 97–8, 99
    Nagel on 104fn22
    Toulmin on 98–9
medicine
    Margolis on 163–4
    Miller Brown on 164
    values in 148
Megill, Allan
    on dialectical objectivism 110, 111
    on disciplinary objectivism 108

    on methodological objectivism 107–8
mental causation, and coh 36fn65
metaphors, in science 154–5
Miller Brown, W. 163
    Boorse
        bad medicine charge 164
            reply 164–7
        covert normativism charge 144
            reply 144–5
    on disease 164
    on medicine 164
Millikan, Ruth, on EFN 176
mixed evolutionary functional naturalism 188–9
    definition 188
moral values, and psychoanalysis 50–51

Nagel, Ernest 148
    on mechanism 104fn22
naturalism
    Boorse on 13–14
    and coh 14–19
    definitions 13, 19, 28
naturalists
    coh 3
    definition ix
Neander, Karen, on EFN 177–8
Nesse, Randolph, and George Williams
    on allergies 201
    on bacteria 198
    on sickle cell anemia 203, 204
Nezelof, Christian 140, 165, 166
Nissen, Lowell, on function 181–2
nominalists, vs realists ix
Nordenfelt, Lennart, on coh 1–2
normal distribution
    Kuzma on 16
    meaning 16
    serum albumin example 16–18
normativism
    Agich on 3
    Boorse on 39–40
        thick/thin distinction 49fn30
    descriptive 41
    functional
        Boorse on 54–6
        Lennox on 53–4
        meaning 53
    moral
        Boorse on 51–3
        definition 50

Margolis on 50–51
Parsons on 3–4
strong 40
    allergy example 41–2
    Boorse on 42–5
    tobacco example 42fn14
    varieties 39, 40
weak 40, 41, 45–6
    allergy example 46
    Boorse on 46–9
    Engelhardt on 45–6
    meaning 45
normativists
    coh 3
    definition ix
norms
    epistemic 151, 152
    metrical 40–41
    quantitative 40

objectivism
    Boorse on 112–15
    dialectical 95, 107, 110–12
    disciplinary 95, 107, 108–10
    metaphysical 95, 107, 113
    methodological 95, 107–8, 113
objectivist, Boorse as 107–15
Ockham's razor, and units of selection 213
ontologists, vs physiologists ix
osteoporosis
    EHCH case 205–9
    and intercellular homeostasis 205–6

Pargetter, Robert *see* Bigelow, John
Parsons, Talcott
    definition of health 3–4, 24
    on normative coh 3–4
part-functionalism 103–4
    allergy example 104
    Boorse on 104–7, 136, 193
    definition 103
    Glennan on 103fn20
    Virchow on 139
pathology
    Boorse on 164–5
    definitions 140–41
    and disease 166
    surgical, Cote and Taylor on 166–7
philosophers, analytic
    criticism of 5–6

Rosenberg on 5
philosophy
    biology example 7
    and coh 5–7
    of health, disciplines xi
physiologists, vs ontologists ix
Poincaré, Henri, on science 146–7, 151
Preston, Beth, on EFN 180
Profet, Margie, on IgE system 200
propensity functional naturalism 183–9
    Bechtel on 184
    Bigelow and Pargetter on 183, 184, 185–6, 187
    criticisms 185–8
    definition 184
    McLaughlin on 187–8
psychoanalysis, and moral values 50–51
Purtilo, David, on Down's syndrome 202

realists, vs nominalists ix
Ridley, Mark, on group selection 216, 217
Robbins, Stanley L. 140, 141
Roberts, M.B.V. 32
Rosenberg, Jay, on analytic philosophers 5
Rubin, Emanuel 141
Ruse, Michael
    on epistemic values 152–3
    on evolutionary biology 153
    on evolutionism 151
    on metaphors in science 155
    on naturalist coh 3
Ryle, J.A. 24–5

Scadding, J.B., Boorse, circularity charge 126
    reply 126–7, 131
Schrödinger, Erwin, on entropy 109
science
    constructivism 146
    descriptivism 146–7
    Lacey on 147
    Longino on 146
    metaphors in 154–5
    particular value 148
    Poincaré on 146–7, 151
    and pursuit of truth 148
    values in 145–50, 154
Sedgwick, Peter, on disease and illness 43–4
Seemayer, Thomas A. 140, 165, 166
Seidel, Charles 190

shock therapy 52
sickle cell anemia
    effects 203
    EHCH case 202–5
    Nesse and Williams on 203, 204
Skinner, B.F. 59
Sontag, Susan, on description of cancer 154
species design, Boorse on 23, 157
standard deviation 16fn10
Stempsey, William, Boorse, criticism of 139–40, 141, 142
Sterelny, Kim 21

Taylor, Clive *see* Cote, Richard
Thung, P.J. 156, 157
thyroid example, reference class coh 117, 118
tobacco, example of strong normativism 42fn14
tooth decay, and statistical mean 19
Toulmin, Stephen, on mechanism 98–9
tuberculosis
    and bacteria evolution 198
    cause 196–7
    decline 197
    ECHC case 196–9
    Hays on 197
    immune system response 198

units of selection
    Boorse on 136, 210–11
    Gammelgaard on 210fn82
    genes as 137, 211, 212
    groups as 210–11
    and Ockham's razor 213
    *see also* group selection

values
    epistemic 149–50
        Ruse on 152–3
    in science 145–50
van der Steen, Win J. 156, 157
    Boorse, bad biology charge 159–60
        reply 160–61
Virchow, Rudolf, on part-functionalism 139
visibility argument, Gould 211, 212–13

Wakefield, Jerome C.
    Boorse
        bad biology charge 161
            reply 162–3
    on evolutionism 161
WHO (World Health Organization)
    definition of health 2
Williams, George *see* Nesse, Randolph
Wilson, Edward O., advice to scientists 148–9
Wright, Larry 9, 176
    on function 58–63, 93, 162, 174
    Boorse's reply 63–84
Wynne-Edwards, V.C. 214–15

Made in the USA
Columbia, SC
31 May 2023